4200
99¢

Disorders of the Skull Base Region

Nobel Symposium 10

Disorders of the Skull Base Region

Proceedings of the Tenth Nobel Symposium
Stockholm, August 1968

Edited by

CARL-AXEL HAMBERGER and JAN WERSÄLL

Professor of Otolaryngology
Karolinska Sjukhuset
Stockholm, Sweden

Associate Professor of Otolaryngology
Karolinska Sjukhuset
Stockholm, Sweden

WILEY INTERSCIENCE DIVISION
John Wiley & Sons, Inc. *New York, London, Sydney*

ALMQVIST & WIKSELL *Stockholm*

Printed in Sweden by
Almqvist & Wiksells Boktryckeri AB, Uppsala 1969

Preface

Interest in diseases related to the region of the base of the skull has increased considerably during the last decade. This is especially true of problems connected with the area of the pituitary gland and of the foramen jugulare.

During the last few years particular attention has been paid to diagnostic and therapeutic possibilities of dealing with tumours in the inner auditory meatus. The solution of some of these problems has been discussed and worked out in a few clinics in the U.S.A. and in Europe. Selected areas of the field have been discussed earlier at various meetings. Recently, however, it has been considered of the utmost importance that scientists engaged in basic research as well as those concerned with diagnostic and therapeutic activities within the field should meet in order to summarize their conclusions. Stockholm has been regarded as a suitable place for such a meeting, as Swedish scientists, for example, endocrinologists, neurosurgeons, neuroradiologists, and otologists, have taken a special interest in the development of diagnostic and therapeutic methods for treating diseases of the base of the skull.

We are very pleased that so many distinguished scientists have accepted our invitation to take part in the symposium; and we are most grateful for their excellent contributions with lectures and discussions.

The support given by the Nobel Foundation, the Swedish Cancer Society, the Swedish Medical Research Council, and the Cancer Foundation in Stockholm has been of the greatest importance for the organization of the symposium. The organizing committee wishes to express its sincere gratitude for the generous support of these sponsors and for the facilities provided by the Karolinska Institute.

Carl-Axel Hamberger   *Jan Wersäll*

Contents

Session I. Acoustic neuroma 1

Session II. Acoustic neuroma 2

Session VII. Trauma of the skull base

Nobel Symposium Committee

Ståhle, Nils K., chairman, Executive Director of the Nobel Foundation
Hulthén, Lamek, Professor, member of the Nobel Committee for Physics
Tiselius, Arne, Professor, chairman of the Nobel Committee for Chemistry
Gustafsson, Bengt, Professor, secretary of the Nobel Committee for Medicine
Gierow, Karl Ragnar, Ph.D., Permanent Secretary of the Swedish Academy
  (literature)
Schou, August, Director of the Norwegian Nobel Institute (peace)

Organizing Committee

C.-A. Hamberger (chairman)
J. Wersäll (secretary)
C.-M. Eneroth
T. Gejrot
I. Klockhoff

List of participants

H. C. ANDERSEN, Department of Otolaryngology, Århus Kommunehospital, *Århus,* Denmark

H. ANDERSON, Department of Audiology, Karolinska Sjukhuset, *104 01 Stockholm 60,* Sweden

J. ANGELL JAMES, Litfield House, Clifton Down, *Bristol 8,* Great Britain

M. ARSLAN, Clinica Otorinolaringoiatrica nell'Università, Viale Diaz 9, *35100 Padova,* Italy

G. ASCHAN, Department of Otolaryngology, Regionsjukhuset, *581 85 Linköping,* Sweden

E.-O. BACKLUND, Department of Neurosurgery, Karolinska Sjukhuset, *104 01 Stockholm 60,* Sweden

B. BARR, Department of Pediatric Audiology, Karolinska Sjukhuset, *104 01 Stockholm 60,* Sweden

G. BATEMAN, 55 Harley Street, *London W.1.,* Great Britain

P. BERDAL, Department of Otolaryngology, Rikshospitalet, *Oslo,* Norway

M. BERGSTEDT, Department of Otolaryngology, Sahlgrenska Sjukhuset, *413 45 Göteborg,* Sweden

H. BJÖRK, Skepparebrinken 1 A, *Helsingfors* (*Helsinki*), Finland

J. E. BORDLEY, Department of Otolaryngology, The Johns Hopkins Hospital, *Baltimore,* Maryland 21205, U.S.A.

S. BRÜNNER, Department of X-ray Diagnosis, Københavns Amts Sygehus i Gentofte, Niels Andersensvej 65, *Hellerup,* Denmark

K. BURIAN, Filialstation der Universitätsklinik für Hals-, Nasen- und Ohrenkrankheiten, Alserstrasse 4, *1090 Wien,* Austria

H. J. DENECKE, Friedrich-Ebert-Anlage 12, *Heidelberg,* Germany

H. DIAMANT, Department of Otolaryngology, Lasarettet, *901 87 Umeå,* Sweden

C.-M. ENEROTH, Department of Otolaryngology, Karolinska Sjukhuset, *104 01 Stockholm 60,* Sweden

H. ENGSTRÖM, Department of Otolaryngology, Akademiska Sjukhuset, *750 14 Uppsala 14,* Sweden

U. Engzell, Department of Otolaryngology, Karolinska Sjukhuset, *104 01 Stockholm 60,* Sweden

F. Escher, Universitätsklinik für Ohren-, Nasen- und Halsleiden, *3000 Bern,* Switzerland

U. Fisch, Kantonsspital, Otorhinolaryngologische Klinik der Universität, Rämistrasse 100, *8006 Zürich,* Switzerland

E. Fluur, Department of Otolaryngology, Karolinska Sjukhuset, *104 01 Stockholm 60,* Sweden

S. Franzén, Department of Radiopathology, Karolinska Sjukhuset, *104 01 Stockholm 60,* Sweden

R. Frykholm, Department of Neurosurgery, Södersjukhuset, *100 64 Stockholm 38,* Sweden

T. Gejrot, Department of Otolaryngology, Lasarettet, *291 00 Kristianstad,* Sweden

M. E. Glasscock, III, Otologic Medical Group, 2122 West Third Street, *Los Angeles,* California 90057, U.S.A.

B. Grahne, Department of Otolaryngology, Helsingfors Universitets-Centralsjukhus, Haartmansgatan 4 E, *Helsingfors 29 (Helsinki 29),* Finland

T. Greitz, Department of Neuroradiology, Karolinska Sjukhuset, *104 01 Stockholm 60,* Sweden.

A. Grepe, Department of Neuroradiology, Karolinska Sjukhuset, *104 01 Stockholm 60,* Sweden

B. Gustafsson, Secretary of the Nobel Committee for Medicine, Department of Medical Symbiosis Research, Karolinska Institutet, *104 01 Stockholm 60,* Sweden

S. Haglund, Department of Otolaryngology, Karolinska Sjukhuset, *104 01 Stockholm 60,* Sweden

O. Hallén, Department of Otolaryngology, Sahlgrenska Sjukhuset, *413 45 Göteborg,* Sweden

B. Hamberger, Department of Histology, Karolinska Institutet, *104 01 Stockholm 60,* Sweden

C.-A. Hamberger, Department of Otolaryngology, Karolinska Sjukhuset, *104 01 Stockholm 60,* Sweden

G. Hammer, Västra Frölunda Sjukvårdscentral, Box 138, *421 22 Västra Frölunda 1,* Sweden

G. Herberts, Department of Otolaryngology, Sahlgrenska Sjukhuset, *413 45 Göteborg,* Sweden

L. HERLIN, Department of Neurotraumatology, Karolinska Sjukhuset, *104 01 Stockholm 60,* Sweden

W. E. HITSELBERGER, Neurologic Surgery, 2202 West Third Street, *Los Angeles,* California 90057, U.S.A.

L. HOLMGREN, Department of Audiology, Karolinska Sjukhuset, *104 01 Stockholm 60,* Sweden

W. F. HOUSE, Otologic Medical Group, 2122 West Third Street, *Los Angeles,* California 90057, U.S.A.

L. B. W. JONGKEES, Department of Otolaryngology, Wilhelmina Gasthuis, Eerste Helmersstraat 104, *Amsterdam (Oud-West),* The Netherlands

A. S. KETCHAM, Surgery Branch, National Cancer Institute, N.I.H., Bldg. 10, Rm 10N116, *Bethesda,* Maryland 20014, U.S.A.

S. KHECHINASHVILI, 82 Barnov Street, *Tbilisi 79,* U.S.S.R.

I. KLOCKHOFF, Department of Audiology, Akademiska Sjukhuset, *750 14 Uppsala 14,* Sweden

H. KOCH, Department of Otolaryngology, Lasarettet, *220 05 Lund 5,* Sweden

Z. KRAJINA, Voćarsko Naselje 30, *Zagreb,* Yugoslavia

S. LANDIN, Department of Neurology, Karolinska Sjukhuset, *104 01 Stockholm 60,* Sweden

T LAURÉN, Department of X-ray Diagnosis, Kronprinsessan Lovisas Barnsjukhus, Polhemsgatan 30, *112 30 Stockholm,* Sweden

R. LUFT, Department of Endocrinology, Karolinska Sjukhuset, *104 01 Stockholm 60,* Sweden

N. LUNDBERG, Department of Neurosurgery, Lasarettet, *220 05 Lund 5,* Sweden

P. G. LUNDQUIST, Department of Otolaryngology, Karolinska Sjukhuset, *104 01 Stockholm 60,* Sweden

H. MENNIG, Universitätsklinik für Gesichts- und Halschirurgie Charité, Schumannstrasse 20/21, *104 Berlin,* D.D.R.

O. MEURMAN, Department of Otolaryngology, Universitetssjukhuset, *Åbo (Turku),* Finland

A. MIEHLKE, Universitätsklinik für HNO-Krankheiten, Geiststrasse 10, *34 Göttingen,* Germany

T. R. MILLER, Pack Medical Group, 139 East 36th Street, *New York,* N.Y. 10016, U.S.A.

A. MOBERG, Department of Pathology, Karolinska Sjukhuset, *104 01 Stockholm 60,* Sweden

G. MOBERGER, Department of Radiopathology, Karolinska Sjukhuset, *104 01 Stockholm 60,* Sweden

B. MÅRTENSSON, Department of Otolaryngology, Karolinska Sjukhuset, *104 01 Stockholm 60,* Sweden

H. H. NAUMANN, HNO-Klinik der Freien Universität, Städt. Krankenhaus Westend, Spandauer Damm 130, *1 Berlin 19,* Germany

G. NORLÉN, Department of Neurosurgery, Sahlgrenska Sjukhuset, *413 45 Göteborg,* Sweden

G. NOTTER, Department of Radiotherapy, Regionsjukhuset, *701 85 Örebro,* Sweden

C. O. NYLÉN, Familjehotellet Gandvik, Vendevägen 5 B, *182 61 Djursholm,* Sweden

J. H. OGURA, Department of Otolaryngology, Washington University, School of Medicine, 517 S. Euclid, *Saint Louis,* Missouri 63110, U.S.A.

H. OLIVECRONA, Department of Neurosurgery, Karolinska Sjukhuset, *104 01 Stockholm 60,* Sweden

I. PADOVAN, Institute for the scientific research and protection of the ear and respiratory tract, Vinogradska 29, *Zagreb,* Yugoslavia

T. PALVA, Department of Otolaryngology, Universitetssjukhuset, *Uleåborg (Oulo),* Finland

V. PAVLOW, Clinique d'ORL VMI, Rue G. Sofiiski No. 1, *Sofia,* Bulgaria

M. PORTMANN, Clinique universitaire d'ORL, 86 Cours d'Albret, *33 Bordeaux,* France

N. A. PREOBRASHENSKY, Department of Otolaryngology, I-st Medical Institute, ul. Rossolimo 15, *Moscow G-21,* U.S.S.R.

N. RISKAER, Department of Otolaryngology, Københavns Amts Sygehus i Gentofte, Niels Andersensvej 65, *Hellerup,* Denmark

U. SIIRALA, Department of Otolaryngology, Helsingfors Universitets-Centralsjukhus, Haartmansgatan 4 E, *Helsingfors 29 (Helsinki 29),* Finland

B. SJÖGREN, Department of Medicine IV, Sahlgrenska Sjukhuset, *413 45 Göteborg,* Sweden

T. Sjöstrand, Dean of the Medical Faculty, Department of Clinical Physiology, Karolinska Sjukhuset, *104 01 Stockholm 60,* Sweden

E. Wedenberg, Department of Audiology, Karolinska Sjukhuset, *104 01 Stockholm 60,* Sweden

J. Wersäll, Department of Otolaryngology, Karolinska Sjukhuset, *104 01 Stockholm 60,* Sweden

H. Wullstein, Universitätsklinik für HNO-Kranke, Josef-Schneider-Strasse 2, *8700 Würzburg,* Germany

J. Wågermark, Department of Pathology, Danderyds Sjukhus, *182 03 Danderyd 3,* Sweden

S. Zehm, Universitätsklinik für HNO-Kranke, Josef-Schneider-Strasse 2, *8700 Würzburg,* Germany

A. Änggård, Department of Otolaryngology, Karolinska Sjukhuset, *104 01 Stockholm 60,* Sweden

Welcome and opening address

By Torgny Sjöstrand

Department of Clinical Physiology, Karolinska Sjukhuset, Stockholm, Sweden.

This Symposium on Disorders of the Skull Base Region has been made possible by grants from the Nobel Foundation. On behalf of the Medical Faculty of the Karolinska Institute, it is a pleasure for me to extend the sincere thanks of the faculty to the Nobel Symposium Committee for its financial support of the symposium. I direct my thanks to the chairman of the committee, Mr. Ståhle. The realization of the symposium is the result of very extensive and self-sacrificing work on the part of the organizing committee, and I should like to extend the thanks of the faculty to the chairman of the committee, Professor Hamberger, and to the other members of the committee, especially its secretary, Dr. Wersäll.

The sponsorship of the Nobel Foundation, the skilful work of the organizing committee and the participation of so many distinguished scientists are a guarantee that the symposium will fulfil the function of the Nobel symposia, which is to be media for the exchange of information internationally in order to promote further progress in important fields of medicine. On behalf of the Medical Faculty of the Karolinska Institute, I express our best wishes for a successful symposium and extend a welcome to all participants, first and foremost to our foreign guests.

Notes on the history of acoustic tumor operations

By Herbert Olivecrona

Department of Neurosurgery, Karolinska Sjukhuset, Stockholm, Sweden

The foundation for rational treatment of acoustic tumors was laid by Folke Henschen in his monograph on Cerebello-Pontine Angle Tumors, 1910. In this important work he classified the different tumors occurring in this region and showed that acoustic neuromas were by far the most common lesion. He also clarified the anatomy of the acoustic neuromas and showed that their point of origin was almost exclusively in the lateral end of the vestibular nerve. His observation that acoustic neuromas very often cause an enlargement of the porus has become an important aid in the diagnosis of these tumors.

Although encapsulated and benign as well as located in an accessible region, the acoustic tumors long baffled the general surgeons, who tried to remove them. Ever since the first operations for this lesion were made in the late eighties, the mortality remained extremely high, usually 90% or even more and the few survivors were frequently left with serious defects.

It remained for Harvey Cushing to realize that acoustic tumors could not be completely removed with the technical resources present at that time, and he therefore introduced the method of intracapsular removal of most of the content of the tumor leaving the capsule *in situ*. In his monograph of 1917 he showed that with this method the mortality could be reduced to 20%. In his last series published by List, the mortality was reduced to 4%. In spite of this low primary mortality the 5-year mortality became as high as 45% due to recurrence of the tumor, which usually occurred within 3–4 years. The next contribution was made by Walter Dandy, who in 1922 published his method of complete removal of acoustic tumors after first doing an intracapsular evacuation of the content of the tumor and then removing the capsule. In his first series the mortality was still fairly high, but his last series, published by Revilla, showed in the last 40 consecutive cases only 1 death and this superb record of surgical skill remains unsurpassed to this day.

The early radical operations for acoustic tumors were all followed by complete facial paralysis. The late Hugh Cairns was the first to show in 1931 that the facial nerve could be saved by careful dissection of the capsule during its removal. Probably a great many attempts have been made to save the facial nerve in radical operations for acoustic tumors, but there are practically no statistics showing the results. In my own material it has been possible to save the anatomical continuity of the nerve in about 50 % and in the very large tumors even less. Complete or nearly complete facial paralysis is practically always present immediately after operation due to traumatization of the nerve during its dissection. Regeneration occurs in about 60 % of the cases, where the continuity of the nerve has been maintained, but in the remaining cases regeneration is prevented by scar tissue, particularly if the porus is coagulated to destroy possible remnants of the tumor in this location.

The difficulties of operations for acoustic tumors were for a long time greatly increased because of lack of reliable methods of anesthesia. This problem was not solved until the introduction of intratracheal anesthesia after intubation. Fluothane as anesthetic agent and several minor technical improvements now make it possible to administer a smooth and controllable anesthesia, this probably being the most important technical improvement in the conventional methods of operating on acoustic tumors.

The next important contribution to the surgery of acoustic tumors was Atkinson's observations published in 1949 that nearly all fatalities following removal of acoustic tumors were due to ligature of important branches of the anterior inferior cerebellar artery. In small tumors the artery can be identified and its destruction avoided, but in the large tumors the artery is concealed by the mass and therefore impossible to identify. This problem, as well as saving the facial nerve, therefore still remains with us and referring to the anterior inferior cerebellar artery MacKenzie in 1956 made the remark that there probably was an irreducible minimal mortality in radical operations for acoustic tumors of about 10–12 %.

The last important contribution to acoustic tumor surgery was made by the House group in Los Angeles, who revived the old translabyrinthine operation and added two variations of this operation, the transtemporal operation and the combined translabyrinthine and occipital operation after ligature of the sigmoid sinus. With refined technique using an operating microscope and diamond burrs, they were able to show that removal could be accomplished with a very low mortality and with conservation of the facial nerve and sometimes also of hearing in a large number of small tumors. This group also introduced a number of refinements in testing hearing and vestibular function, as well as function of the trigeminal and facial nerves, thereby improving the chances for an early diagnosis.

The situation today is that small tumors up to the size of a hazelnut can be safely removed with sparing of the facial nerve by the conventional method as well as by one of the otological methods. Probably the chance of saving the continuity of the facial nerve is somewhat better in the trans-temporal or translabyrinthine method of House. The large tumors still present a serious problem, and I doubt if any of the methods in use today will be the solution.

As long as the majority of tumors admitted to neurological clinics are large, the mortality will remain fairly high, perhaps around 10 % in the large tumors, and the real problem is to diagnose and treat the tumors while they are still small. With the present methods an early diagnosis is perfectly possible in practically all cases. The trouble is that many patients do not bother about unilateral loss of hearing and unless the patient is lucky enough to have vertiginous attacks that bring him to a specialist in an early stage of the disease, many patients are likely to go on until serious symptoms, indicating a large tumor, are present.

Education of the doctors, general practioners and otologists, who are likely to be the first to see patients harboring acoustic tumors, will probably be the most important factor in improving the results of surgery.

The vestibulo-cochlear nerve

By Hans Engström

Department of Otolaryngology, Akademiska Sjukhuset, Uppsala, Sweden

The vestibulo-cochlear nerve contains two functionally and structurally separate portions, the acoustic or cochlear nerve and the static or vestibular nerve. The cochlea and the cochlear nerve are phylogenetically late developments from the vestibular labyrinth and its nerve fibres. The vestibulo-cochlear nerve contains a varying number of fibres, which propagate impulses from, but also towards, the cochlea. The major number of fibres are of afferent nature, meaning that they lead impulses from the sense organ to acoustic and vestibular centres. There is, however, also a small number of fibres which propagate impulses from the brain stem towards the labyrinth. These fibres, which number about 500–600 to the cochlea (Rasmussen, 1953) and approximately 200 to the vestibular labyrinth (Gaçek, 1960), have been much discussed in recent years.

According to A. Rasmussen, the total number of cochlear nerve fibres is 35,000–50,000 in man. The number of vestibular fibres is lower, 14,200–24,000, but the number of nerve fibres seems to vary not only between different individuals, but there also seems to be a different proportional distribution to different parts of the labyrinth. A high number of cochlear fibres may be the result either of a dense innervation in each segment or of an elongation of the cochlea as a whole. The pattern of cochlear innervation and also the length of the cochlea have recently been described by Engström, Ades and Andersson (1966) and by Bredberg (1968).

The two main divisions of the vestibulo-cochlear nerve both contain myelinated nerve fibres with bipolar ganglion cells (Fig. 4). There are, however, also rather many unmyelinated fibres, running between the myelinated ones.

The cochlear nerve forms a connexion between the organ of Corti and the cochlear nuclei in the brain stem. In its peripheral portion, the cochlear nerve also contains efferent fibres from the contralateral superior olive and from the homolateral part of the medulla. A major portion of the nerve fibres lead impulses from nerve endings at the bases of cochlear sensory cells to the ventral and dorsal cochlear nuclei.

The afferent fibres have bipolar ganglion cells, located to the helical spiral

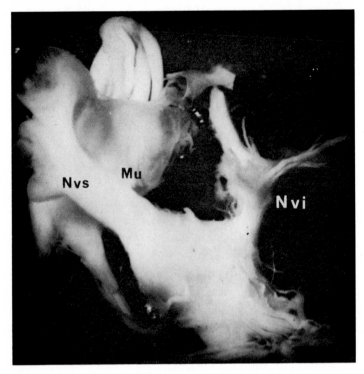

Fig. 1. Vestibular nerve with the upper branch (Nvs) and the lower branch (Nvi).The nerve to the macula utriculi at Mu. Cat.

ganglion. The total number of ganglion cells is estimated at about 31,000 in man. A recent monograph by Kellerhals, Engström and Ades contains a description of the main features of these ganglion cells.

There is a considerable variation in the diameter of the nerve fibres; 1–9 μ in man (Engström and Rexed, 1940). There is also a very characteristic difference between two types of neurons in the spiral ganglion. Thus 90 % of the ganglion cells are much larger than the remaining 10 %. The former group of ganglion cells also has a thick myelin coating, containing many layers of myelin lamellae. This myelin can be densely packed or have a more or less loose arrangement (cf. Kellerhals, Engström and Ades, 1968). The ganglion cells of the smaller group have only a single or sometimes double layer of Schwann cell or satellite cell cytoplasm around the perikaryon, and they can be easily distinguished from the larger myelinated cells, especially in the guinea-pig.

The fibres of the acoustic nerve have a highly characteristic somato- or tonotopical arrangement in the nerve. Thus, the whole nerve is slightly twisted, but fibres from the top of the cochlea mainly have a central position in the nerve, while fibres from the base of the cochlea are arranged in the peripheral layers of the nerve during its course in the inner acoustic meatus.

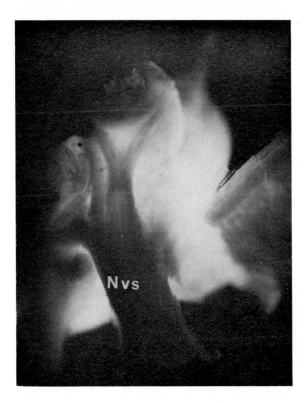

Fig. 2. The upper vestibular nerve branch (Nvs) to the anterior and lateral ampulla. Cat.

The arrangement of the blood vessels is also similar, as pointed out recently by Axelsson. As there is considerable evidence that high-frequency perception is located chiefly to the basal end of the cochlea, this means that fibres with a best frequency of, for instance, 4000 H_z should be found preferably in the peripheral portion of the acoustic nerve.

The acoustic nerve has one portion of "peripheral" and one portion of more "central" type with a "glial cone" forming the border between these two parts. This arrangement has been much discussed in relation to several different diseases, such as syphilis, psammomas and also in relation to acoustic neuromas.

Although the efferent fibres of the acoustic nerve have been much discussed in recent years, we still know relatively little about their function. They are, as stated earlier, rather few as compared to the larger number of afferent fibres, and their peripheral endings are nevertheless very imposing both in size and number (cf. Engström, 1958, Smith and Sjöstrand, 1961). It is mainly believed that the efferent fibres form a regulatory feed-back system (cf. the discussion at the CIBA Symposium 1967).

The vestibular nerve is situated behind the cochlear nerve. The nerve has two major divisions, the superior and the inferior vestibular nerve (Fig. 1). The

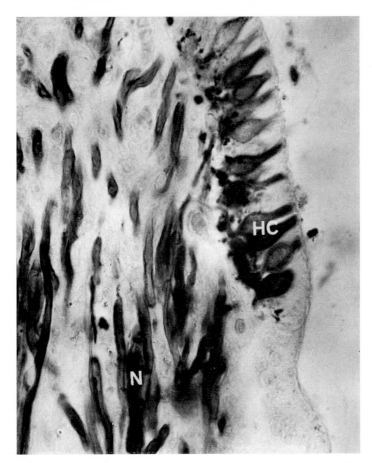

Fig. 3. Vestibular sensory cells (HC) and nerve fibres in a crista ampullaris of a guinea-pig. Maillet stain. Light microscopy.

upper branch sends or receives fibres from the lateral and superior ampullae, from the macula of the utricule and from a small portion of the macula sacculi (Figs. 2 and 3). The lower vestibular branch contains fibres from the posterior ampulla and from the major portion of the macula sacculi. The diameter of the nerve fibres ranges from 1 to 13 μ.

The vestibular nerve contains in its proximal part also the efferent fibres to the cochlea. Further out, these fibres pass to the cochlear nerve to form the intraganglionic bundle.

While both cochlear and vestibular nerve fibres have bipolar ganglion cells, the former are located to the bony canal of Rosenthal in the cochlea, whereas the latter lie in the internal auditory canal itself. The ganglion vestibuli (Scarpae) consists of one ganglion in mammals. The ganglion cells are considerably larger in the vestibular ganglion than in the cochlear (Figs.

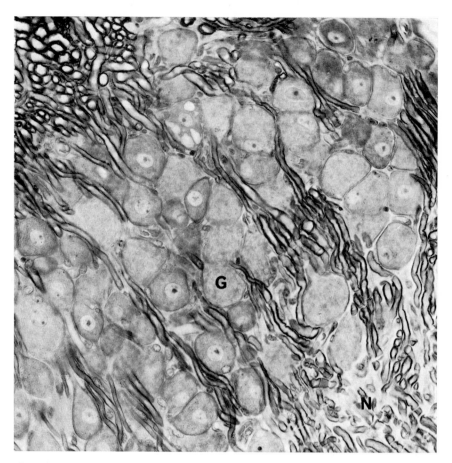

Fig. 4. Ganglion cells from the vestibular ganglion (G) and many nerve fibres (N). Guinea-pig. Phase-contrast microscopy.

4 and 5). Also in the vestibular ganglion, there are two kinds of distinctly different cells, one richly myelinated (Fig. 6) and one practically without coating. While those in the cochlear nerve form about 10 % of the total number, they are only about 3–5 % in the vestibular nerve.

The myelin coating of the richly myelinated cells may vary considerably in structure from one cell to the next, but also around individual cells (Ballantyne and Engström, 1969).

There has been considerable discussion about how different vestibular sensory regions are projected inside the nerve, inside the vestibular ganglion and in the proximal portion of the vestibular nerve. Lorente de Nó strongly advocated that there is a distinct somatotopic or tonotopic organization inside the vestibular nerve, and also inside the ganglion and the secondary vestibular ganglion cells. Lorente de Nó (1926) also pointed out that the

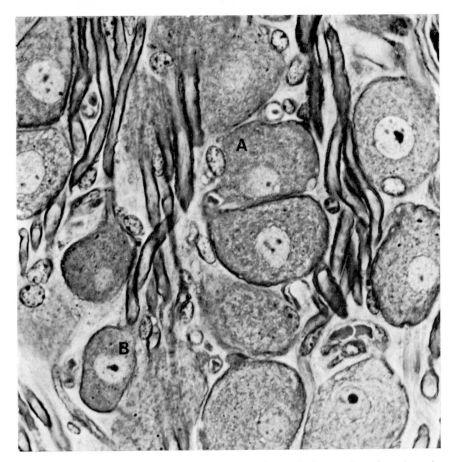

Fig. 5. Different sizes of ganglion cells (A and B) in the vestibular ganglion of a guinea-pig. Phase-contrast microscopy.

vestibular ganglion cells have a varying diameter in different portions. It is very evident that the ganglion cells vary in size, but a distinct regional subdivision is not easy to find, and this finding has recently been debated by several authors. It is of great interest from the point of this symposium that the region of the vestibular ganglion could very well also be the region of origin of acoustic neuromas. In this region there is normally a very wide range of disorderly arrangement of the myelin sheath around the ganglion cells, and many different kinds of cytoplasmic organization can be normally observed in the satellite cells.

There is still some confusion regarding the distribution of the vestibular nerve fibres (Fig. 7) in the brain stem and in the cerebellum. Reference is made to the excellent book by Brodal *et al.* (1962), and to the recent publication by Pompeiano (in press).

The efferent vestibular nerve fibres are few, but they still form a rich

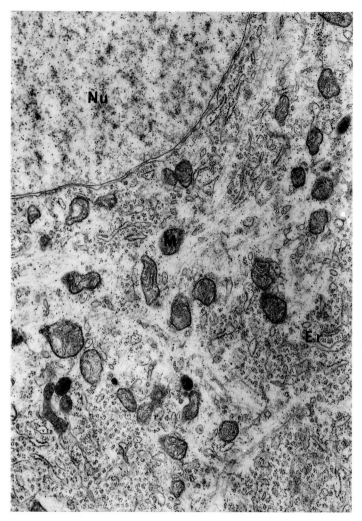

Fig. 6. Electron-microscopic picture of a vestibular ganglion cell. Nu is the nucleus, N one of many mitochondria and Er the endoplasmic reticulum.

network in the lower part of the sensory epithelium. They form rich contacts with both sensory cells, nerve chalices and sensory cells. Many of these contacts seem to be "en passant synapses" from the widespread efferent plexus.

References

Axelsson, A., *Acta Otolaryng.* (Stockholm), Suppl. 243 (1968).
Ballantyne, J. & Engström, H., *J. Laryng., 83,* 19 (1969).
Bredberg, G., *Acta Otolaryng.* (Stockholm), Suppl. 236 (1968).
Brodal, A., Pompeiano, O. & Walberg, F., *The vestibular nuclei and their con-nections,* Ramsay Henderson Trust Lecture. Oliver Boyd, Edinburgh (1962).

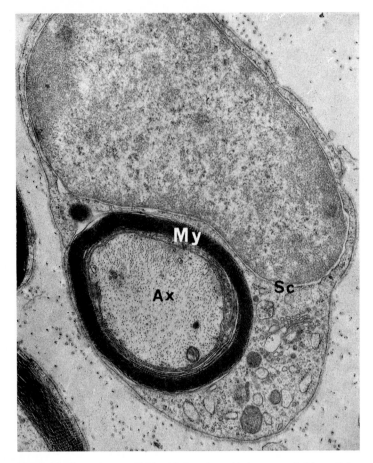

Fig. 7. Myelinated nerve (My) with axoplasm (Ax) surrounded by a Schwann cell (Sc). The section through the Schwann cell passes in this case through the nucleus (upper half of the micrograph). Electron microscopy. Magnification 20,000 x.

Engström, H., *Acta Otolaryng.* (Stockholm), *49,* 109 (1958).

Engström, H., Ades, H. W. & Andersson, A., *Structural pattern of the organ of Corti,* Almqvist & Wiksell, Stockholm (1966).

Engström, H. & Rexed, B., *Mikr. Anat. Forsch., 47,* 448 (1940).

Gaçek, R. R., *Efferent component of the vestibular nerve. Neural mechanisms of the auditory and vestibular systems.* Ed. by Rasmussen, G. L. & Windle, W., Springfield (Ill.), 276 (1960).

Kellerhals, B., Engström, H. & Ades, H. W., *Acta Otolaryng.* (Stockholm), Suppl. 226 (1968).

Lorente de Nó, R., *Études sur l'anatomie et la physiologie du labyrinthe. Travaux du laboratoire de recherches biologiques de l'université de Madrid* (Ramon y Cajal) (1926).

Pompeiano, O., *NASA Symposium,* Pensacola (Fla), in press.

Rasmussen, A. T., *Laryngoscope, 50,* 67 (1940).

Rasmussen, G. L., *J. Comp. Neurol., 99,* 61 (1953).

Smith, C. A. & Sjöstrand, F. S., *J. Ultrastruct. Res., 5,* 523 (1961).

The normal anatomy of the cerebello-pontine angle as studied radiologically

By Arne Grepe

Department of Neuroradiology,
Karolinska Sjukhuset, Stockholm, Sweden

The normal anatomy, as seen at pneumoencephalography, of the coarser structures in the basal cisterns has long been well known, and was thoroughly investigated by Liljequist (1959). The more delicate structures, such as the cranial nerves, have on the contrary been more difficult to discern at X-ray examination. This is due to the superimposed bone, and this applies especially to the cerebello-pontine angle. Progress in operative technique in this region has, however, made it imperative to gain more information about these less accessible structures, i.e., to improve the technique of cisternography. Cisternography has been performed with both positive and negative contrast media. Water-soluble contrast media are contraindicated because of their toxic effects. In recent years, cisternography has been carried out with oily contrast media (Baker, 1963, Gass, 1963, Scanlan, 1964, Reese and Bull, 1967). However, due to their physical properties, these media are less suitable when the aim is to study minor anatomical details. Moreover, a complete evacuation of the contrast medium is impossible. Air does not have any of these disadvantages, but due to its low contrasting capacity, some authors consider it inadequate for the study of the cranial nerves. However, the recent development of equipment that enables tomographic studies to be performed during all stages of pneumoencephalography offers new possibilities, and this has encouraged us to attempt to study minor anatomical details in the basal cisterns with air.

In order to be able to identify these details at pneumoencephalography *in vivo,* a postmortem study with special regard to the normal anatomy of the cranial nerves was deemed necessary. After developing a suitable technique for postmortem cisternography, this examination was performed in 8 cadavers without earlier known brain or cranial nerve disorders. The basal cisterns were filled with a suspension of barium sulphate in a gelatin solution (1/10 of Micropaque in 9/10 of a 10% solution of gelatin). The distribution of contrast medium after percutaneous injection into the basal cisterns is shown in Fig. 1. The basal part of the brain, together with the skull base,

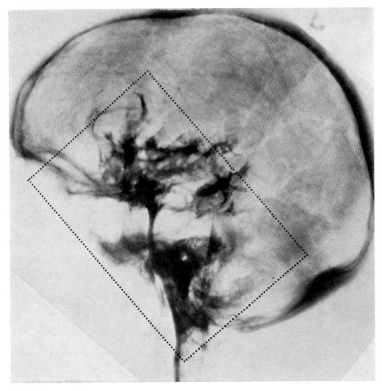

Fig. 1. Basal cisterns in a cadaver filled with contrast medium. Dotted lines indicate size of specimen removed *en bloc*.

was then removed in one piece for further radiological and anatomical examination. Tomographic cuts were made and the specimens were sliced in the same planes.

The postmortem tomogram in Fig. 2 permits a close study of the normal anatomy of the VIIth and VIIIth cranial nerves in their cisternal course.

As I reported in a paper read at the VIIIth Symposium Neuroradiologicum in Paris 1967, these postmortem examinations have facilitated the identification of cranial nerve structures at pneumoencephalography *in vivo*. Such a comparative postmortem and encephalographic study had not been performed before, and the normal anatomy of the nerves in the cerebellopontine cistern was incorrectly described by Epstein in his monograph of 1966.

In our encephalographic studies, we found convincing evidence that the facial and statoacoustic nerves can be seen in the frontal projection at pneumoencephalography *in vivo* (Fig. 3). The nerves are seen surrounded by air in the cistern, in the porus, and in the meatus. Although the nerves are superimposed, even with this limitation it should be possible to get an

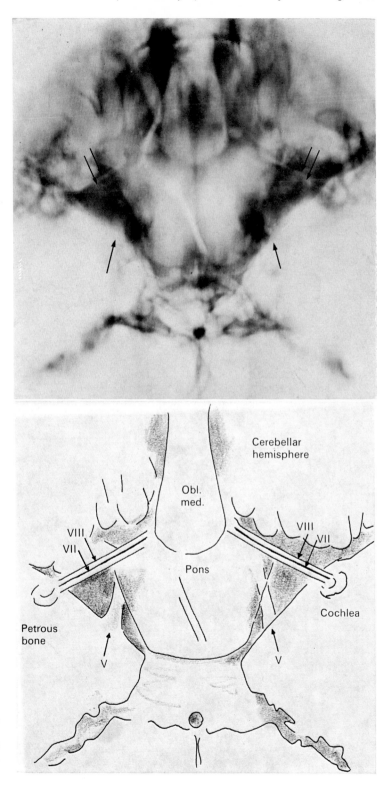

Fig. 2. A postmortem
tomogram almost parallel
with the skull base. The
cerebello-pontine cisterns
are roughly triangular in
shape.

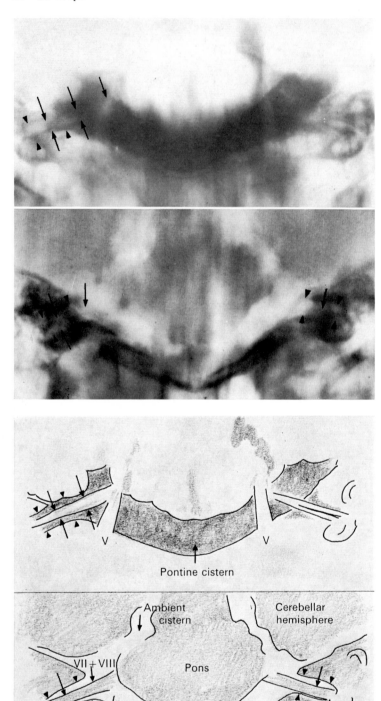

Fig. 3. Above, the Vth and VIIIth cranial nerve are seen in a postmortem examination. Below, the facial and statoacoustic nerves are seen at pneumoencephalography *in vivo*. The nerves are seen in the cistern, in the portus and in the internal meatus surrounded by air.

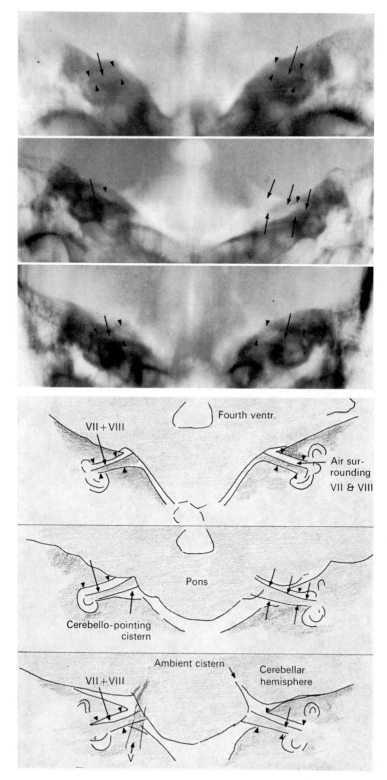

Fourth ventr.

VII + VIII

Air sur-
rounding
VII & VIII

Pons

Cerebello-pointing
cistern

Ambient cistern

Cerebellar
hemisphere

VII + VIII

g. 4. In these three dif-
ent pneumoencephalo-
ams, the VIIth and
IIth cranial nerves are
en in the cistern, in the
rus, and in the internal
atus surrounded by air.

idea of whether or not a small neuroma is present. In their intracanalicular courses, these nerves can almost always be seen, but how much of their cisternal course that can be followed depends on the size of the cistern (Fig. 4).

Concerning the other nerves in the cerebello-pontine cistern, I showed in the aforementioned comparative study that the trigeminal nerves can often be studied in a frontal projection at pneumoencephalography in tomograms cut parallel with these nerves. On the other hand, it has only seldom been possible to discern the glossopharyngeal and vagal nerves.

We await a water-soluble contrast medium that can be tolerated by neural tissue, and that will give optimal detail at cisternography. In the meanwhile, we believe that pneumoencephalography with the tomographic facilities now available can sometimes give as much information about the cranial nerves as do oily contrast media, and sometimes more.

References

Baker, H. L., Jr., *Radiology, 81,* 791 (1963).

Epstein, B. S., *Pneumoencephalography and cerebral angiography,* Year Book Medical Publishers Inc., Chicago (1966).

Gass, H., *Amer. J. Roentgen., 90,* 1197 (1963).

Grepe, A., *Encephalographic and postmortem studies of the optic chiasm and the acoustic nerves.* Transactions of the VIIIth Symposium Neuroradiologicum Paris 1967. Résumé des communications, 36 (1967).

Liljequist, B., *Acta Radiol.* (Stockholm), Suppl. 185 (1959).

Reese, D. F. & Bull, J. W. D., *Amer. J. Roentgen., 100,* 650 (1967).

Scanlan, R. L., *Arch. Otolaryng.* (Chicago), *80,* 698 (1964).

Diagnosis of vestibular system disorders

By Gunnar Aschan

Department of Otolaryngology, Regionssjukhuset, Linköping, Sweden

The theme of this session is acoustic neuroma, and it seems me for a certain reason a good choice to start with the vestibular aspects of the symptoms and the diagnostic procedure aimed at an early diagnosis so essential for radical surgery, and as few as possible lasting postoperative losses.

Henschen's observation (1910–1915) that the acoustic neuromas primary developed from the vestibular branch of the VIIIth cranial nerve must have the clinical consequence first to ask for vestibular symptoms and to perform a vestibular examination. The clinical picture is, however, not as simple as that. In slowly developing vestibular lesions, peripheral as well as central, the *subjective* symptoms are more or less ruled out by compensatory processes of central origin. The literature gives little information about what symptoms first take the patient to the doctor, vestibular disturbances or auditory. Judging from a material of 30 patients it seems that about 50 % of them started with not too disturbing vestibular symptoms. Both the patient and often the examining doctor will, however, take a hearing loss more seriously.

The *objective* vestibular findings are, on the contrary, not ruled out by the central compensatory process, and here the caloric test is the absolutely dominating diagnostic aid, and also gives the most constant objective findings. This can be inferred from the literature. House, despite a changing technique for calorization, had 96 % positive caloric findings, Dix and Hallpike (1960) give, with their consequent technique, 100 % asymmetric caloric findings, 93 % being of the canal paresis type. In my own material of 30 cases, all had a canal paresis, 23 being completely without caloric reactions on the affected side.

In larger materials, less than 10 % of the patients showed a directional preponderance, and I think that this must be in accordance with Henschen's statement mentioned not being 100 % valid. Less than 10 % of the neuromas develop medial to the internal acoustic meatus, as Dix and Hallpike discussed in 1966. The value of the caloric test must also be judged against Johnson's presentation (1966) of the House material. Only 118 of 163 patients had so much hearing left that refined audiological tests could be performed. In the same material, 30 patients were classified as having "small tumours". Only 7 had significant audiological findings indicating acoustic neuroma. It seems to me thus worth pointing out that before a patient has a hearing loss, and also later when he has completely or nearly completely lost his hearing, the caloric test is the diagnostic tool that might indicate an acoustic neuroma. In Sweden, often the latter situation is the more common, 18 of 30 patients were so deaf that no refined audiological tests could be performed.

Unilateral nerve deafness is for every otologist a rather common observation. The problem is to screen out such patients who might have an acoustic neuroma which, on the other hand, compared to unilateral nerve deafness of varying degrees is very rare. Our national insurance gives some interesting figures. In one year, more than 10,000 patients had an X-ray of the internal acoustic meatus, but only 40 patients were operated on for acoustic neuroma (Sweden has 7.5 million inhabitants), and we may hope that the indication for those X-rays at least had a unilateral hearing loss as a motivation.

My point is that the aim of the otologist must be to achieve better clinical screening of the patients before they are referred for X-ray of the internal acoustic meatus. The combination of pure tone audiogram and caloric testing can be made in practically every ENT unit, even small ones, and only patients with caloric asymmetries should be referred for X-ray examinations. Such a procedure should be fairly safe, and if the X-ray departments are not overrun by clinically not too well motivated examinations, they could use the time spared for such patients in whom the internal meatus is not enlarged, and the diagnosis can be made only by advanced neuroradiology. We will probably hear much more about that later, but I think that the otologist must be the one who devises that better screening.

I said otologist because, despite the subspecialization within otology, such a clinical screening demands for vestibular as well as audiological examinations judged as a whole which can be compressed in a slogan "No caloric test without a pure tone audiogram, but also no unilateral nerve deafness without a caloric test".

Let me say a few words about the vestibular examination technique. I hope that all of you know that vestibular nystagmus is decreased in intensity or disappears completely if the patient can fixate. This is valid both for nystagmus as a spontaneous symptom, or nystagmus induced by vestibular stimuli such as calorization. Here, electronystagmography comes into the picture as a diagnostic tool. Merely closing the eyelids is enough to increase the intensity of vestibular nystagmus of all kinds up to 10 times, and the objective record gives several additional parameters for example, duration of calorically induced nystagmus, on which to base the quantitative analyses.

This use of electronystagmography is especially important when searching for acoustic neuromas, because nystagmus as a spontaneous sign is present in up to 50% of the patients. If in these patients this spontaneous nystagmus is inhibited by fixation, this may be a severe source of error in quantitative analysis of the caloric responses. Electronystagmography eliminates this, because the intensity of the nystagmus present before calorization will serve as the reference.

Summing up my points of view on early diagnosis of acoustic neuroma, neither vestibular nor audiological examinations used singly will give a reasonably safe clinical screening of the patients before referring them for X-ray examination. The *otologist* has to operate with both, and judge both examinations together as a whole. Regarding the vestibular examinations, the electronystagmograph will give much safer results, serving in a way similar to the audiometer, when performing audiological examinations.

General discussion

C. O. Nylén
First, I would like to express my sincere thanks for the kind words addressed
to me by the chairman, Professor Jongkees.

After listening to the lecture of Professor Olivecrona, I would like to point
out that with him, Antoni, Sahlgren and I—starting about 50 years ago and
lasting for many years—had a very good cooperation in diagnosing the
tumours of the brain, some of which were acoustic tumours.

Dr. Aschan pointed out in his paper the importance of the caloric examination and electronystagmography. I would like to add that there are also
many other vestibular examinations, such as positional nystagmus, galvanic
and rotatory tests, that ought to be performed before the diagnosis is
established from the vestibular point of view.

Moberg to Engström
Did your slides represent material from human beings or animals? Are there
any differences in this respect between human beings and animals?

Engström to Moberg
The main principles in the arrangement of the nerve fibres and ganglion cells
of the statoacoustic nerve seem to be the same in those higher mammals we
have studied. In all animals with a coiled cochlea, there is a certain coiling
of the nerve as a whole, with fibres from the apex centrally, and fibres from
the base of the cochlea peripherally. In the vestibular nerve there is, in all
the mammals we have studied, a fairly systematic and corresponding arrangement of the nerve fibres and ganglion cells, although species variations
are found, as described by de Burlet, by Weston and several others.

Jongkees to Aschan
Dr. Aschan gave a very clear survey of the vestibular examination and its
value for the diagnosis of acoustic neuromata, and I agree with him that the
caloric test is extremely important. I only cannot agree to the use of the
expression *canal paresis* for hyporeactivity to caloric stimulation.

In acoustic neuroma, the canal is not "paretic" (whatever a paretic canal
may mean).

Khechinashvili to Aschan
Dr. Aschan has spoken about the necessity of a careful investigation in each
patient with vestibular symptoms. I think that this is right, and vestibulometry
should be as detailed as possible. We always perform EEG studies simultane-

ously with ENG studies. It gives a better understanding of the vestibular function, especially in cases where central nervous system involvement is possible.

Bergstedt to Aschan

It was interesting to listen to Aschan's excellent presentation. I agree completely with him about methods. I should like to take the opportunity of stressing the importance of performing both cold and warm water syringing in the caloric vestibular test. The occurrence of a preponderance to the healthy side otherwise masks an abnormality.

Arslan to Aschan

In very early cases of acoustic neuroma, an excellent diagnostic tool is the galvanic test, since galvanic stimulation is specific only to the vestibular fibres.

Caloric stimulation, on the contrary, acts for both, receptors and fibres; this is the reason why, in a very early stage of the disease, the caloric test can often give only a doubtful response; in these cases, the galvanic test is very helpful.

Fisch to Aschan

A question to Dr. Aschan regarding the parameters used in the analysis of ENG recordings in acoustic neuroma. In Zurich, we have operated on 9 acoustic tumours of less than 2.5 cm maximal diameter. In all these cases, the caloric response was impaired on the side of the lesion. The reduction in the caloric response in one case was, however, only apparent following the analysis of the velocity of the slow component, and not in the study of the duration. Did you observe similar cases?

Aschan to Jongkees

I agree that the term *canal paresis* is inadequate. Nevertheless, everyone knows what it means, and I doubt if much is gained by changing the nomenclature. The title of this session is just as inadequate. We say acoustic neuromas when the term should be vestibular neurinoma.

Aschan to Arslan

I have practically no experience of the galvanic test. For some unknown reason, there seems to be a border in the middle of Europe for this method.

Aschan to Fisch

We have seen that other parameters, such as the eye speed, total amplitude and number of beats, indicate a canal paresis, but not the duration.

Audiologic diagnosis of acoustic neuroma

By Ingmar Klockhoff

Department of Audiology, Akademiska Sjukhuset, Uppsala, Sweden

Hearing loss in cases of acoustic neuroma is devoid of specific characteristics; that is to say, there is no tone audiogram typical of nerve-fibre deafness. It is only when the residual hearing is tested with various kinds of supra-threshold stimuli—tones as well as speech—that pathophysiologic features become evident—which are specific enough to serve as a means of distinguish between nerve-fibre deafness and end-organ deafness.

Even with stimulation just above the threshold, the pathologic tone threshold discloses what is usually referred to as *tone threshold decay* or pathologic adaptation. This phenomenon is most easily demonstrated by means of an ordinary tone audiometer, pathologic decay being considered to be present if an initially slightly suprathreshold tone needs constantly to be increased for the tone sensation to be maintained. With a Békésy audiometer, the same phenomenon can be observed by Jerger's method, when it is manifested as a significant tone threshold drop with continuous tonal stimulation compared with if the tone is presented interrupted—a so-called Jerger type III or IV.

Lack of recruitment of loudness is, however, the characteristic of nerve-fibre deafness which is by far the best known. With Fowler's classical alternate binaural loudness balance test, much stronger sound stimuli are required on the affected than the unaffected ear to attain equal loudness, if such a sensation can be obtained at all within the limits of the available tone intensities.

In objective recruitment examination with the acoustic stapedius reflex test, as originally suggested by Metz, the results are in close agreement with those of the Fowler test in cases of recruitment. In view of this it would be expected in nerve-fibre deafness that the lack of recruitment would be manifested in an elevation of the reflex threshold equal to that of the tone threshold of the affected ear. Just what actually happens here has been examined closely by Henry Anderson, who will later on be giving an account of the properties of the acoustic stapedius reflex in retrocochlear lesions.

Another characteristic of nerve-fibre deafness is a *speech discrimination loss* that is disproportionally large in relation to the tonal hearing loss; when this is still only moderate a speech discrimination score close to zero is by no means uncommon.

In nerve-fibre deafness the *directional hearing acuity,* too, has been found to be *reduced* significantly more than in hearing loss of more peripheral origin. The insufficiency is manifested by a pathologically reduced precision in repeated location of tonal sound sources placed in different positions in an echofree chamber.

The fact that in a fairly large proportion of acoustic tumour cases the phenomena characteristic of nerve-fibre deafness cannot be demonstrated with acceptable reliability by the common psychoacoustic test battery does not necessarily imply an inadequacy of the tests as such. This may be due to the fact that the pattern of destruction due to the tumour is complex and, because of circulatory disturbances, also may involve cochlear structures. In addition, there is the familiar fact that cochlear lesions of different origin are fairly common in the adult and increase with age. Since there may be an uncertain component of cochlear deafness, either due to the tumour or independently of it, one must be prepared for confusing cochlear symptoms. This means that audiologic examination should be looked upon as a screening for indications, where no one of the tests mentioned can definitely be ranked above the others.

Clinical practice

Of the predominantly unilateral perceptive deafness that is of relevance in this connection, tumour of the acoustic nerve is a comparatively uncommon cause. In Sweden with a population of about 8 millions, only some 40 cases are diagnosed in a year, and for several of these, audiologic tests are not applicable because, by the time a tumour is suspected, the loss is already too great. Still, every otolaryngologist must have a routine clinical procedure that may be considered acceptable for the immediate object, namely of reliably ascertaining that the deafness in question is *not* due to an acoustic tumour. The very fact that the patient consults the physician for a perceptive hearing loss that has appeared suddenly or worsened rapidly, with subsidiary symptoms such as tinnitus, distortion, and reduced sound tolerance, suggests another genesis than acoustic neuroma; for this usually appears to result in a less noticeable deterioration in the hearing; that may be one reason why the hearing loss is sometimes not recognized until other symptoms have prompted a consultation.

As regards testing in practice, it would seem that the best approach is first to try to obtain an impression of the degree of recruitment. This is most simply accomplished by means of the Fowler test, with an ordinary tone audiometer, to ensure that strong tones within the frequency range of the hearing loss produce a sensation equal to that obtained in the unaffected ear. Such evidence of complete recruitment practically rules out the possibility of an acoustic tumour. On the other hand, if there is incomplete recruitment, or remarkably poor discrimination for conversational or telephoned speech, further tests are indicated. Tests of vestibular function and corneal sensibility do not formally belong to the strict audiologic diagnosis, but it might not be out of place to recall that where there is the slightest uncertainty such tests should be included in the initial examination. Only where the results of these tests are uncertain would it seem necessary to refer the patient to a more well-equipped place for further audiologic examination, such as regular speech audiometry and tests of the acoustic stapedius reflexes and the decay phenomenon. There are, of course, a variety of other hearing tests, especially for recruitment, that can be applied for the same purpose, according to personal inclination and conviction. This final audiologic examination might conveniently be carried out parallel with further medical examination of CSF protein, cranial reflexes, etc., and, finally, in the case of pathologic indications, an X-ray examination covering the internal auditory foramen, and encephalography as a basis for a final assessment.

Of the application of the audiological tests, it may finally be said that pure nerve-fibre deafness is easily distinguished from pure end-organ deafness. Difficulty in interpretation arises, however, in the various cases of hearing loss, where pathophysiologic retrocochlear features are found to be concomitant with dominant cochlear symptoms, but where no retrocochlear lesion can be identified. This suggests that in predominantly cochlear deafness there are not infrequently elements of a retrocochlear nature, the character of which remains uncertain, because of the natural difficulty of obtaining simultaneous histologic evidence.

The clinical necessity of being able to recognize the relatively few acoustic tumours has undoubtedly constituted an effective spur to the development of a multifacetted test battery. However, these expanding resources are extremely important not only from the aspect of tumour diagnosis, but also because they improve our prospects of distinguishing different patterns of sensory-neural defects. A better differential diagnosis in such respects would put us in a better position to deal with the ever present yet difficult questions relating to the cause of the injuries, their pathogenesis and prognosis.

In such a context, the case of acoustic tumour provides a particularly rewarding object for study, since here the presence of nerve-fibre damage is safely established.

Intra-aural reflexes in retrocochlear lesions

By Henry Anderson, Bengt Barr and Erik Wedenberg

Department of Audiology, Karolinska Sjukhuset, Stockholm, Sweden

This study concerns the possibilities that are provided by the acoustically elicited reflexes of the intra-aural muscles for making an early diagnosis in cases of retrocochlear hearing impairment, especially in cases of tumours affecting the acoustic nerve.

Methods for recording the reflex activity of the intra-aural muscles have with the years assumed increasing importance in clinical diagnosis of various forms of hearing defects. These methods of investigation which are often referred to as impedance measurements are based on electro-acoustic registration of the activity of the intra-aural muscles as manifested in the sound-reflecting properties of the tympanic membrane. Various technical arrangements have been proposed for this purpose and references on this subject are found in the bibliography.

The acoustic reflex measurement can be used for obtaining answers to a number of problems in hearing diagnosis; of interest in the present context are the responses that can be recorded when the inner of the two intra-aural muscles, the stapedius muscle, is induced to contract. This muscle is the effectuating organ in a reflex arc whose afferent pathway consists of the sensory cells of the cochlea and the acoustic nerve. In sound stimulation of moderate intensity a reflex contraction is elicited in the stapedius muscle and the degree of contraction increases with the intensity of the stimulus within a fairly large dynamic range (Fig. 1). The reflex response can thus be used as a measure of the afferent inflow through the sensory-neural system of the ear at supra-threshold levels.

By ascertaining the lowest intensity for which recordable responses are obtained at different test frequencies—just as for the usual hearing threshold audiogram—a reflex threshold curve is recorded (Fig. 2). If then the stimulus tone is presented at definite levels above this reflex threshold a relative measure of the strength of the muscle contraction in the form of response amplitude is obtained. These functions are thoroughly examined in earlier studies, where certain pathologic criteria also have been formulated.

Another interesting feature of the reflex response is its persistance on prolonged acoustic stimulation. Fig. 3 shows a representative recording in a normal ear; the test was performed at 500, 1000, 2000 and 4000 Hz

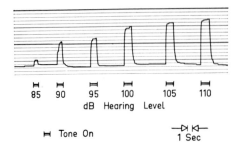

H   H   H   H   H   H
85 90 95 100   105   110
        dB Hearing Level

H Tone On   —▷◁ K◁—
                           1 Sec

Fig. 1. Increase in response amplitude
as a function of stimulus tone intensity.
Stimulus frequency 1000 Hz.

at a level of 10 dB above the reflex threshold and with a stimulus duration
of 10 seconds. For the lower test frequencies no fatigue at all is observed
in this period; at 2000 Hz a small but significant reduction in the response
amplitude is noted, and at 4000 Hz this reduction is marked. This phenomenon has been termed "reflex decay"; it is quantified as the time (in seconds)
for the response amplitude to be reduced by 50 per cent.

Fig. 4 shows the mean persistence of the response for 50 ears of young
subjects with normal hearing. In no one of the subjects any reduction of
response amplitude was observed for the lower test frequencies, whereas
the median "half-life" of the responses for 2000 and 4000 Hz was 14 and
7 seconds, respectively.

A natural question in this connection is whether the cause of this fatigue
is to be sought in the motoric or sensory part of the reflex arc. The very
fact that the reflex decay is dependent on the stimulus frequency suggests
that the fatigue lies on the afferent side. Moreover, this is readily confirmed

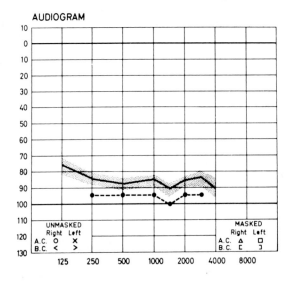

AUDIOGRAM

Fig. 2. Median and semi-
interquartile range (shaded)
for the normal reflex threshold. — — — denotes lower
limit for pathologic threshold values.

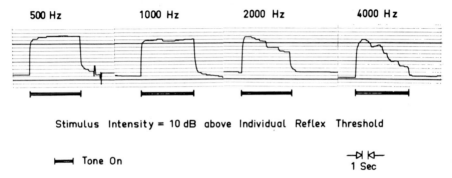

| 500 Hz | 1000 Hz | 2000 Hz | 4000 Hz |

Stimulus Intensity = 10 dB above Individual Reflex Threshold

▬ Tone On

—▷| |◁—
1 Sec

Fig. 3. The reflex response on prolonged stimulation recorded in a normal ear.

experimentally. For even in the fatigue phase the full amplitude of the response is readily recovered by inserting complementary acoustic or tactile stimuli.

The object of this study was to examine primarily the reflex threshold and the reflex characteristic in a series of established disorders of the acoustic nerve at as early a stage as possible. Cases of such confirmable lesion are very rare and to enable other differential diagnostic hearing tests

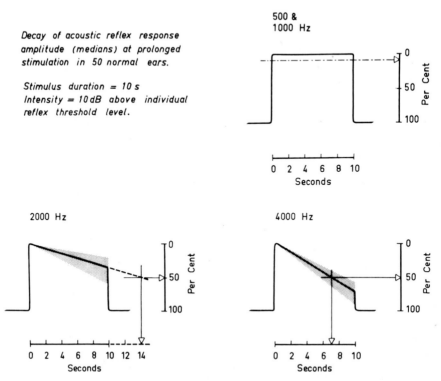

Decay of acoustic reflex response amplitude (medians) at prolonged stimulation in 50 normal ears.

Stimulus duration = 10 s Intensity = 10 dB above individual reflex threshold level.

500 & 1000 Hz

2000 Hz

4000 Hz

Fig. 4. Half-life points of responses indicated by continuous arrows; dash-dotted arrow is limit of recording accuracy. Shaded area: Semi-interquartile range.

Table 1. *Result of differential diagnostic hearing tests (12 acoustic tumours, 5 posterior fossa tumours)*

	Speech discr.	Fowler's test	Threshold decay
Tested	17	14	16
Positive	8	9	8
Proportion of positive tests	47%	64%	50%

to be applied reliably it was stipulated that the hearing loss should not exceed 60 dB, a requirement that further restricted the choice of subjects. Since the study was begun in 1964 we have succeeded in finding 17 such patients, 12 of whom had acoustic nerve tumours (10 confirmed surgically and 2 by neuro-radiography) and 5 cases of posterior fossa tumours so located as to affect the acoustic nerve. All but 1 of these 5 were confirmed at operation, and in the 5th, where no operation could be performed, the site was confirmed radiographically.

The hearing threshold of the affected ear in about one half of the cases was better than 20 dB (the mean for 500, 1000 and 2000 Hz); in no case was the hearing loss greater than 60 dB. The hearing threshold curve was usually sloping or flat; it should be noted that no less than 6 of the subjects displayed a quite normal hearing threshold in the range 250–4000 Hz, due account being taken of age, sex and occupation.

The results of the traditional hearing tests used in differential diagnosis, namely speech discrimination, Fowler's test and the hearing threshold decay test, are found in Table 1. These tests were positive in only about 50 per cent of the applications, a degree of unreliability that is a well documented feature.

As regards the results of the reflex measurements the reflex threshold was pathologically elevated in all 17 cases, in 7 cases so much that the reflex could not be elicited even at maximum available sound stimulus (120 dB hearing level).

In the 10 cases where the reflex threshold could be attained, however, there was yet another interesting feature in the reflex response, namely an abnormally rapid fatigue on prolonged stimulation. As has been shown earlier, there is normally no measurable reflex decay for the frequencies 500 and 1000 Hz. For the tumour group there was a marked reflex decay, the response amplitude for these frequencies being halved in about 3 seconds; for none of the subjects, at any of the test frequencies, was the halving-time longer than 5 seconds. (Fig. 5).

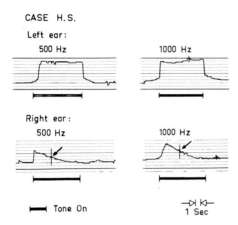

CASE H.S.

Left ear:
500 Hz   1000 Hz

Right ear:
500 Hz   1000 Hz

◼━━ Tone On   ━▷◀ ◀┤━
                       1 Sec

Fig. 5. Recording of reflex decay in one of the acoustic tumour cases. In left, normal ear no reflex decay is observed and the response has here the characteristic rectangular configuration; in the affected right ear the reflex decay is clearly seen: the half-life of response (indicated by arrows) is in the order of 4 seconds.

From the standpoint of reflex measurement there are thus two properties that are distinctive of the tumour group, namely, an elevated reflex threshold and the described abnormally rapid decay in the reflex response.

As regards unilateral elevation of the reflex threshold this sign is not exclusively pathognomonic for retrocochlear lesions of this particular type: although very rarely encountered, such elevation may be observed, for instance, in certain forms of sudden deafness. It is thus evident that even though a unilateral pathologic elevation of the reflex threshold is not entirely specific for expansive lesions involving the acoustic nerve, it should always arouse suspicion of the presence of such a process.

As regards reflex decay a different situation obtains. During the years that this study has been going on the reflex decay test has been performed in more than 600 patients where the clinical picture has pointed to the possibility of a retrocochlear process—that is to say the greater part of the patients referred to our department for thorough otoneurologic examination. In this biased material of sensory defects where a disproportionate number of retrocochlear lesions would be expected only 6 more cases of definitely pathologic reflex decay were found. In none of these cases, however, did the further medical examination disclose any signs of an expansive process. The traditional differential diagnostic hearing tests in these 6 cases were indicative of retrocochlear hearing impairment in two thirds of the application—that is to say, a slightly higher proportion than in the group of verified tumours. There can be hardly any doubt that these cases, too, actually had some forms of impairment of the acoustic nerve although it was of a less specific nature.

Three cases of multiple sclerosis with hearing loss as one of the features of the pathologic picture are of special interest. In these patients, too, reflex decay was noticed, but the halving time was on average slightly longer than

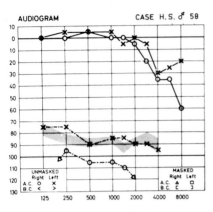 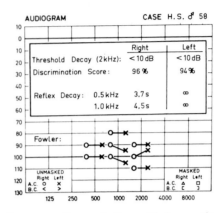

Fig. 6. Result in one of the cases, male 58 years, with surgically verified acoustic tumour on the right side. The hearing threshold (left upper curve, circles) of the affected ear is quite normal with respect to age nor did the threshold decay test, speech discrimination test or Fowler's recruitment test reveal any abnormality in the hearing function. Distinct positive for retrocochlear affection were the elevated reflex threshold (left, lower curve) and the pronounced reflex decay on this side.

for the tumour group—6.2 against 3 seconds. Since the cause of any hearing defect in multiple sclerosis is considered to be located in the nerve trunk, this observation constitutes further evidence that the reflex decay phenomenon is associated with lesion to the acoustic nerve.

It would seem justified to infer from the results of this study that where an elevated reflex threshold and pathologic reflex decay are recorded in spite of slight or moderate unilateral hearing loss it is highly probable that there is a retrocochlear affection due to an expansive process. In severe hearing loss—subtotal deafness—however, the validity of the observations is open to discussion and it is still too early to say whether the tests can be of any value in such cases.

The tests would appear to be particularly valuable in clinical diagnosis for in the first place they have been positive in every case where they could be applied, and, not the least important, the elevated reflex threshold and pathologic reflex decay would appear to be the earliest observable audiologic signs of a retrocochlear affection; this is borne out by a few extreme cases where the hearing threshold was entirely normal and where none of the other differential diagnostic hearing tests disclosed the presence of a retrocochlear lesion (Fig. 6).

In view of the introduction of new surgical methods for early operation of acoustic tumours, these tests may be expected by virtue of their simplicity to assume decisive importance for the early audiologic diagnosis of such disorders.

References

Anderson, H. & Barr, B., *Acta Otolaryng.* (Stockh.), *62*, 171 (1966).

Anderson, H. & Barr, B., *Laryngoscope, 77,* 1825 (1967).

Anderson, H. & Wedenberg, E., *Acta Otolaryng.* (Stockh.), *65,* 535 (1968).

Jepsen, O., *Studies on the acoustic stapedius reflex in man.* Thesis, Universitetsforlaget, Aarhus (1955).

Johnson, E. W., *Arch. Otolaryng.* (Chic.), *84,* 247 (1966).

Klockhoff, I., *Acta Otolaryng.* (Stockh.), Suppl. 164 (1961).

Roentgenological diagnosis in acoustic neuroma

By Torgny Greitz

Department of Neuroradiology,
Karolinska Sjukhuset, Stockholm, Sweden

This paper can by no means give a complete survey of the radiological examination of acoustic neuroma. It will only touch on the diagnosis of bone
changes and will not deal with tomography of the internal meatus, which is
the subject of the following presentation. It will not include cisternography
with oily contrast media, because in Sweden we have no experience of this
technique.

According to most authors, acoustic tumours can be diagnosed radiologically on the basis of bone erosion in about 60 % of cases. In an additional
20 %, changes are present that make the diagnosis highly probable. In 15
to 20 % there are no changes. As a screening procedure, radiological examination of the internal meatus is therefore inferior to careful refined
otoneurologic examinations, and analysis of the CSF protein content. These
clinical methods are all positive in more than 90 % of cases. The roentgenological examination has the advantage of giving a specific diagnosis, but
is a rather time-consuming procedure that should be restricted to cases in
which diagnosis is supported by a careful clinical investigation.

In the last decades, there has been continuous progress in the encephalographic diagnosis of acoustic neuroma, based on alternating improvements in
technique and anatomical knowledge. The normal anatomy of the basal
cisterns and their changes in acoustic neuroma have been studied extensively
by Liliequist (1959). We are now at a point where very refined structures
may be studied with encephalography (Grepe, 1967, 1968). The technique
used for encephalography at the neuroradiological department of Karolinska
Hospital is essentially the same as that of Robertsson and Lindgren, with
minor modifications made possible through improved facilities for tomography (Fredzell et al., 1968). In our opinion, pneumoencephalography, not
ventriculography, is the method of choice especially in the diagnosis of extra-
cerebral tumours, because pneumoencephalography allows examination of
the ventricular system and of the basal cisterns as well. In the presence of
increased intracranial pressure or in a patient with signs of an extensive
tumour, burr holes are made before the procedure, to allow an immediate

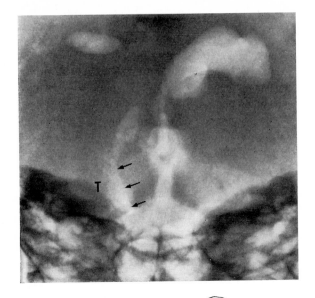

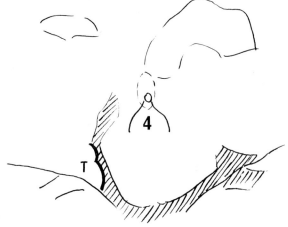

Fig. 1. Acoustic neuroma in right pontine angle deforming the brain stem by displacing its surface (arrows). Cerebello-pontine cistern dilated on the side of the tumour (T). Fourth ventricle (4) is not deformed.

ventricular puncture in the case of acute herniation. Immediate operation following pneumoencephalography is preferable in most cases. These facts call for close cooperation between the neuroradiologist and the neurosurgeon.

Small acoustic neuromas are seen at pneumoencephalography as a filling defect just outside the meatus, and in most cases the surface of the pons is displaced away from the petrous bone by the tumour. This causes a dilatation of the cistern medial to the tumour, which is a very typical finding (Fig. 1). Small neuromas cause no deformity of the fourth ventricle. Consequently, they cannot be diagnosed by ventriculography. In most cases, however, the fourth ventricle is deformed. It is elevated on the side of the tumour. It is then said to be rotated. In the air-filled cerebello-pontine cistern, only that part of the neuroma which grows in the cistern can be assessed. The remain-

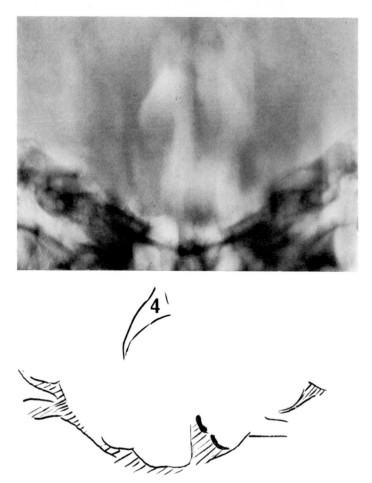

Fig. 2. Large acoustic neuroma on the left side (arrows). The fourth ventricle (4) is considerably displaced and deformed, indicating intrapontine invagination. The tumour is larger than expected from evaluation of its cisternal part.

ing portion of the tumour may be invaginated into the pons. From the displacement and the deformity of the fourth ventricle, it is possible to evaluate whether the tumour is more extensive than judged from its cisternal part. In order to obtain a correct idea of the size of the tumour, it is therefore essential to fill the ventricular system (Fig. 2). This means that ventriculography may be deemed necessary in cases with non-filling of the ventricular system at pneumoencephalography. In order to tell whether the tumour is extra- or intra-axial and to diagnose small tumours, the cisterns have to be examined. In the majority of cases with acoustic neuromas, a deformity of the brain stem on the tumour side has been present. This was the case in all acoustic neuromas published by Liliequist. If we are going to operate on the very small tumours, we cannot rely on displacement of

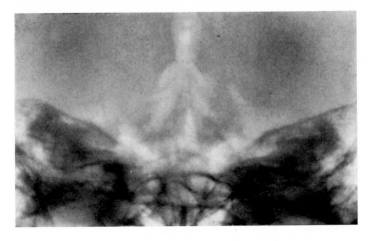

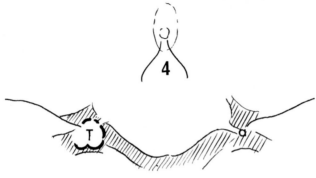

Fig. 3. Small neuroma (T) on right side without deformation of brain stem and without displacement of fourth ventricle (4). Medial portion of normal acoustic nerve (a) can be seen on the left side.

structures adjacent to the tumour. We must be able to demonstrate the tumour itself. And, as a matter of fact, we are able to diagnose small tumours which do not cause any deformity of the brain stem (Fig. 3).

In recent years, oily contrast media, such as Pantopaque and Myodil, have been used in an attempt to increase the diagnostic accuracy, especially in small tumours (Scanlan, 1964, Reese and Bull, 1967). We have no personal experience of this method. Judging from the reports and the illustrations which have been published, the tumours so far diagnosed are not significantly smaller than those seen at encephalography with air. As a matter of fact, the smallest radiologically diagnosed acoustic neuroma that we have seen is a case presented by Siew *et al.,* and this patient was examined with air. As demonstrated by Grepe, even the normal acoustic nerve can be seen at pneumoencephalography, especially when this method is combined with tomography. This, of course, is a promising fact with regard to the possibilities of visualizing very small tumours. But nevertheless, it is obvious that a

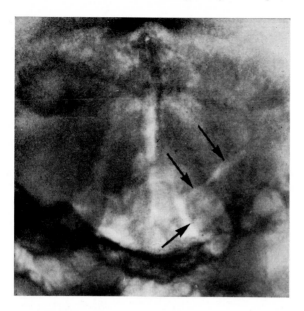

Fig. 4. Meningioma of left pontine angle. The tumour has a square shape.

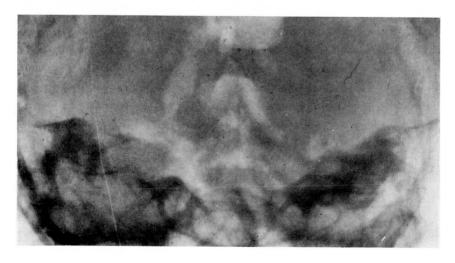

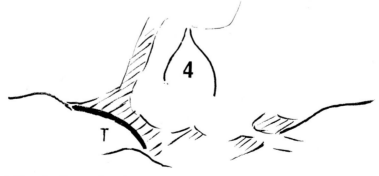

Fig. 5. Extradurally growing cholesteatoma causing a flat indentation in cerebello-pontine cistern.

62   *T. Greitz*

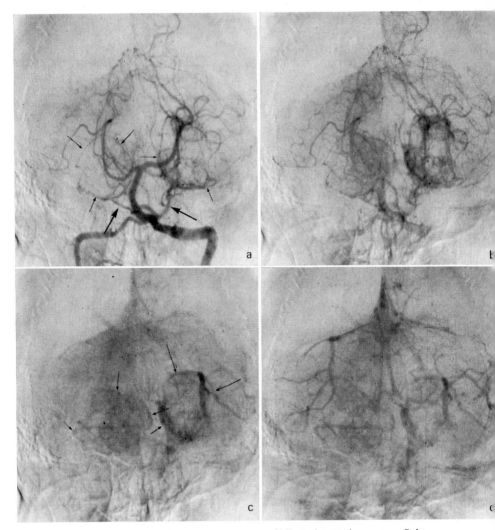

Fig. 6. Serial angiography of vertebral artery in a case of bilateral acoustic neuroma. Subtraction films. Tumour blush is apparent in b) and c). Small arteries (small arrows) mainly emerging from the anterior inferior cerebellar arteries (big arrows) and veins of cerebello-pontine angle (small arrows in c) encircle the tumours.

higher contrast than that obtained with air is desirable. Our hope is for a contrast medium with better physical and biological properties than Panto-paque, for example a non-neurotoxic water-soluble contrast medium, and we feel confident that such a medium will be available in the not too distant future.

The acoustic neuroma is the commonest tumour in the cerebello-pontine angle. Other tumours that have to be taken into consideration are neuromas of different origins, meningiomas, cholesteatomas, chordomas, and chon-dromas. The encephalographic picture in these tumours is often different

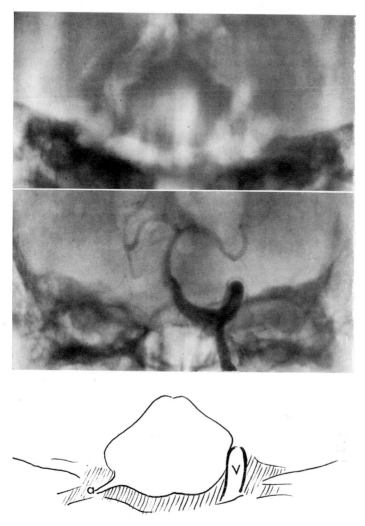

Fig. 7. Filling defect in left cerebello-pontine cistern caused by ectatic vertebral artery (V) as evidenced by angiography. Normal acoustic nerve on right side (a).

from that of an acoustic neuroma. The acoustic neuroma has, as a rule, a spherical or conical shape. Meningiomas usually have a more square appearance (Fig. 4). A cholesteatoma growing extradurally has a smooth surface but is rather flat (Fig. 5).

For successful removal of the tumour, it is of benefit to the surgeon to know, not only the extra-axial nature of the tumour, but also its relation to the surrounding vessels. Preoperative information in this respect is obtained by vertebral angiography. A homogeneous, faint staining of a round tumour is typical of neurinoma, and allows an exact determination of the size of the tumour. The relation between the neuroma and the surrounding vessels can be exactly determined, both with regard to the anterior inferior cerebellar artery and the veins of the cerebello-pontine angle, including the petrosal vein (Fig. 6). The small arteries adjacent to the tumour are stretched and curved around it. The veins of the cerebello-pontine angle are usually displaced in an arched fashion around the tumour (Greitz and Lindgren, 1961). This venous displacement is frequently more helpful than the arterial displacement.

Vertebral angiography is of great value in the differential diagnosis of tumours. Expanding lesions in the cerebello-pontine angle also include vascular abnormalities, such as arterial aneurysms and arteriovenous malformations. With vertebral angiography, the true nature of these lesions can be revealed (Fig. 7).

To sum up, radiological investigation of acoustic neuroma should include examination of the internal meatus and the basal cisterns. As a preoperative measure, vertebral angiography is desirable.

References

Fredzell, G., Greitz, T., Grepe, A. & Holmström, L., *Mimer III and rotating chair. Acta Radiol. (Diag.), 7, 543 (1968).

Greitz, T. & Lindgren, E., *Cerebral angiography in Abrams Angiography, vol. I. Little, Brown & Co., Cambridge, Mass. (1961).

Grepe, A., *Encephalographic and postmortem studies of the optic chiasm and the acoustic nerves.* Transaction of the VIIIth Symposium Neuroradiologicum Paris 1967. Résumé des communications, 36 (1967).

Grepe, A., *The normal anatomy of the cerebello-pontine angle as studied radiologically.* This symposium.

Liliequist, B., *Acta Radiol.* (Stockholm), Suppl. 185 (1959).

Liliequist, B., *Acta Radiol.* (Stockholm), Suppl. 186 (1959).

Lindgren, E., *Acta Radiol.* (Stockholm), *31,* 161 (1949).

Reese, D. F. & Bull, J. W. D., *Amer. J. Roentgen., 100,* 650 (1967).

Robertsson, E. G., *Further studies in encephalography,* Macmillan, Melbourne (1946).

Scanlan, R. L., *Arch. Otolaryng.* (Chicago), *80,* 698 (1964).

Siew, F. G., Kricheff, I. & Chase, N. E., *The diagnosis of small acoustic neuromas using contrast material.* Transaction of the VIIIth Symposium Neuroradiologicum Paris 1967. Résumé des communications, 44 (1967).

Tomography in acoustic tumors

By Sam Brünner

Department of X-ray Diagnosis, Gentofte Hospital, Copenhagen, Denmark

As in the case of other tumors in the organism, it is extremely important to make an early diagnosis in cases of acoustic tumors. The surgical treatment is much easier when the tumor is small, and of course more complicated in cases of more widespread involvement. The diagnosis of an acoustic neuroma situated in the internal acoustic canal is no longer solely of secondary interest, as early diagnosis can be followed by surgical removal using a translabyrinthine approach (House, 1961, 1964).

Today, it is possible to make a diagnosis of acoustic tumors down to a size of 3–4 mm by using improved roentgen diagnostic procedures, and in this way to ensure early oto- or neurosurgical treatment before hearing or the facial nerve is impaired.

Roentgen technique

Different methods have been employed to make a roentgen diagnosis of acoustic tumors, as shown in Fig. 1. Frequently, conventional roentgen examinations are made, often giving unsatisfactory results unless the destructive process is large.

Pneumoencephalography with cisternography is one of the ideal methods of studying the basal cisterns and the region close to the internal acoustic porus. By employing tomography, evaluation of the cisternography is simplified. In addition to this, vertebral angiography can help in making a diagnosis. By using tomography, it is possible to visualize the whole internal auditory canal, especially with the help of apparatus that gives a good coefficient of distinctness, e.g. the Polytome, which permits cuts of 1 mm thickness by using a hypocycloid movement (Brünner et al., 1961).

Different tomographic projections can be used to visualize the internal auditory canal, as shown in Fig. 2.

1. antero-posterior projection
2. lateral projection
3. Stenvers' projection
4. axial projection

RADIOLOGICAL EXAMINATION

1) Conventional radiography

2) Pneumoencephalography
      a) Cisternography
      b) Cisternography + tomography

3) Tomography of the auditory canal

4) Vertebralis angiography

5) Opaque cisternography + tomography

Fig. 1. Differential type of roentgenological examinations of the internal auditory canal.

Of these, the frontal projection is the best and at the same time the easiest, as it permits a simultaneous evaluation of both internal auditory canals. The lateral tomography shows the internal acoustic canal in cross-section. Stenvers' projection is seldom used to evaluate the porus. Axial tomography is only infrequently used.

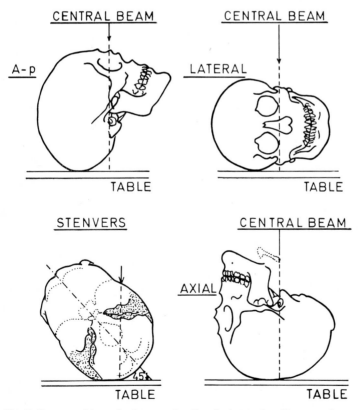

Fig. 2. Tomographic projections to visualize the internal auditory canal.

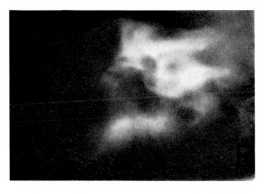

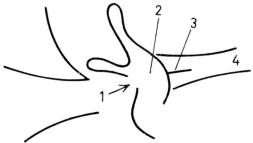

Fig. 3. Antero-posterior tomography of the internal auditory canal. 1. vestibular window, 2. vestibule, 3. crista falciformis, 4. internal acoustic canal.

Roentgen anatomy

The internal auditory canal forms a right angle to the sagittal plane of the skull and an angle of about 45° to the long axis of the petrous pyramid. The medial opening is *the porus,* with its maximum diameter in the same axis as the petrous pyramid. The posterior, superior and inferior lips of the porus are prominent and made up of dense bone, while the anterior lip is usually poorly demarcated, so that the anterior wall of the canal blends smoothly with the postero-medial wall of the petrous apex. The lateral end of the canal is closed by a vertical plate (the lamina cribrosa).

Arising from the lamina cribrosa is a horizontal crest (the crista falciformis), which is very well shown on the tomographic cut (Fig. 3). The internal auditory canal contains the facial nerve, the nervus intermedius, the acoustic nerve and the internal auditory branch of the basilar artery. The internal auditory canal in cross-section usually has an oval shape, with its vertical diameter slightly larger than its horizontal diameter.

Many authors have made measurements to show the variation in the normal acoustic canal. Some of the best of these are from the University Clinic of Chicago.

As seen from Table 1, the shapes were classified in 3 types after measurement taken just medially to the lamina cribrosa at the termination of the posterior wall, and at the point of greatest variation, if any, between these

Table 1. *Shape of the internal acoustic canal.*

University of Chicago (Valvassori) series.

Shape		Bilateral comparison of shape	
Straight	51 %	Same	90 %
Narrowed medially	30 %	Different	10 %
Narrowed laterally	—		
Oval	19 %		

two points. The canal was considered straight when there was no more than 1 mm difference in the diameter anywhere in its length. As seen in the table, 51 % of the cases were in this group.

The canal was considered narrower medially when the diameter of the medial end was at least 1 mm smaller than any other portion of the canal. 30 % of the cases were in this group. The canal was considered oval when the diameter of its mid-portion exceeded by more than 1 mm the medial and lateral ends. 19 % of the cases were in this group. As seen from the table, the variation in shape between the internal auditory canals of the same subject occurred in only 10 %, which should suggest a further investigation.

Table 2 shows the vertical diameter height measured in a plane perpendicular to the long axis of the canal. As seen from the table, comparisons between the two sides of the same subject showed 99 % of the patients with only 1 mm or less difference between the two sides. A variation from 1–2 mm is considered questionable, and a variation above 2 mm between the two sides is considered abnormal. Table 2 also shows that any canal with a vertical diameter below 2 mm or above 9 mm should be considered abnormal.

The length of the posterior wall was measured from the lamina cribrosa to the deepest portion of the concave lip of the posterior wall. As seen in Table 3, the greatest length was 11 mm, the shortest was 4 mm and the average length 8 mm. A variation in the length of the posterior wall between the two sides up to 2 mm is considered significant, a variation from 2–3 mm is considered questionable and a variation over 3 mm is abnormal.

By employing the different criteria, as shown in Table 4, it is possible to suspect the presence of an acoustic tumor in cases of pathological changes. As mentioned earlier, it is of course easier the larger is the tumor.

Table 2. *Vertical diameter (height).*

University of Chicago (Valvassori) series.

Diameter		Bilateral variation	
Maximum	8.0 mm	Up to 1.0 mm	99 %
Minimum	2.0 mm	1–2 mm	1 %
Average	4.0 mm	2–3 mm	—

Table 3. *Posterior wall length.*

University of Chicago (Valvassori) series.

Length		Bilateral variation	
Maximum	11.0 mm	Up to 1.0 mm	86 %
Minimum	4.0 mm	1–2 mm	13 %
Average	8.0 mm	2–3 mm	1 %

In cases of small tumors, tomography does not always lead to a correct diagnosis (Valvassori mentions 75 % of all cases), and supplementary examinations with positive contrast media, e.g. Pantopaque (Iophendylate), can be performed (Pulec *et al.*, 1965, Scanlan, 1964, Valvassori, 1966).

The examination is especially necessary, as it excludes very small tumors, when complete filling of the acoustic canal is seen, in cases where symptoms indicate an acoustic neuroma.

The technique will now be described briefly.

The study is performed under fluoroscopic control by TV. Lumbar puncture is performed with the patient lying on the side to be examined, with the head elevated and slightly flexed towards the opposite side. 4–5 ml of Pantopaque is introduced under TV visualization. By tilting the table in a Trendelenburg position, the opaque column is moved to the upper cervical canal, where it pools, because of the lateral flexion of the head. By lowering and at the same time extending the patient's head, the contrast medium is allowed to flow through the foramen magnum, filling the pontine cistern and pooling in the dependent cerebello-pontine cistern. The patient is then moved to a prone position, and by rotating the head approximately 45°, it is possible to get the contrast medium into the internal auditory canal. It is extremely important to fill a canal to its lateral extremity, which can be identified by the vestibule. The patient is then rotated to the frontal position, the table is lowered, and tomograms in the frontal projection are made. The patient's head is then rotated towards the opposite side, and the asymptomatic side is examined in the same way. After completion of the examination, the patient stands upright, allowing the contrast medium to collect in the lumbar region, and then it is withdrawn.

Table 4. *Differential-diagnostic criteria in tomography of the internal auditory canal.*

1. Variation in shape between the internal auditory canal of the same subject.
2. Dilatation of the medial end 1 mm more than the lateral end.
3. A variation of the vertical diameter between the two sides of the same patient over 2 mm is considered abnormal.
4. The concave medial lip of the posterior wall should always be distinct and smooth.

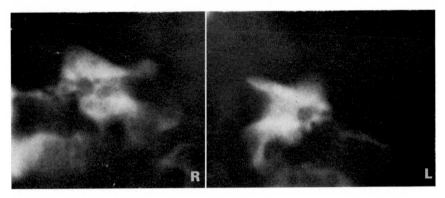

Fig. 4. *Case 1. Antero-posterior tomography.* Woman, 43 years old, with a large left acoustic neuroma. The left internal auditory canal shows widening of the medial end and funneling. The right side is within normal limits.

I shall now give a few examples of tomographic findings in cases examined with positive contrast medium.

Case 1, a woman, 43 years old

Ten-year history of headaches, fainting spells, left facial neuralgia. Admitted with papilledema, violent headaches, neck pains.

Showed neurosensory hearing deficit on the left. Stiff neck and too dizzy and ataxic to sit or stand.

Tomography. The left internal auditory canal showed widening of the medial end, "funneling or trumpeting" (Fig. 4).

The right side is regarded as being within normal limits.

Operation. Very large acoustic neuroma, approximately the size of a lemon, was found.

This case emphasizes the important aspect of the radiographic features of acoustic tumors. The changes in the canal itself may be relatively minimal, and yet there may be a large associated intracranial component.

Case 2, a man, 56 years old

Progressive hearing loss, vertigo, and continuous tinnitus of high-pitched variety of the right ear for about 2 years.

On examination, decreased ice-water calorics on the right side. Sensory neural deafness on right side. The patient was considered to have Ménière's disease.

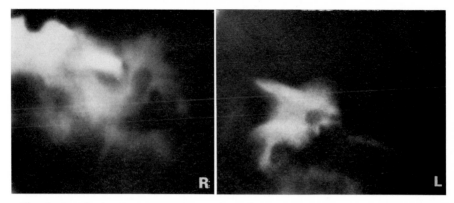

Fig. 5. *Case 2. Antero-posterior tomography with Pantopaque.* Man, 56 years old, with a history of progressive hearing loss, vertigo and tinnitus. The internal auditory canal is normal with Pantopaque as far as the vestibule.

Polytome examination with Pantopaque. The result was regarded as being entirely within normal limits. The canal is filled with Pantopaque as far as the vestibule (Fig. 5).

Case 3, a woman, 56 years old

She complained of a buzzing noise in the left ear for 3 years. This was associated with dizziness, and a loss of hearing on the left side.

Polytome examination with Pantopaque. Contrast medium on the right side inside the canal. This is entirely within normal limits.

The left side is abnormal. There is widening at its medial end. Moreover, the contrast medium does not enter the canal, and a filling defect measuring approximately 2 cm in diameter is clearly seen (Fig. 6).

Operation. Acoustic neuroma.

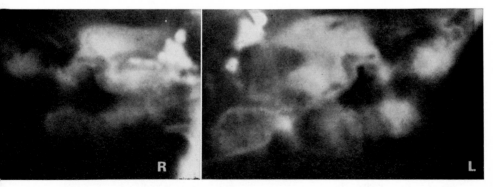

Fig. 6. *Case 3. Antero-posterior tomography with Pantopaque.* Woman, 56 years old, with hearing loss on the left side and dizziness.
Normal right side. The left side shows widening of the medial end of the internal acoustic canal. The contrast medium does not enter the canal.

Case 4, a woman, 54 years old

She presented with a right-sided neurosensory hearing loss of 1 year. Tinnitus, unsteadiness on feet, absent corneal reflex, loss cold caloric, positive tone decay.

Tomography. Normal left internal auditory canal.

The right internal auditory canal is larger than the left.

Polytome examination with Pantopaque. The contrast medium reaches the porus or medial end of the right internal auditory canal. No contrast is visualized in the canal itself.

The features are those of an acoustic neuroma confined mainly to the canal.

Operation. Acoustic neuroma.

Discussion

"Porus roentgen examination" of earlier times gave a positive diagnosis of acoustic tumor in only 50% of cases where a tumor was present. The reason is that only larger tumors projecting through the porus or situated close to the internal porus can be expected to give osseous changes. The advanced oto-surgical technique of recent years demands an earlier and more exact diagnosis. By thin-section tomography with modern apparatus giving cuts of 1 mm thickness, e.g. the Philips Polytome, it is possible to better the roentgenological diagnosis by comparing the internal auditory canals of the two sides. By measurement and comparison, a diagnosis is easier to arrive at. In some cases the tumor is so small, and situated so far laterally in the internal auditory canal, that it has become necessary to supplement one's examinations with positive contrast examinations with contrast filling of the internal auditory canal, a method that in nearly all cases leads to a correct diagnosis.

Conclusion

In this way tomography, complemented by positive contrast examination, has increased the roentgenological diagnostic possibilities enormously and thus made it possible to supply the earlier and more exact diagnosis that recent years' operative improvements have demanded.

Frontal tomography, the best projection, is easy to perform and permits a quick simultaneous evaluation of both internal acoustic canals.

Summary

The roentgenological tomographical changes in normal and pathological internal acoustic canals, especially in cases where an acoustic tumor is suspected, are reviewed.

In doubtful cases, the necessity of supplementary examinations with positive contrast medium (Pantopaque) is stressed.

References

Brünner, S., Petersen, Ø. & Stocksted, P., *Amer. J. Roentgen., 86,* 281 (1961).
House, W. F., *Laryngoscope, 71,* 1363 (1961).
House, W. F., *Arch. Otolaryng.* (Chicago), *80,* 599 (1964).
Pulec, J. L., Baker, H. L. & Miller, R. H., *Laryngoscope, 75,* 1572 (1965).
Scanlan, R. L., *Arch. Otolaryng.* (Chicago), *80,* 698 (1964).
Valvassori, G. E., *Laryngoscope, 76,* 1104 (1966).
Valvassori, G. E. & Pierce, R. H., *Amer. J. Roentgen., 92,* 1232 (1964).

Cerebrospinal fluid diagnosis in cases of acoustic neuroma

By Sven Landin

Department of Neurology, Karolinska Sjukhuset, Stockholm, Sweden

Analysis of cerebrospinal fluid (CSF) in cases of cerebral tumours has a limited diagnostic value in comparison with other investigation. Both the protein content and the cell count are usually normal. There are, however, exceptions, i.e., tumours closely connected to the cerebrospinal fluid space. In these cases, the protein content of the CSF is often raised and electrophoresis of the CSF proteins tends to come closer to that of serum. Above all, increased gamma globulin in CSF electrophoresis can be observed.

The acoustic neuromas have a direct connection to the CSF space. One might say that these tumours are "bathing" in the CSF. For this reason, the CSF often shows pathological changes:

1. Increase in the total protein content is very common. In Table 1 you can see the frequency of different symptoms (in %) on admission to hospital. Two groups of subjects are presented, Edwards–Paterson (157 cases) and 50 personal cases from the Karolinska Hospital. Next to impairment of hearing, the increase in total protein content of the CSF is the most common symptom.

2. In cases of acoustic neuroma the CSF is often yellow. This can be the result of the increase in protein or the presence of bilirubin.

Cellular elements are generally normal.

However, the most important is the increase in protein in CSF. Fig. 1 shows the CSF protein in 47 of our 50 patients. Values over 40 mg/100 ml are pathological with our method. Many very high values were noted, and the mean value was 187 mg/100 ml. In a survey of 345 patients with acoustic neuroma from different clinics, the mean value was 153 mg/100 ml.

Our opinion is that in cases of suspect acoustic neuroma, lumbar puncture should be done earlier and more frequently than to-day. It is probable that increased protein in CSF will be found in a very high percentage of subjects, and also in cases with small tumours. Lumbar puncture may be dangerous in cases with tumours in the posterior fossa, and this investigation

Table 1. *Symptoms on admission* (%).

	Edwards–Paterson 157 cases	Neurolog. Clin., K. S. 50 cases
Impairment of hearing	99	100
Tinnitus	52	—
Caloric reaction, extinguished	83	} 88
impaired	15	
normal	2	12
Vertigo	42	64
Loss of balance, ataxia	77	82
Nystagmus (Brun's nystagmus)	92 (50, 9)	70 (44)
Corneal hyporeflexia	87	86
Dilated internal acoustic meatus	—	62
Sensory disturbance of face	62	44
Facial weakness or palsy	63	22
Headache	84	70
Papilloedema	76	20
Raised protein content of C. S. F.	97	94

ought to be done where neurosurgical service can be offered quickly. It can probably be said, however, that lumbar puncture is without any risk if a so-called Sise-Antoni needle is used, and in cases with a small tumour where papilloedema and other signs of intracranial hypertension are lacking.

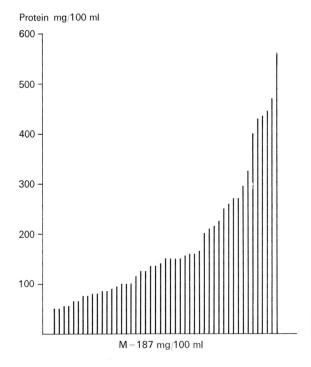

Protein mg/100 ml

M = 187 mg/100 ml

Fig. 1. Protein content of C. S. F. 47 cases.

Histopathology of the stato-acoustic nerve

By *Anders Moberg*

Department of Pathology, Karolinska Sjukhuset, Stockholm, Sweden

and Henry Anderson & Erik Wedenberg

Department of Audiology, Karolinska Sjukhuset, Stockholm, Sweden

Sensory neural retrocochlear hearing defects of unknown aetiology are not uncommon—about 10 %—in audiologic practice, and in many of these cases an acoustic neuroma is suspected. The known incidence of acoustic neuroma, however, is very low. According to the Swedish Cancer Registry, about 35 acoustic neuromas are found annually in living subjects and at autopsy (population 7.5 million). This gives an incidence of 0.0005 per thousand. There is a great discrepancy between this figure and the higher incidence that could be suspected from audiological practice and from the investigation of Hardy and Crowe (1936). After serial sectioning of the VIIIth nerve obtained at autopsy, they found 5 minute acoustic neuromas in 250 subjects.

The purpose of this study was to determine the incidence of acoustic neuromas and to search for other pathological findings in the VIIIth nerve that could serve as a basis for sensory neural retrocochlear hearing defects.

Material and methods

At autopsy, the skull was opened and the brain removed in the ordinary manner. The bony canal of the VIIIth nerve was opened and the nerve taken out. The average length of the nerves obtained for microscopical examination was 13 mm, of which about 3 mm represented the intracranial part of the nerve.

The nerves were fixed in 10 % neutral formalin, embedded in paraffin in the usual manner, and sectioned transversely at about 1-mm intervals. The sections were stained with the van Gieson connective tissue stain.

The material was collected at consecutive autopsies and comprises the right and left nerves from 105 subjects, 53 males and 52 females. The average age was 65.0 years (range 24 to 92). Specific audiological or vestibular data were not available for any of the patients.

Table 1. *Histopathology of 105 pairs of the VIIIth nerve.*

| Finding | No. of subjects | Location | | | Age (yrs) |
		Right	Left	Bilat.	
Neuroma	2	2			78, 90
Neuroma (?)	1		1		60
Metastatic carcinoma	1			1	60
Cholesteatoma	1	1			78
Blood clot*	1	1			37
Nests of capillary vessels	3	2	1		50, 56, 68
Fibrosis	14	4	6	4	64.8 (mean)
Normal	83				65.0 (mean)

* Fibrosis was observed in the left nerve.

Results (Table 1)

Two right-sided neuromas with a typical microscopical appearance were encountered in the series. In one of the subjects—a 78-year-old woman with ovarian carcinoma—the neuroma could be followed from the vestibular ganglion to the internal auditory meatus. It appeared to be uniform in thickness with a cross-section of 1.5×1.0 mm (Figs. 1 and 2). The other tumour—a 90-year-old woman who died of pulmonary embolism—was seen in only one of the middle sections of the nerve, which means that the length of the tumour could not have been more than 2 mm. It measured 1.1×0.7 mm in cross-section.

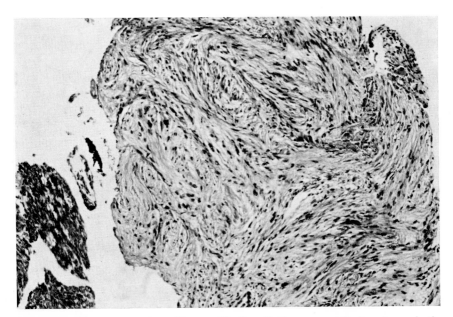

Fig. 1. Acoustic neuroma, about 80 × magnification. Ordinary nerve structure is seen in the left lower corner.

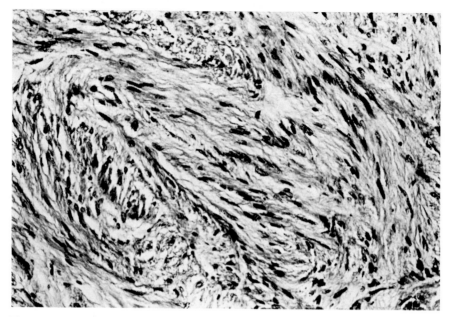

Fig. 2. Detailed enlargement (210 ×) of Fig. 1.

A third subject—a 60-year-old man with bronchial carcinoma—had a left-sided tumour-like condition, with interlacing nerve fibres and oedema that contrasted with the ordinary nerve structure (Fig. 3). No fibrosis or palissading of the cells was observed. The lesion measured 1.6 × 1.6 mm and was present in only one of the middle sections. It is debatable whether the lesion

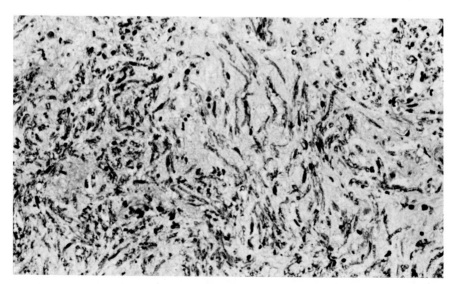

Fig. 3. Neuroma or neuromatous tumour-like nodule. Total disorganization of the nerve fibres. 210 ×.

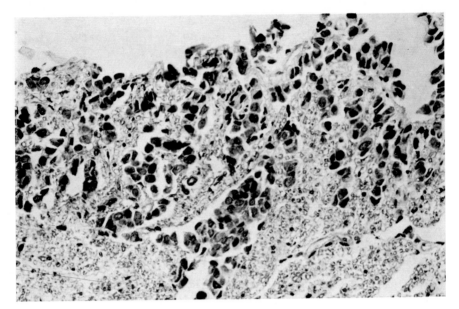

Fig. 4. Metastatic carcinoma. 210 ×.

should be classified as a true neuroma or as a neuromatous tumour-like nodule.

Carcinomatous metastases were present bilaterally in the nerves (Fig. 4) of a 60-year-old woman with carcinoma of the urinary bladder. The patient had metastases to the liver and vertebrae, but the brain was macroscopically unaffected and normal for the age.

In one subject, a cholesteatoma compressed the right nerve and was partly incorporated in it (Fig. 5). This patient was a 78-year-old man who died of a ruptured aortic aneurysm. Clinical information as to previous diseases of the ear was not available.

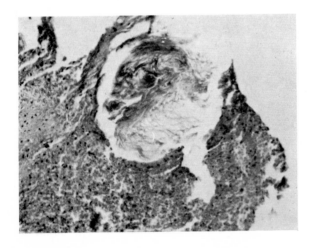

Fig. 5. Cholesteatoma incorporated in the nerve. About 80 ×.

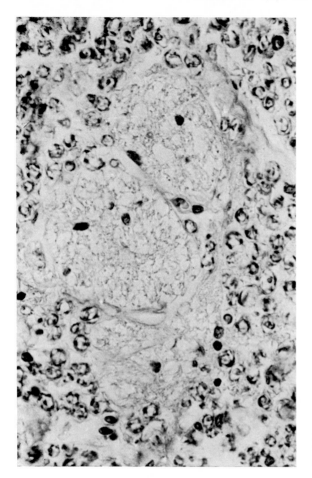

Fig. 6. Nests of capillary vessels in central parts of the nerve. 530 ×.

A partly organized blood clot compressed the right nerve in a 37-year-old woman who died of pulmonary embolism. The macroscopical examination of the brain revealed no major pathological features, and there were no signs of micro-thromboembolism in other organs.

In three nerves, a nest of small capillary vessels was noted in central parts of the nerve (Fig. 6). The vessels had a diameter of about 0.1 mm, but since they contained only coagulated fluid, it could not be determined whether the vessels were of haemangiomatous or lymphangiomatous nature.

Fibrosis was observed in many instances, but was difficult to evaluate, since fibrosis proved to be a constant feature in the vestibular ganglion. Whether this ganglionic fibrosis is part of the ageing process or a pathological feature cannot be judged from the present material. Definite fibrosis of the nerve—not in the ganglionic area—was observed in 14 subjects; 4 bilateral, on the right side in 4 and on the left in 6. A left-sided fibrosis was observed in the patient—mentioned above—with a blood clot compressing

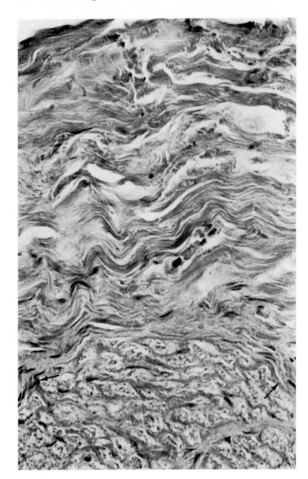

Fig. 7. Massive perineural fibrosis (from top to arrows). In this enlargement (530 ×), the ordinary perineurium is about 100 times thinner.

the right nerve. The fibrosis was located within the nerve in 15 nerves and in the perineurium in 3 (Fig. 7). There was no difference in sex or mean age between those with fibrosis (64.8 years, range 37 to 78) and the material as a whole (65.0 years, range 24 to 92). The microscopical appearance gave no indications of the aetiology of the fibrotic process.

Discussion

In this consecutive series of 105 patients there were two, possibly three, typical but very small acoustic neuromas. The results are then consistant with those of Hardy and Crowe (1936)—the only comparable study—who found 5 neuromas in 250 subjects.

This incidence of neuromas—about 2% in unselected autopsy series—is some ten thousandfold the incidence given for entire populations (e.g. the Swedish Cancer Registry). The conclusion from these two series is that the incidence of acoustic neuromas in the ageing population is sufficiently high to be seriously entertained as a diagnostic alternative under appropriate circumstances, and is not merely a rarity.

Small capillary vessels were noted in central parts of the nerve in 3 subjects. This finding, too, is consistent with the results of Hardy and Crowe (1936), who found an angiomatous network in 7 of 250 subjects. The clinical significance of this finding is unknown, as well as the possible relation to haemorrhage or ultimate fibrosis in and around the acoustic nerve.

Carcinoma metastases were observed bilaterally in a subject who died in an advanced stage of metastazing carcinoma. It is generally believed that neurological disturbances associated with carcinoma appear late in the course of the disease. This is not always the case, however, since Moberg and v. Reis (1961) found that in 6 of 8 patients with meningeal carcinosis, the first sign of the tumour was the neurological disturbances. In meningeal carcinosis, cranial nerve disorders are common, and it could well happen that the first sign of a carcinoma might be acoustic or vestibular symptoms.

Audiological and vestibular data were not available for this series of patients. It would be of interest to repeat an investigation of this type on a series of patients for which relevant clinical data are available. This seems to be the only possibility of evaluating the aetiology and significance of pathological changes in the VIIIth nerve, such as vascular abnormalities, fibrosis and ganglionic fibrosis.

Summary

The VIIIth nerves obtained from 105 consecutive autopsies were step-sectioned for microscopical examination. Pathological changes were noted in 22 patients, 2 of whom had typical acoustic neuromas. This finding—consistent with the results of Hardy and Crowe—permits the conclusion that acoustic neuromas in the ageing population should not be counted in fractions of per thousand but in per cent of the population.

References

Hardy, M. & Crowe, S. J., *Arch. Surg., 32*, 292 (1936).
Moberg, A. & v. Reis, G., *Acta Med. Scand., 170*, 747 (1961).

General discussion

Palva to Klockhoff
Two things have emerged clearly during this meeting. Dr. House just pointed out one of them. Acoustic neuroma as such, even if arising in the nerve, causes both neural and cochlear symptoms. Secondly, there is no single test that would tell you clearly what part of the system is involved. The loudness balance test, for instance, may be negative or incomplete if there is a lesion of both external and internal hair cells. Similarly, the tone decay test may show a very pronounced loss in cochlear as well as neural cases. We have to employ a test battery in each case of suspected neuroma but even then, the evidence is only suggestive, and we must use our skill as clinicians to make the diagnosis. I congratulate Dr. Klockhoff on his very clear presentation of the situation.

Bordley to Klockhoff
I would like to ask Dr. Klockhoff if he has had experience in "conduction time" studies of the VIIIth nerve where there is a neuroma. Such studies have been performed in our clinic by Dr. Shimizu. He studied the time of appearance of cortical potentials after acoustic stimuli by use of a summating computer. He found prolonged conduction time of the nerve in the patients he had studied with such tumours, where there were very few other diagnostic signs.

House to Klockhoff
Neural and vascular changes are both involved in early acoustic neuroma.

Klockhoff to Palva
Since I fully agree with your points of view, I only want to thank you for your comments.

Klockhoff to Bordley
No such experience at all.

Klockhoff to House
My formulations about the possibility of a complex ear pathology with a combination of end-organ and nerve-fibre symptoms were made with respect to your points of view, with which I agree.

Palva to Anderson
I should like to ask one particular question. Mr. Anderson showed a case of proven acoustic neuroma with normal audiograms. Nevertheless, the stapedial

muscle reflex was much beyond the normal average 80 dB sensation level. Can he explain how this arises? Can the result be just inside the normal distribution curve (inside 3 SD:s) or is it due, for instance, to reversed recruitment?

Anderson to Palva

The reflex threshold of the affected, right ear is far above the outer limit of normal distribution, and elevated to an extent that we regard as definitely pathological; in the audiogram demonstrated, it appears most strikingly in comparison to the reflex threshold of the normal ear.

There is not a simple relation between the psycho-acoustic conception recruitment and reflex threshold elevation; in the case in question, for instance, no abnormality in the loudness function was found with Fowler's test, in spite of the elevated reflex threshold.

Portmann to Greitz

Why does Dr. Greitz not use Pantopaque—does he think that it is more dangerous than pneumography? We use this method (2 cc only) in Bordeaux without any serious trouble hitherto.

Brünner to Greitz

I am interested to know why you do not work with Pantopaque examinations in Sweden. Are there any prohibitions from the government to work with this type of contrast? I would also like to stress that the first thing is to make a complete clinical examination before the patient is sent for X-ray examination.

Fisch to Greitz

We have performed 75 Pantopaque studies without complications in $1\,^{1}/_{2}$ years. The method used has been that of the minimal amount (1 to 2 cc) described by Dr. William House.

House to Greitz

Does Dr. Greitz use Pantopaque in the study of intervertebral discs? If not, why not? If so, why not use it in the cisterns?

Greitz to Portmann, Brünner and House

Drs. Portmann and Brünner have asked me why I do not use Pantopaque. One reason is the fact that Pantopaque always produces an arachnoiditis which can be seen at subsequent myelography. This is admitted by most people who work with this medium, but it is said to be of no clinical significance. However, the medical government in Sweden feels so strongly about it that Pantopaque is not marketed in Sweden, and can be used in clinical practice only after special permission.

In answer to Dr. House: I do not use Pantopaque in the spinal canal, because I feel that it is an inferior contrast medium from the purely technical point of view. The only situation in which it is advantageous from the diagnostic point of view is in the diagnosis of root compression by intravertebral discs in the cervical area. But with regard to the diagnosis of acoustic neuromas, I cannot be convinced that Pantopaque offers any advantages. As a matter of fact, Dr. Brünner showed us very clearly that Pantopaque does not always penetrate into the normal meatus. Hence, it does not show us the anatomy, and therefore I think that it is a bad contrast medium.

Frykholm to Brünner

Regarding Pantopaque myelography: I have seen at least 10 patients with severe cauda syndromes after Pantopaque myelography, and have explored 5. In all these cases, the cauda equina was simply baked into a massive fibrous scar tissue, in which small drops of oil could be discerned. Nothing could be done to the local condition. All patients suffered from intractable severe pain, and one patient committed suicide. I have never seen any similar pathological changes, except after myelography with Pantopaque.

All patients came from areas where doctors maintain that they never have seen any disadvantage of Pantopaque myelography, or that complications are "extremely rare". According to my experience, therefore, I think that it is very wise of the Swedish medical authorities to have forbidden the use of Pantopaque in this country.

Palva to Landin

Normally, in electrophoretic studies, the spinal fluid albumin is immunologically different from serum albumin, showing a faster mobility in the electrophoretic field. Has the speaker done any studies comparing the CSF albumin mobility in neuroma cases with that of serum albumin? This might help us to get better information about the mechanism of the albumin increase, whether it is synthetized in the CSF space, or whether it just seeps through the capillary walls due to venous stasis.

Hitselberger to Landin

We have found normal protein in 6 of 7 cases of primary cholesteatoma. Is there any explanation for this?

Burian to Landin

Is there a difference in the CSF protein content when you do a lumbar or suboccipital punction?

Glasscock to Landin

In our series, we have found a correlation between size of tumour and protein content of CSF. In our smaller tumours, the protein is normal and as the tumours enlarge, the protein increases.

Landin to Palva

No I have not. But your question is very interesting, and I should like to do the investigation you are proposing.

Landin to Hitselberger

I do not know, but perhaps because they are not rich in blood vessels.

Landin to Burian

I cannot answer that. We never do any suboccipital punctures in these cases. (Normally, the CSF proteins are quantitatively and qualitatively different in suboccipital and lumbar CSF.)

Landin to Glasscock

In our 50 cases no tumour has, as far as I can remember, been smaller than a hazelnut. I do not know how big the tumours were in Edwards–Paterson's cases. The reason for the high CSF protein in these cases is not known. If the background to the increased CSF protein is damage to the barrier between blood and CSF, then it is perhaps not so astonishing that the bigger tumours, rich in blood vessels, give the highest CSF protein values. But I think that even a small acoustic neuroma might give a barrier damage.

Bordley to Moberg

Dr. Moberg's excellent paper is very opportunely timed. We should give more consideration to the marked variation in the growth rate of these tumours. The slow growth rate of some tumours was mentioned this morning by Dr. Olivecrona. In a paper written many years ago by Drs. Cushing, Crowe and Guild, 7 VIIIth nerve tumours were reported in a review of serial sections of the temporal bones of about 250 patients, with normal audiograms, normal speech audiometry and normal vestibular studies, employing the less accurate vestibular test methods of that day. Studies of consecutive autopsies will certainly show old people with small tumours which have caused no difficulty in life. Small tumours may not be always dangerous in old people.

Wersäll to Moberg

I want to express my appreciation to Dr. Moberg for his excellent contribution. I hope that, in the future, a co-operation between the Ear Clinic and the Pathology Department will make it possible to study the morphology of the auditory and vestibular nerves in people in whom audiograms and vestibular function studies have been made. Maybe, however, we need about 1000 cases before the actual statistics of acoustic nerve pathology are known.

Engström to Moberg

You called some nerves in your material "normal", but we know from our studies on the human cochlea that there are hardly any normal human nerves in that age group.

Moberg to Bordley

The neuromas found in this series were in aged people. The mean age of the total material was high (65.0 years) and the age distribution of patients with neuromas did not differ from that of the total material. The demonstration of a small tumour in an old person gives no inkling of its rate of growth.

Moberg to Engström

It is quite correct that some nerves were called "normal". It might have been better—and perhaps more adequate—to state that the nerves had "no major abnormalities".

Moberg to Wersäll

It would be very interesting to cooperate with the otologists to obtain more knowledge about these problems, but some 1000 cases seem to be a bit Utopian.

Chairman's summary of session I

L. B. W. Jongkees

For a summary of the excellent papers of this morning's session, I would like to start by quoting a daring statement made by the defendent of a thesis in my city. He said: "Acoustic neuroma is not a neurological disease any more but an otological problem." Surely an optimist, this young doctor and, though I appreciate his point of view, I should like to put it in a slightly different way. The problems of acoustic neuromas, or better of tumours of the cerebello-pontine angle and inner-ear canal, are typical problems for a group—for teamwork (audiologists, vestibular specialists, otologists, neurologists, etc.). The enormous progress in the diagnostic and surgical possibilities, the

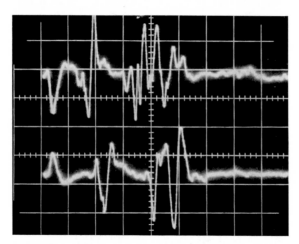

Fig. 1. Provoked myograms of frontal muscles in a patient with a left-sided tumour of the pontine angle. Not race of facial paralysis.
Upper curve: right side, lower curve: left side.
The curves should be read from left to right and begin at the moment of the mechanical stimulus.
The first reaction is a systematic artefact, the second one is the muscular response.
Latency time: right side: 13 msec, left side: 19 msec.

work of the House group is, above all I think, that we have been alerted. And also that we have the task of referring the patients with small tumours to the surgeons, in order that they can give the patient the best chance to survive, above all, to live. The diagnosis remains difficult, and the case history is extremely vague, especially in the beginning. Progressive hearing loss in one ear, perhaps some tinnitus, a slight dizziness (from the merest sensation of unsteadiness to, but very rarely, a Ménièriform attack) is in general all.

The doctor, at this moment already, must be careful. If it is a progressive perceptive deafness, he has to proceed to more sophisticated examinations of the hearing function. Not only tone audiogram but also speech audiogram. An excessive loss of understanding, a loss of discrimination, even in a normally hearing ear, Békésy audiograms showing Jerger's type IV curves, excessive adaption, are reasons for alarm. And since, this morning, we heard from Mr. Anderson about the stapedius reflex decay and its diagnostic value. The examination of the vestibular functions should never be omitted. A complete bilateral caloric test with warm and cold stimulation is absolutely necessary, and only very seldom is the caloric test symmetrical. ENG will show us a spontaneous or positional nystagmus in nearly all cases. In our department, van Saane has found that hyperventilation and the Valsalva test are very helpful in eliciting spontaneous nystagmus in cases of peripheral lesion, and therefore in tumours of the VIIIth nerve. As regards the galvanic test, Pfaltz made some interesting observations indicating that superthreshold

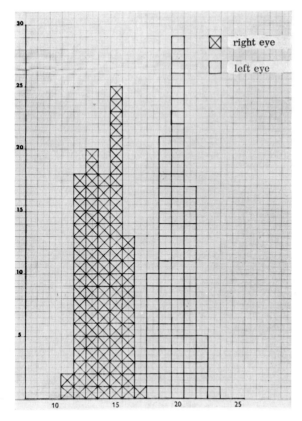

Fig. 2. Spread of the latency time in the test on the patient in Fig. 1. Number of responses tested on the ordinate, latency time in msec on the abscissa.

measurements could help in finding acoustic tumours. Let us hope that it will lead to important information. There is one thing I missed in this morning's session, and that is the importance of the function of the facial nerve. Forgive me if I ride my hobby horse for a moment, but it is possible to find very slight differences in the conduction time of a mechanic stimulus and the provoked muscular contraction, if the stimulus, provoked with a little hammer falling between the two eyes, is measured by electromyographical recording in the two frontal muscles. Even if the face seems perfectly symmetrical at rest and during movements, a difference between the conduction time on the two sides may indicate hypofunction of the facial nerve (Pelz) (Figs. 1 and 2). It seems that in some instances a decreased lacrimal secretion and a lowering of the taste perception (electrogustrometry) may be of importance too.

X-ray investigations are of great importance, but should be performed at the right moment, with the right questions with the best technique. If I may put it in a very strong way (much too strong): Do not ask the radiologist whether there is a tumour, ask him where the tumour is and how big it is.

Routine X-rays, like Stenvers' projection, skull base, transorbital may be of help but are generally insufficient. In my opinion, epicycloid tomography, and vertebral arteriography are the most valuable to us. I must confess, however, that I am a very lucky man, having in Amsterdam at my disposal the X-ray department of the father of both epicycloid tomography and subtraction arteriography, Ziedses des Plantes. And he is more than a good X-ray man, more even than an artist, he is a sorcerer.

Eventually pneumo- and/or opaque cisternography will outline the tumour for us. As regards the neurological symptoms, I point to the statement at the beginning of this summary. There should be no other neurological symptoms! If there are, we are really too late (though I must say that even in small tumours, the cerebrospinal fluid may sometimes have a high protein content).

In conclusion: There is not one test that proves the presence of an acoustic tumour. We need the whole battery. If we use it intelligently, we shall be able to find them early. It is our duty to find them early. It is not our duty to have them all operated on. In many instances they grow very slowly, and I do not think that in very old people, in those who are already in bad general health etc., we should operate on the tumour.

As doctors, we must try to know, but above all we should apply our knowledge with care, in order to offer our patients the best chance of living as happily as possible.

ACOUSTIC NEUROMA 2

Transtemporal bone removal of acoustic neuromas

By William F. House

Otologic Medical Group, Los Angeles, California, U.S.A.

Acoustic neuromas have assumed a major role in the practice of otology. By now, far more time is being spent in searching for these tumors than is being spent in their surgical removal. This is as it should be.

In 1917, Cushing published his monograph outlining his series of 30 cases accumulated over a period of four years. These patients were frightfully ill, two of them being blind, six could only perceive shadows and 18 had far advanced papilledema. The symptoms resulting from increased intracranial pressure were so overwhelming in these patients that it was not until he reviewed all 30 cases that he realized hearing loss was usually the first symptom, and that it preceded other symptoms by several years.

Through Cushing, the acoustic tumor syndrome of steady progression of symptoms from hearing loss to death from elevated intracranial pressure and cranial nerve deficit, became recognized. Cushing also lowered the operative mortality from an appalling 80 per cent to 20 per cent. He did this through wide bilateral suboccipital decompression and intracapsular removal of the tumor. He was often not sure preoperatively which side the tumor was on, so this bilateral approach also allowed both angles to be explored.

Through popularization of the acoustic tumor syndrome by Cushing, Dandy in 1925 was able to operate on smaller tumors. He advocated a unilateral approach with partial cerebellar removal. He also strongly advocated a primary total removal with sacrifice of the facial nerve since recurrence surgery resulted in a much higher mortality.

Very little in the nature of surgical technique was contributed for many years after Dandy. In the 1950's, however, it became common to diagnose acoustic neuromas when they were small enough to only have symptoms connected with the 8th nerve.

A serious dichotomy between early diagnosis and early removal developed, since the techniques usually resulted in loss of the facial nerve. Olivecrona (1940) seemed to be the only surgeon making a serious effort at this time to preserve the facial nerve. He was able to do this in 65 per cent of his cases.

It seemed to me that the application of microsurgical temporal bone techniques to acoustic tumor surgery would be beneficial, and in February, 1961,

Table 1.

Case 46	Pre-op.	Post-op.
SRT	40 dB	35 dB
PB	48 %	64 %
SISI	0 %	60 %
Bekesy	IV	IV

Table 2.

Case 55	Pre-op.	Post-op.
SRT	15 dB	10 dB
PB	14 %	98 %
SISI	0 %	60 %
Bekesy	III	I

the first acoustic neuroma was operated using these techniques. In the ensuing seven years, 200 unilateral acoustic neuromas have been operated. These cases are reviewed in detail in a monograph to be published in the December, 1968, issue of the Archives of Otolaryngology.

Three basic surgical techniques have been developed:

1. The middle fossa approach for small tumors, that is, those confined to the internal auditory canal.

2. The translabyrinthine approach for medium tumors, that is, those extending beyond the internal auditory canal but not causing any symptoms other than those related to the 8th nerve.

Table 3.

Case 138	Pre-op.	Post-op.
SRT	20 dB	15 dB
PB	96 %	100 %
SISI	95 %	75 %
Bekesy	II	II

Table 4.

Case 145	Pre-op.	Post-op.
SRT	15 dB	15 dB
PB	92 %	88 %
SISI	85 %	100 %
Bekesy	II	II

Table 5.

Case 146	Pre-op.	Post-op.
SRT	45 dB	
PB	40 %	Dead Ear
SISI	100 %	
Bekesy	II	

Table 6. *Preservation of Facial Nerve.*

141 Survivors, 1 Year Follow Up
102 (72 %) Intact
 32 (23 %) Partial Weakness
  7 (5 %) Total Loss

Table 7. *Ataxia.*

187 Survivors — 6 Cases (3.2 %) of Ataxia

3. The transsigmoid approach for large tumors, that is, those tumors associated with 5th or other cranial nerve involvement, and for cerebellar involvement and/or elevated intracranial pressure.

The ideal time to operate on an acoustic neuroma is when it is still confined to the internal auditory canal. In our series of 200 cases, we have had 5 such cases. We have been able to save the hearing in 4 out of 5 cases. Tables 1 through 5 summarize the pre- and postoperative hearing in these cases.

Table 8. *Recurrences.*

Cases	Time Since Surgery	Number of Partial Removals	% of Partial Removals	Number of Recurrences
1–50	4–7 years	22	44 %	8
51–100	2½–4 years	21	42 %	4
101–150	1–2½ years	6	12 %	1
151–200	1–present	7	14 %	0
Totals		56	23 %	13

Table 9. *Causes of Death.*

	Number
Pulmonary embolism	2
Postoperative hemorrhage	4
Postoperative edema	3
Anterior inferior cerebellar artery infarction	3
G. I. hemorrhage, myocardial infarction	1
Extradural hematoma	1
Total	14

Table 10. *Fatalities.*

```
  5 Small Tumors         –   0 fatalities
131 Medium-sized Tumors  –   3 (2.2 %) fatalities
 64 Large Tumors         –  11 (17 %) fatalities
```

Preservation of the facial nerve

Facial nerve function is often temporarily impaired following microsurgical removal of acoustic neuromas. For this reason, I have listed the status of the facial nerve function in those cases that are one year or more postoperative.

Ataxia

Ataxia in this series has occasionally resulted from hemorrhage into the cerebellar hemisphere. In one case having a suboccipital approach, the ataxia was due to removal of cerebellar tissue. Table 7 summarizes our total experience with ataxia.

Recurrences

Out of 200 cases there were 56 partial removals. Twelve of these cases have undergone surgery for recurrent tumors. The recurrence rate, according to length of postoperative period, is summarized in Table 8.

Fatalities

There have been 11 fatalities in primary acoustic surgery, or 5.5 % of the series. Three additional cases have died following surgery for recurrence, for an overall mortality rate of 7 %. Table 9 summarizes the causes of fatality. Table 10 breaks down the fatality according to tumor size.

Summary

I believe these statistics say one thing quite clearly. Early diagnosis and removal of acoustic neuromas saves lives and prevents permanent disability.

References

Cushing, H., *Tumors of the Nervus Acousticus and the Syndrome of the Cerebellopontine Angle,* Saunders, Philadelphia (1917).
Dandy, W. E., *Surg. Gynec. Obstet., 41,* 129 (1925).
Olivecrona, H., *J. Neurol. Psychiat., 3,* 141 (1940).

Management of the large acoustic tumor

By William E. Hitselberger

Otologic Medical Group, Neurosurgery, Los Angeles, California, U.S.A.

I would like to deviate somewhat from my prepared presentation in order to say a few words in favor of the use of pantopaque in the posterior fossa for the diagnosis of cerebellopontine angle tumors. It is my opinion that it is the single best diagnostic test available at this time for the accurate delineation of these tumors. Needless to say, we have relied heavily on this technique.

Fluoroscopic iophendylate (pantopaque) examination

Initially a fluoroscopic iophendylate examination was performed in these cases using the technique described by Scanlan (1964). This procedure was, and still is, satisfactory in the delineation of the large angle tumor (Fig. 1). Unlike the air contrast study, this examination utilizes a hyperberic contrast material (iophendylate). Because of the high specific gravity of the contrast material, that portion of the tumor which is dependent and approximates the posterior surface of the petrous bone is outlined most accurately. The delineation of that portion of the tumor which is adjacent to the brain stem, or indents the superimposed cerebellum, is not ideal. Unfortunately, this portion of the tumor is not outlined satisfactorily by any of the current radiologic techniques. The primary reason for this is a dense neuro-fibrovascular layer, impervious to contrast material, that exists in this plane.

Pneumoencephalography

In our experience, pneumoencephalography has not been consistently reliable in the demonstration of cerebellopontine angle tumors. Ten percent of the patients in the current series of 200 cases of acoustic tumors had previously taken pneumoencephalograms which were interpreted as normal. Pneumoencephalography is also painful for the patient, being associated with considerable headache and backache following the procedure. Finally, there is a recognized danger to the introduction of air into the lumbar subarachnoid space in the face of elevation of intracranial pressure caused by a posterior

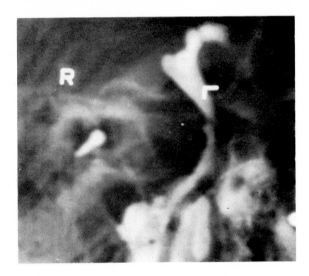

Fig. 1. Fluoroscopic panto-paque study of the posterior fossa. A large acoustic tumour is seen protruding from the internal auditory canal indenting the contrast column. Note the position of the vertebral artery near the medial border of the tumour. A metalic marker has been placed in the external auditory canal.

fossa tumor. I do not feel that this danger is lessened by the placement of air into the ventricular system from above. Indeed, this may accentuate a critical pressure balance that exists at the incisural notch. At this level, in the adjacent mesencephalon and upper pons, the centers controlling blood pressure and respiration exist. The effect of upward or downward herniation of the brain in this region can be disastrous, regardless of whether the herniation is due to pressure release from above or below. This was dramatically impressed on us in a recent case. After cannulation of the lateral ventricle in a patient with marked elevation of intracranial pressure, there were almost immediate deleterious changes in blood pressure and respiration with near fatal outcome.

Polytome-iophendylate examination

The smaller acoustic tumors confined to the internal auditory canal or only slightly protruding into the posterior fossa have not been accurately demonstrated using iophendylate with the conventional fluoroscopic technique. The reason is that these small tumors require demarcation in reference to the surrounding bony landmarks of the temporal bone, such as the internal auditory canal, the vestibule, and the semicircular canals. Unfortunately, with fluoroscopy, this bony detail is lost and the exact situation and contour of the tumor cannot be accurately determined.

The polytome x-ray unit allows x-ray sections to be taken through the temporal bone in almost any direction. The bony detail is superb. By combining the polytome x-ray with a small amount of contrast material, accurate delineation of these small tumors is possible. A one cc. quantity of iophen-

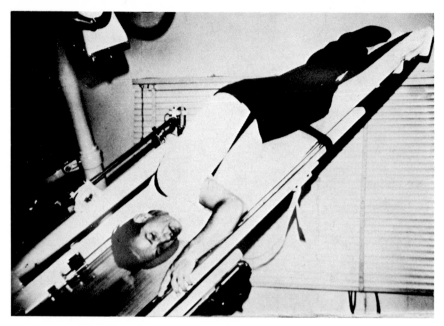

Fig. 2. Position of a patient prior to exposure of the polytome x-ray. The downward tilting of the table allows the hyperberic pantopaque to gravitate cephalad into the lateral recess of the posterior fossa where it fills the internal auditory canal.

dylate is sufficient for the examination. This can be placed in the lumbar subarachnoid space with a small bored $\neq$ 24 needle. The use of a small bored needle usually prevents a dural-arachnoid tear and results in a low incidence of complications such as headache and backache (less than 5 %). By placing the patient in the lateral decubitus position with the involved side lower-most, and tilting the cephalad end of the x-ray table downward (Fig. 2), the contrast material will gravitate superiorly into the cerebellopontine angle and internal auditory canal on the involved side. Although the internal auditory canal does not appear to be the most dependent portion of the dried skull in this position, in a living patient it apparently is. Because of this, small tumors may be demonstrated with a minute amount of contrast material and proper positioning of the patient with fluoroscopic guidance (Hitselberger and House, 1968).

Evolution of the transsigmoid operation

For the removal of the large acoustic tumor extending below the level of the jugular bulb, and associated with multiple cranial neuropathy or increased intracranial pressure, the translabyrinthine and suboccipital operations both have deficiencies. Basically, a procedure has been needed which would allow access to the inferior pole of the tumor, decompression of the posterior fossa, and preservation of the facial nerve with total tumor removal.

The suboccipital operation allows access to the inferior pole of the tumor and decompression of the posterior fossa, but usually only after retraction or resection of a portion of the lateral cerebellar hemisphere with subsequent postoperative ataxia. In addition, this method gives the least opportunity to preserve the facial nerve whether or not the posterior lip of the internal auditory meatus is removed. The translabyrinthine operation has been ideally suited for the removal of those tumors extending out of the internal auditory canal into the posterior fossa, but not below the level of the jugular bulb. In this situation, access to the inferior pole of the tumor is limited using the translabyrinthine approach. A great advantage of this operation, however, is that it allows early identification and preservation of the facial nerve. This is accomplished without cerebellar retraction or resection. A total removal, a shortened period of convalescence and early return to a useful life are obvious advantages.

We have felt that the management of the large acoustic tumor would best be achieved by a technique that would take advantage of some of the features of both procedures. An operation has been devised in which the translabyrinthine opening has been carried posteriorly over the sigmoid sinus. The lateral subocciput is removed. The sigmoid sinus is ligated and the dura is opened forward to the internal auditory meatus. The dura over the cerebellum is not disturbed. This operation allows exposure of the inferior pole of the tumor and identification of the IXth, Xth, and XIth cranial nerves as in the suboccipital operation. Bony decompression of the posterior fossa, total removal of the tumor and early exposure and separation of the facial nerve from the tumor can be obtained. If changes in blood pressure or respiration occur during attempts of removal of the tumor and are persistent, the procedure is terminated (Hitselberger and House, 1966).

Ligation of the sigmoid sinus

As the tumor grows in the posterior fossa and becomes a large space-occupying lesion associated with elevated intracranial pressure, venous collateral builds up from the vast potential venous drainage net that usually lies dormant in the tentorium, posterior fossa dura, and dura overlying the clivus. One needs only to look at a venogram in this region to realize the enormous potential for venous collateral flow that exists (Fig. 3). Cushing recognized this fact, but to him the excessive collateral existing in the posterior fossa dura and around the foramen magnum was a hazard which had to be dealt with in approaching these tumors through the subocciput. We have now taken

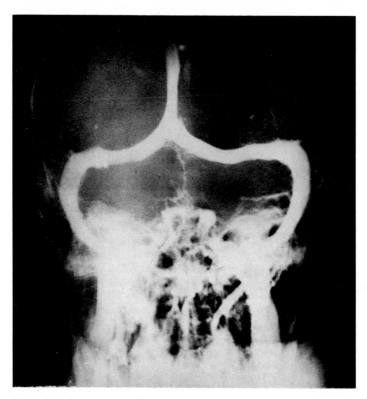

Fig. 3. Jugular venogram showing bilateral patency of the lateral and sigmoid sinuses. Note the extensive venous collateral which exists around the foramen magnum and at the base of the skull.

advantage of the extensive venous collateral circulation to gain exposure of the tumor and lessen the risk of damage to surrounding normal neurologic structures.

With the development of a reliable technique for jugular venography, we have usually carried out this procedure prior to a transsigmoid operation. This is done to ascertain the patency of both lateral sinuses and to determine the existence of adequate venous collateral flow along the base of the skull. In every patient harboring a large acoustic tumor in whom jugular venography was carried out, bilateral filling of the lateral and sigmoid sinuses was obtained with a unilateral contrast injection.

More important than the contrast demonstration of bilateral sinus patency with jugular venography prior to surgery, is the patient's response at operation to clamping off of the sigmoid sinus. If when a clamp is placed over the sigmoid sinus there is a sudden rise in the pressure of underlying brain contents, manifest by tightening of the dura, it is recommended that this sinus be left intact. In this situation, the venous drainage to this sinus is important for the drainage of blood from the brain. An interruption of this pathway could conceivably lead to further deleterious elevation of intra-cranial pressure. This situation occurred in one patient in the present series. In this case, a total removal of the tumor was accomplished by combined suboccipital translabyrinthine approach with forward displacement of the sinus that allowed increased exposure in the cerebellopontine angle. This patient was the only one in the present series in whom ligation of the sinus had an adverse effect. In one case, bilateral sinus ligation was carried out at separate procedure with an interval of six months between operations. In this patient, bilateral acoustic tumors were removed with preservation of hearing and facial nerves.

Staged procedures

Initially the removal of large acoustic tumors was carried out as a two-stage procedure. The first stage consisted of removal of the lateral subocciput and bone over the sigmoid sinus forward to the internal auditory meatus. A large spring clamp was placed over the sigmoid sinus. At the second stage, the sinus was ligated and the tumor was removed. The operation was performed in two stages because of the length of the total procedure (8–10 hours), and the necessity to ascertain if sinus ligation would be tolerated. We have now improved our own operating technique to the point where the whole procedure is carried out in from 4 to 6 hours. In addition, we have not noted any neurologic deficit that could be attributed to sinus ligation; i.e., papilledema, headaches, or neurologic defects.

Analysis of cases

A combined approach to the cerebellopontine angle with ligation of the sigmoid sinus was not undertaken until 1965. Since that time 33 patients with large acoustic tumors have undergone this procedure as their primary operation. Total removal of the tumor was obtained in 22 cases (66%). There were three fatalities. Facial nerve function has returned in 24 patients (72%).

Summary

In evaluation of the patient with a large acoustic neuroma, we feel that radiologic techniques using a positive contrast material (iophendylate) are to be preferred over the traditional pneumoencephalograms. Delineation of the tumor has been consistently accurate. The procedure is associated with less discomfort to the patient and does not necessitate a commitment to an operative procedure subsequent to the termination of the study. For the diagnosis of the small acoustic tumor, we have used the polytome x-ray unit and a small quantity of contrast material (1 cc).

Thirty-three patients in this series of 200 patients had large acoustic tumors removed through a combined suboccipital, translabyrinthine approach to the cerebellopontine angle with ligation of the sigmoid sinus. This procedure was initially carried out as a two-stage operation, but it is now accomplished in a single stage. The procedure allows the widest exposure of any of the operations now used for removal of these tumors. The suboccipital craniectomy allows the exposure of the inferior pole of the tumor and the IXth, Xth, and XIth nerves. The translabyrinthine access allows early identification and preservation of the facial nerve. In this series a total removal of the tumor was carried out in 22 patients (66%). There were three fatalities. The facial nerve was preserved in 24 patients (72%).

References

Hitselberger, W. E. & House, W. F., *Arch. Otolaryng.* (Chicago), *84,* 267 (1966).
Hitselberger, W. E. & House, W. F., *J. Neurosurg.,* *29,* 214 (1968).
Scanlan, R. L., *Arch. Otolaryng.* (Chicago), *80,* 698 (1964).

General discussion

Norlén to House

In our 14 cases of small tumours, or middle-sized, according to Dr. House's nomenclature, we have no operative mortality. From the first slide (Fig. 1) you can see the age distribution in our entire series, and the number of small tumours is indicated in black. I will return later to the age distribution in discussing mortality in the large tumours. The next slide (Table 1) demonstrates clinical findings in the small tumours, and the following one (Table 2) demonstrates the pre- and postoperative facial nerve function. In only one case, the facial nerve could not be saved, but in this case the nerve could be resutured in the posterior fossa with very good functional recovery. The only two cases in which the functional result was poor were those in which, already preoperatively, paresis was present.

In our total series, we have no operative mortality under the age of 40. After that age, the mortality rate rises slowly, so that our total mortality rate under the age of 60 is 11 %. In the older age groups, the mortality rate is high, especially in the male. The female patients seem to stand the operation much better. The indications for surgery must therefore be seriously considered in a patient around the age of 70 years. I ask Dr. House if he has made any correlation concerning age, sex and mortality in his series.

Miehlke to House

I feel that all of us have to be very grateful to Dr. William House for his pioneering work in the discovery of the contents of the internal meatus.

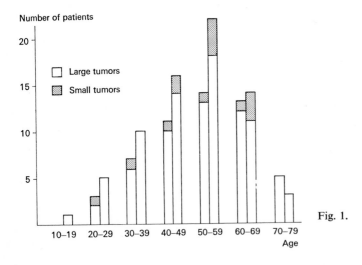

Fig. 1.

Table 1. *Pre- and postoperative clinical findings in 14 cases of small acoustic neuromas.*

Corneal reflex			CSF protein		
Normal	12		Under 50 mg %	6	
Uncertain	1		Above 50 mg %	4	
Absent	1		Information lacking	4	
Hearing	Preop.	Postop.	*Caloric response*	Preop.	Postop.
Totally deaf	2	13	Normal	4	—
Diminished	12	1	Diminished	8	1
			Absent	2	13
Porus widening	14				

Table 2. *Pre- and postoperative facial nerve function in 14 cases of small acoustic neuromas.*

No preoperative paralysis	12
Partial preoperative paralysis	2
Anatomical continuity preserved at operation	13
Postoperative	
good function	10
some function	2
no function	2

Above all, this holds true for facial nerve surgery. I believe that, in the very near future, we will have definite indications for attacking the facial nerve in the internal meatus.

In cases of transverse fracture of the petrous bone, for instance, the facial nerve is often torn off or shorn off in the internal meatus. In other cases, only some bone chips from the fractured roof of the labyrinth have been found embedded in the VIIth nerve. In contrast to past procedures, we should nowadays carefully expose such fractures via the middle cranial fossa approach according to Dr. House's technique (Figs. 1–5).

Brünner to House

How many of your patients have had contrast examinations and do you have any complications in your material? Did any of your patients in the group operated on 5 years ago have any complications?

Olivecrona to House

I should like to say something about this magnificent presentation. With regard to pneumoencephalograms, we never had any trouble about those, in the first place because we do not do pneumoencephalograms in tumours causing raised intracranial pressure. In small tumours without any pressure, we never had any trouble with pneumoencephalograms and, as Professor

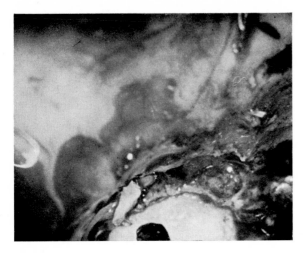

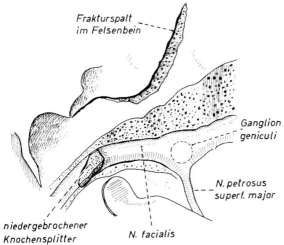

Fig. 1. Transverse fracture of the petrous pyramid with a bone splinter depressed into the facial nerve.

Greitz has shown earlier today, we get very good pictures outlining the tumour, and we know exactly how big it is. Concerning the surgical technique, I think I agree with Dr. House that the access to the lower pole of the tumour is somewhat better after ligating the sigmoid sinus. However, in a conventional operation, access to the lower pole is quite good; it is access to the superior pole which is one of the real difficulties in removing acoustic tumours. Last year I suggested that perhaps it would be practical to do first a temporal operation and dissect the facial nerve free and free the tumour from its attachment to the porus, and then a week later remove the tumour by the conventional suboccipital approach, which should be easier, as the tumour will be mobile after its attachment to the porus has been freed.

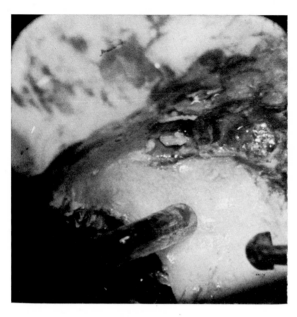

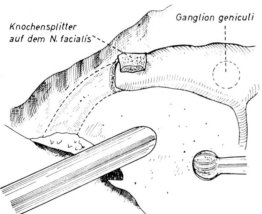

Knochensplitter
auf dem N. facialis

Ganglion geniculi

Fig. 2. Between cochlea and vestibular portion of the labyrinth the bone is thinned out in the direction of the internal meatus.

House to Brünner

At the present time, we are performing more and more positive contrast studies of the posterior fossa. We inject 1 cc of dye into the subarachnoid space, and position the patient so that the dye runs into the posterior fossa. We then examine the internal auditory canals by means of Polytome techniques. We now perform about 5 such examinations for every positive one. I am not aware of any more serious complications with this technique than would be expected with a similar number of spinal taps. The most serious complication to date has been the need, in several cases, to hospitalize the patient for several days because of post-spinal headache. In addition, some

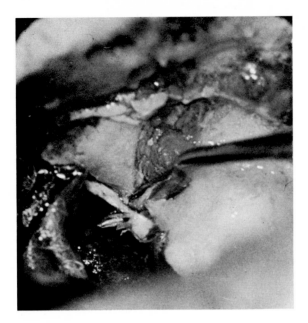

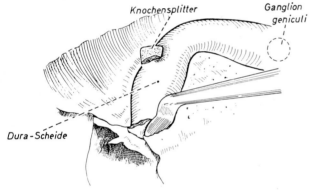

Knochensplitter

Ganglion geniculi

Dura-Scheide

Fig. 3. The dural sheath of the internal auditory meatus is exposed from above by removing of the last layer of covering bone.

patients have discomfort down the back of their legs for periods up to a month or two. These have not, however, been persistent nor are they considered to be serious or disabling. This apparently is related to a reaction from the Pantopaque. I am not aware of any complications from Pantopaque used as long ago as 5 years.

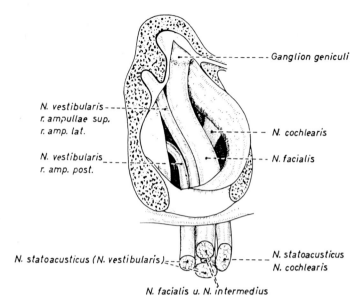

Fig. 4. Splitting of the dural sac with a diagrammatic view of the contents of the internal auditory meatus.

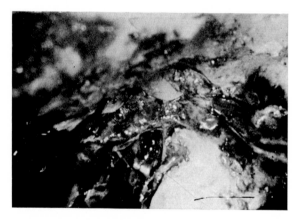

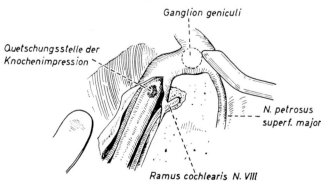

Fig. 5. View of the contents of the internal auditory meatus from above the facial nerve is bruised by a depressed bone splint.

Results of total and subtotal removal of acoustic neuromas

By Nils Lundberg

Department of Neurosurgery, University of Lund, Sweden

This paper concerns a personal series of unilateral acoustic neuromas. The series consists of 93 consecutive cases operated upon between 1947 and 1966. Four patients were operated on twice, 3 because of a recurrence after partial removal; in the 4th case the first operation could not be completed because of intractable brain swelling. The tumour was later totally removed under hypothermia. The total number of operations was thus 97.

Operative technique

The cerebello-pontine angle was exposed by a lateral suboccipital approach. The technical routine was mainly conventional, and there is no need to describe it in detail. However, in some respects it differed from what may be regarded as the usual procedure.

Thus, during the last 10 years, in 47 patients the intracranial pressure was monitored by continuous recording of the ventricular fluid pressure before, during, and after the operation. Preoperatively, fluid was drained under pressure control as soon as there was reason to suspect that the intracranial hypertension could damage the brain or optic nerves. The ventricular cannula was also used for ventriculography, for tapping of fluid at the beginning of operation, and for early diagnosis of postoperative haematoma. When the ventricular fluid pressure rose after operation, fluid was drained only if a postoperative clot could be excluded.

Routine measures intended to improve the access to the cerebello-pontine angle were: lateral position of the patient, a linear retromastoid incision, extending far down the neck, partial exposure of the sinuses, making it possible to retract the sinus border forwards and upwards, and resection of the lateral pole of the cerebellar hemisphere.

The intrameatal part of the tumour was exposed by removing the posterior wall of the porus with a dental drill, and was extirpated under direct vision. The tumour plug was tilted out, and the facial nerve exposed or at least identified by electric stimulation. This procedure has been routinely applied since 1951 and has been used in altogether 53 cases.

Table 1. *Operative mortality.*

Tumour size	No. of operations	Surgical deaths[a]	Per cent
Group 1	7	0	0
Group 2	40	2	5
Group 3	50	4	8
Total	97	6	6.2

[a] Deaths up to 1 month after op.

In those cases where the facial nerve merged in the capsule outside the porus and could not be localized by vision, attempts were made to identify it by electric stimulation, and to cut out and preserve the part of the capsule containing the nerve. Likewise, when the capsule was firmly adherent to the pons, a small fragment of capsule and tumour tissue was left. Furthermore, in a few cases, the intrameatal tumour plug was not completely removed. In this paper, *subtotal removal* (22 cases) is to be understood as radical extirpation of a tumour except for at most such small fragments.

Anaesthesiological procedures

Since 1955, 41 operations were done under hypothermia. Hypothermia was induced by surface cooling with circulating air. Anaesthesia and muscular relaxation were maintained by ether and in most cases the patient was breathing spontaneously. The operation was performed at a rectal temperature of 27–28°C. Rewarming was started before the dura was closed.

Totally 14 operations were done under controlled respiration without hypothermia. The patient was ventilated by an Engström respirator, which was set to give moderate hyperventilation (P_aCO_2 25–30 mm Hg).

One reason why we used hypothermia was to get ample space in the cerebello-pontine angle and to diminish the risk of brain swelling during the operation. Pressure against the cerebellum with a retractor is surely *one* cause of postoperative trouble and should, when possible, be avoided. In

Table 2. *Mortality rates.*

	Operative mortality	Case[a] mortality
1947–1956, 40 operations	10.0 %	23.1 %
1957–1966, 57 operations	3.5 %	5.6 %
Total	6.2 %	12.9 %

[a] Including cases of late death presumably due to postop. sequelae (4) or recurrence (2).

Table 3. *Postoperative working capacity.*

Tumour size	No. of operations	Full or almost full	Moderately impaired	Severely impaired	Semi-invalids	Total invalids	Un-known
1	7	4	2[a]				1[b]
2	38	20 52,6 %	8 21,1 %	4 10,5 %	5 13,2 %	1 2,6 %	
3	45	19 42,2 %	12 26,7 %	8 17,8 %	4 8,9 %	2 4.4 %	
Total	90	43 47,8 %	22 24.5 %	12 13.3 %	9 10 %	3 3.3 %	1 1.1 %
			72.3 %				

[a] By other diseases.   [b] Incapacitated by cerebral haemorrhage 4 months after op.

most cases operated upon under hypothermia, the tumour could be removed without retraction of the cerebellum. Another reason for using hypothermia was the hope that mechanical manipulation and ischaemia would cause less damage to the brain—a hope that is founded mainly on experimental evidence.

Results

The results with regard to mortality, working capacity and function of the facial nerve are accounted for in Tables 1–4. In these tables, the operations or the cases have been grouped according to the size of the tumour, using the same grading as Olivecrona in his recent paper (1967). Group 1 includes small tumours, about the size of a hazelnut and not exerting any pressure on the brain. Medium-sized tumours, about the size of a walnut, are assigned

Table 4. *Facial nerve function.*

Tumour size	No. of operations	Anatom. contin. preserved	No or insignif. paresis	Slight paresis	Moderate paresis	Severe or total paresis	Un-known
1	7	7	3	3			1[a]
2	38	23	8	7	3	12	8
3	45	21	7	8	5	20	5
Total	90	55 61 %	18 20 %	18 20 %	8 9 %	32[b] 36 %	14 15 %
				44 = 49 %			

The figures include 4 cases where the stumps of the severed nerve were adapted end-to-end. Good recovery of function in 1 case, fair in 2 cases.
[a] Postop. function disappeared after reop. with removal of haematoma in the cerebello-pontine angle. Total pareses when discharged.
[b] Anastomosis with the hypoglossus in 24 cases, with the spinal accessory in 1 case.

to group 2. Tumours belonging to this group make an impression in the pons and the cerebellum, but do not cause any appreciable displacement of the brain stem. Large tumours—ping-pong or even golf-ball sized—belong to group 3. These tumours cause a marked dislocation of the brain stem and often protrude upwards through the tentorial notch.

Table 1 shows the overall postoperative mortality.

The causes of postoperative death were:

lesion of the brain stem: 4 cases,

haemorrhage in the central part of the right cerebral hemisphere: 1 case,

sudden cardiac arrest 3 days postoperatively: 1 case.

It should be noted that no death was caused by haematoma in the cerebel-lo-pontine angle.

In *Table 2,* the mortality rates for the two decades between 1947 and 1966 are given separately. The figure 3.5 % represents 2 deaths after a total of 56 operations. In one case the cause of death was cerebral haemorrhage during or soon after the operation in a hypertensive patient. The second patient had one of the largest tumours in the series and advanced intracranial hyper-tension. The preoperative roentgen diagnosis was cerebellar tumour, and consequently the operation was performed without hypothermia. The proce-dure was severely disturbed by intractable brain swelling and profuse bleed-ing, and the patient succumbed without having regained consciousness after the operation. Autopsy was not done.

Table 3 shows the working capacity estimated on the basic of question-naires and outpatient records. The total figure, 90, includes all operations except 6 with a fatal outcome, and 1 which was interrupted because of brain swelling and completed 2 months later under hypothermia.

The impairment of the working capacity in 2 cases belonging to group 1 was due to other diseases (chronic polyarthritis and mental insufficiency). The patient in the same group whose working capacity is classed as unknown would probably have regained her preoperative capacity had she not had a stroke 4 months after operation.

The postoperative function of the facial nerve is given in *Table 4.* The validity of the figures is reduced by the large number of cases labelled "un-known". However, the figure 49 % is probably representative of the number of patients with acceptable function of the nerve.

The figures in Table 4 include 4 cases in which the facial nerve was severed between the porus and the pons, and the ends could be approximated and kept in place by a blood clot. Recovery of function was achieved in 3 of these cases — good in one, fair in two.

As mentioned, small pieces of the tumour capsule with or without frag-ments of attached intracapsular tissue were left behind in 22 cases (subtotal removal). One aim of the present study was to ascertain whether this means an increased risk of recurrence. As seen in *Table 5,* there was one recurrence. In this case, part of the tumour about the size of an almond and attached to the pons was left behind. In the other cases, the pieces left were smaller— usually only small fragments of capsule.

Table 5 also illustrates the well-known high frequency of recurrence after partial (intracapsular) removal. However, it should also be noted that two patients are alive without signs of recurrence 11 and 14 years after intra-capsular evacuation. In 59 cases of total removal, there has so far been no recurrence.

Another purpose of this investigation was to study the effect of different anaesthetic procedures on the operative conditions and the postoperative out-come (*Tables 6–7*). Local anaesthesia was routine from 1947–1951, ordinary intratracheal anaesthesia from 1952–1956. From 1956, controlled respiration without cooling and hypothermia were used alternately.

In Table 7, four parameters (brain swelling during operation, postoperative course, late results with regard to working capacity and facial nerve function) are graded according to a 1–3 scale, the higher figures being less favourable. The figures in the table represent average scores.

The figures in Tables 6 and 7 are certainly biased to some extent and should be judged with caution. Nevertheless, hypothermia appears to have a favourable effect on the operative conditions, the postoperative course and the surgical mortality.

Discussion

When operating upon acoustic neuromas, especially upon large ones, the surgeon sometimes has to choose between (a) leaving behind part of the capsule adherent to the pons or the facial nerve and (b) removing the entire capsule with the risk of injury to these structures. From the figures in Table 3 it appears that leaving such small fragments of tumour tissue does not in-crease the risk of recurrence to such an extent that a total removal should always be aimed at.

It seems difficult to disregard the favourable influence of hypothermia as demonstrated in Tables 6 and 7. Some years ago, I began to use controlled respiration with moderate hyperventilation instead of hypothermia. However, after having experienced a couple of cases with a swollen brain during the operation, I took up hypothermia again. I think that hypothermia is an alterna-tive to the sitting position, which undoubtedly produces optimal conditions for the surgeon, but at the same time increases the risk of postoperative

Table 5. *Recurrences.*

Removal	No. of surviving cases	Operated recurrences	Non op. recurrences	Deaths of recurrence
Partial	6	2[a]	2	2
Subtotal	22	1[b]	0	0
Total	59	0	0	0

[a] 1 pat. alive 16 years after reop. (total removal) with full working capacity.
  1 pat. dead of other disease 2 years after reop. (evacuation of cyst).
[b] Living with moderately impaired working capacity $3\frac{1}{2}$ years after reop. (total removal).

haemorrhage. This is clearly demonstrated by Drake, who reported 4 deaths from postoperative haemorrhage in 30 cases (1967 a).

Finally, I wish to compliment Drs. House and Hitselberger on their amazing series of acoustic neuromas. What I think is particularly amazing is the proportion of small tumours which so conspicuously differs from that in other series. In Olivecrona's material of 349 cases 6% (1967), in the series of Hullay and Tomits 26% (1965), and in the present series 7.5% belong to group 1. Group 1 seems to correspond to the "small" and "medium sized" tumours in the series of House and Hitselberger, which constitute about 70% of the total number.

It is quite clear that the diagnostic work behind these figures is a remarkable achievement, and if they represent what we can arrive at by improving our diagnostic aids, this work may be regarded as a milestone in the history of the treatment of acoustic neuromas. It is a truism to state that early diagnosis makes all the difference.

I am less impressed by the surgical results. For many years, neurosurgeons have removed small acoustic neuromas by the suboccipital route without ap-

Table 6. *Anaesthesiologic procedures.*

	No. of operations	Surgical deaths	Postop. haematoma	Late deaths from postop. sequelae	Recurrences
Local anaesthesia	21	3	1		3
General anaesthesia with spont. resp.	21	1	5[a]	3	
General anaesthesia with controlled resp.	14	2			1
Total	56	6	6	3	4
		11%	11%	5.4%	7.2%
Hypothermia	41	0	0	1	1
				2.4%	2.4%

[a] Induced hypotension in all 5 cases.

Table 7. *Anaesthesiologic procedures.*

	Brain swelling during op.	Postoper. course	Working capacity	Facial nerve function
Local anaesthesia	0.5	0.5	1.5	2.3
General anaesthesia with spont. resp.	0.3	1.2	2.1	3.5
General anaesthesia with controlled resp.	1.1	1.3	2.1	2.6
Hypothermia	0.1	0.3	1.7	2.7

preciable difficulties and with excellent results. The simplicity and safety with which such small neuromas can be radically extirpated and the facial nerve preserved has been pointed out by McKissock in 1954 and recently re-emphasized by Olivecrona (1967) and by Drake (1967 a) and Pool (1966). Although limited, my experience of small tumours is in agreement with these statements. The combined approach which House and Hitselberger use for removal of larger tumours certainly gives good access to the lateral part of the tumour. However, what is important in radical operations on large tumours is the access to the medial and caudal parts, which must be dissected off from the pons and the trigeminal and facial nerves. This access cannot be improved by dividing the sinus or removing the postero-lateral part of the petrous bone, at least not to such an extent as to justify these procedures. Furthermore, removal of the posterior wall of the porus (Dandy, 1925) gives an equally good or even better access to the intrameatal part of the tumour.

In my opinion, Dr. House and Dr. Hitselberger have made an important contribution by improving our means for early diagnosis of acoustic neuromas, but it still remains to be shown that their transtemporal technique, in comparable series, gives equally good or better results than the suboccipital approach.

References

Dandy, W. E., *Surg. Gynec. Obstet., 41,* 129 (1925).
Drake, C. G., *J. Neurosurg., 26,* 459 (1967).
Drake, C. G., *J. Neurosurg., 26,* 554 (1967).
Elliott, F. A. & McKissock, W., *Lancet, 2,* 1189 (1954).
Hullay, J. & Tomits, G. H., *J. Neurosurg., 22,* 127 (1965).
Olivecrona, H., *J. Neurosurg., 26,* 6 (1967).
Pool, J. L., *J. Neurosurg., 24,* 485 (1966).

The surgical anatomy of the so-called internal auditory artery

By Ugo Fisch

Department of Otolaryngology, Kantonsspital, Zürich, Switzerland

The recent developments in microsurgery of the internal auditory meatus and cerebello-pontine angle have created the need for a precise knowledge of the vascular system in this region of the body. The aims of the present investigation were:

1. To study the arterial system of the internal auditory canal in man with particular reference to its surgical approach through the middle cranial fossa.

2. To clarify the still existing confusion in regard to the vascular segment which may be defined as the internal auditory artery.

Consulting the "Nomina Anatomica" prepared by the international nomenclature committee, one will be surprised to find that, officially, the name of the internal auditory artery does not exist! Nevertheless, in the most recent textbooks of otology, the name internal auditory artery is used to define a vessel arising either directly from the basilar trunk or from the anterior inferior cerebellar artery. Commonly, the names of internal auditory and labyrinthine are also used as synonymous terms for the same vessel.

In order to throw some light on these questions, the arterial system of the internal auditory canal in man was investigated in 11 cadavers (22 temporal bones) by the intravascular injection of a silicone rubber compound ("Microfil"—trademark of Canton Bio-Medical Products, Swarthmore, Penna.). The age of the patients ranged from 10 to 91 years (Table 1).

The posterior part of the skull, including both pyramids, the posterior cranial fossa and the intact tentorium, was removed from the cadaver within 12 hours of death. The cerebello-pontine angle of each side was then exposed through an incision in the tentorium, and the basilar artery identified in the region of the clivus. A vessel having a close relation to the VIth or abducent nerve (Cushing, 1910) is seen to take off from the basilar trunk in the direction of the porus acusticus internus of each side. A fine polyethylene tubing is introduced into this artery through its opening in the lumen of the basilar trunk using the magnification afforded by the operating microscope.

Before injection, it is rather difficult to identify the vessels lying around

Table 1. Age and sex of the patients. Investigated side and corresponding number of labyrinthine arteries found in each specimen.

Pat.	Sex	Age (yrs)	Investigated side	Number of lab. art. right	left
I	♂	50	—	left	—	2
II	♂	58	right	left	2	1
III	♂	48	right	left	2	2
IV	♂	75	right	left	2	2
V	♂	10	right	left	2	2
VI	♀	70	right	left	1	1
VII	♀	43	right	left	1	1
VIII	♀	71	right	left	2	1
IX	♀	91	right	left	1	2
X	♂	61	right	left	2	1
XI	♂	83	right	left	1	—

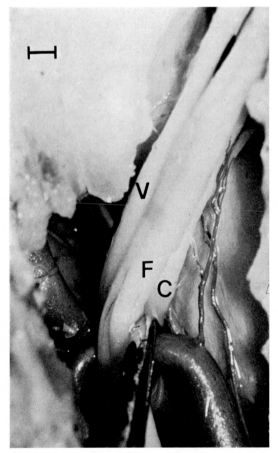

Fig. 1. *Case III: male, 48 years.* View of the left porus acusticus internus following removal of the bony roof of the internal meatus. C = cochlear nerve. V = vestibular nerve, F = facial nerve. Note the difference in size between the cerebellar vessels forming a loop at the porus acusticus internus and the two small arteries taking off for the meatus. The bar in the upper left corner of the figure corresponds to 1 mm.

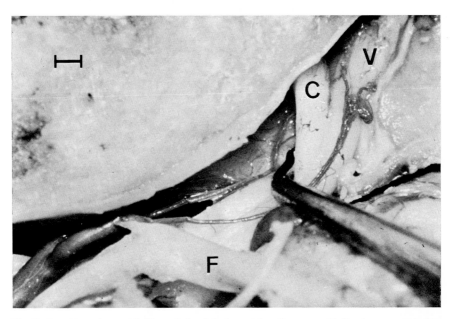

Fig. 2. *Case II: male, age 58.* View of the right internal auditory canal following removal of its bony roof. The facial nerve (F) has been pulled aside. The cochlear (C) and vestibular (V) division of the VIIIth nerve are exposed. Note the two arteries entering the internal auditory canal above and underneath the cochlear nerve. The bar in the upper left corner of the figure corresponds to 1 mm.

the porus. Following injection of the silicone rubber compound—which is accomplished with a maximal pressure of 160 mm of mercury and under direct microscopical control—the vascular pattern at the entrance of the internal auditory canal becomes very apparent. However, in order to determine the exact course of each vessel, the bony roof of the internal auditory canal has to be removed, using the same microsurgical technique employed for its middle cranial fossa approach.

Following this procedure, two or more small arteries—with one exception—have been seen to enter the porus acusticus internus of the specimens under investigation (Figs. 1, 2, 4). These vessels may be divided into:

— arteries concerned with the blood supply of the membranous labyrinth (the *labyrinthine arteries* in the proper sense), and

— arteries bringing blood to the structures lying in the internal meatus itself, i.e., to the cochlear and vestibular division of the VIIIth nerve, to the meningeal membranes and to the periosteum of the bone surrounding the internal auditory canal.

In 9 of the investigated temporal bones (cases II_L, VI, VII, VIII_L, IX_R, X_L, XI_R) a *single labyrinthine artery* was found to enter the internal auditory meatus. In the remaining 11 ears (cases I_L, II_R, III, IV, V, VIII_R, IX_L,

Arteries of the internal auditory meatus

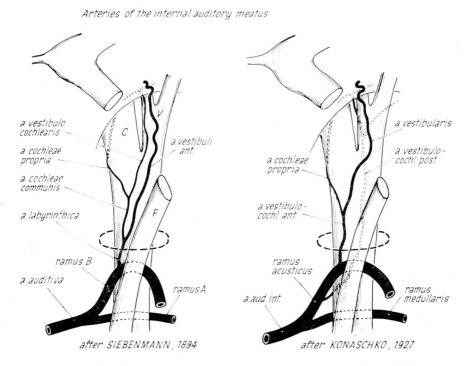

Fig. 3. Ramification of the arteries of the internal auditory meatus according to Siebenmann and Konaschko.

X_R) *two labyrinthine arteries* were present (Table 1). In 5 of 9 cases with successful bilateral injection (cases III, IV, V, VI and VII) the same *mono-arterial* or *bi-arterial* type was observed for both sides (right and left temporal bones) of the same specimen. In the remaining 4 cases (II, VIII, IX and X) the number of labyrinthine arteries varied for one side and the other.

If only one labyrinthine vessel was present, its ramification followed with minor variations the pattern described by Siebenmann in 1894 (Fig. 3) giving origin to the well-known arteria vestibuli anterior, arteria vestibulo-cochlearis and arteria cochleae propria. In those cases with two labyrinthine arteries, the ramification pattern was similar to that observed by the Russian Konaschko in 1927 (Fig. 3). This pattern differs from that of Siebenmann insofar as the arteria vestibulo-cochlearis is not seen as a branch of a single labyrinthine vessel, but is a separate artery, called arteria vestibulo-cochlearis posterior, originating from a larger cerebellar vessel.

In all specimens, the labyrinthine artery or arteries entered the internal auditory canal at the anterior inferior rim of the porus (Figs. 1, 2, 4). In the mono-arterial type, the labyrinthine vessel always lay between the cochlear and facial nerve. In the bi-arterial type, one vessel (the superior) takes the

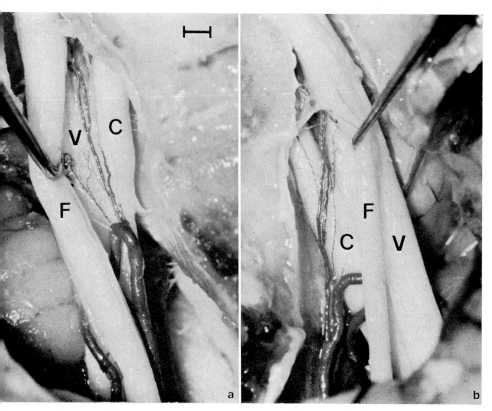

Fig. 4. *Case V: male, age 10.* View of the right (Fig. 4A) and left (Fig. 4B) internal auditory canal. C = cochlear nerve, F = facial nerve, V = vestibular nerve. Note the loop of a branch of the anterior inferior cerebellar artery between facial (F) and VIIIth (C = cochlear division, V = vestibular division) nerve. Three arteries take off from this loop to enter the internal auditory canal. Note the ramification of the larger artery (arteria labyrinthica) in the canal. The bar on the upper right corner of the figure corresponds to 1 mm.

same course as the single labyrinthine artery in the mono-arterial cases between the cochlear and facial nerves giving origin to a cochlear and vestibular branch. The other vessel (the inferior) goes along the bottom of the internal auditory canal, crosses the cochlear nerve at its inferior surface, and follows the inferior branch of the vestibular nerve towards the inferior vestibular area of the meatal fundus (Fig. 2).

In the mono-arterial type, frequently a vessel of about the same size as the labyrinthine artery is seen to enter the meatus, taking a course similar to that of the inferior labyrinthine artery in the bi-arterial cases. This artery will not, however, reach the fundus of the meatus, and its main branches supply the vestibular nerve, particularly the region of Scarpa's ganglion. In all the cases, the arterial vessels reaching the superior and the inferior vestibular areas of the fundus of the meatus are larger than the corresponding vessels directed

Case V: male, age 10

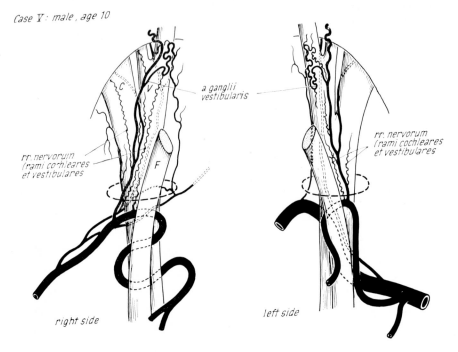

a ganglii
vestibularis

rr. nervorum
(rami cochleares
et vestibulares

rr. nervorum
(rami cochleares
et vestibulares

right side

left side

Fig. 5. *Case V: male, age 10.* Schematic representation of the vascular patterns observed in Fig. 4.

towards the cochlear area. The arterial branch destined to the cochlear area originates in all the cases from a labyrinthine vessel at the superior aspect of the cochlear nerve, and runs in the anterior half of the meatus along and around this nerve covered by the facial nerve (Figs. 2, 4, 5). The subarcuate artery has been found to originate as a separate branch from a cerebellar vessel outside the porus in 14 specimens.

The drawings of Fig. 3 were performed according to Siebenmann's and Konaschko's original descriptions. Only the size of the represented arteries was changed according to the present findings. The vessels penetrating in the meatus acusticus internus do not exceed 150 microns in diameter, and are therefore of nearly arteriolar size; in fact, these vessels are small arteries because, histologically, their media presents with more than one muscular layer. (Baker and Iannone, 1959). Larger cerebellar vessels may be found to form a loop into the meatus. However, this situation was met only twice in the present investigation. Most commonly, the vascular loop of the anterior inferior cerebellar artery or of one of its branches was seen to lie at the porus or outside it.

The reason for the existing confusion about the definition of the internal auditory artery (Nager, 1954) becomes evident if the correct size of the vessels entering the meatus acusticus internus is considered. The artery called

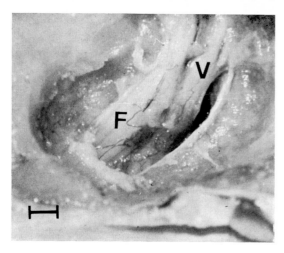

Fig. 6. *Case II: male, age 58.* The right internal auditory canal as seen in the course of the approach through the middle cranial fossa. The dural sac has been opened. The vestibular (V) and facial (F) nerve are clearly visible. Note the vascular pattern in the region of Scarpa's ganglion and the arterial branches for the facial nerve. The bar in the lower left corner of the figure corresponds to 1 mm.

internal auditory by Siebenmann, Cavatorti, Stopford and Konaschko is not primarily involved with blood supply of the inner ear, and is in fact—as Nabeya already stated in 1923—a misconception of a cerebellar vessel, either of the anterior inferior or of an accessory cerebellar artery (Nabeya, 1923, Ferrari-Lelli, 1940, Guerrier and Villaceque, 1949 and Charachon and Latarjet, 1962).

The schematic drawings of Siebenmann, Nabeya and Konaschko (Fig. 3) also convey the false impression that the artery or arteries entering the internal auditory canal only divide into two or three branches for the membranous labyrinth. In fact, these vessels show an *extensive ramification* in order to supply the structures lying in the internal canal itself (Figs. 4, 5). The numerous ramifications of the labyrinthine artery or arteries have been recently observed by Hansen (1967) and were already well known to Nabeya. This author states in his "Study in the Comparative Anatomy of the Blood-Vascular System of the Internal Ear in Mammalia and in Homo (Japanese)": There are many blood vessels in the meatus acusticus internus, innumerable arterial branches are given off by the trunk of the arteria labyrinthica or by the trunks of the arteriae labyrinthicae. Nabeya forgot these branches in his schematic drawings, because his interest was mainly focused on the blood supply of the internal ear.

As seen in Figs. 4 and 5, numerous arterial branches in the internal meatus are concerned with the vascularization of the VIIIth and facial nerves, and may therefore be called *rami nervorum*. Smaller branches also go to the dural sac of the internal meatus (Fig. 5). These dural vessels supply the dura, as well as the periosteum of the bone surrounding the meatus. The involvement of these vessels by the development of an acoustic tumour may be the cause of the enlargement of the internal auditory canal observed without evidence of increased intrameatal pressure.

The arterial system of the internal auditory meatus

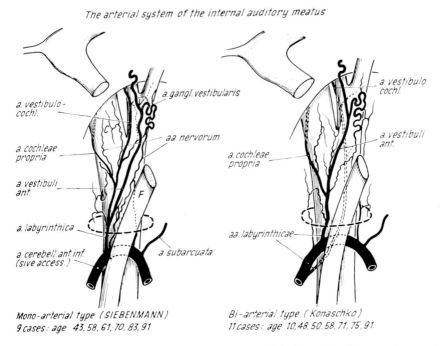

Fig. 7. Schematic representation of the arterial system of the internal auditory meatus according to the present investigation.

The largest arterial vessel of the internal meatus not primarily concerned with the blood supply of the internal ear is a branch given off by the superior vestibular artery for the region of Scarpa's ganglion (Figs. 2, 5), which may therefore be called arteria ganglii vestibularis. The arteria ganglii vestibularis forms numerous glomerula-like convolutions around the superior vestibular ganglion, receives anastomotic branches from the inferior vestibular artery and other vessels lying in the posterior, inferior aspect of the internal meatus, and also provides smaller rami for the facial nerve.

The arteria ganglii vestibularis is of particular surgical importance, because it is the first vessel visualized in the meatus in the course of its approach through the middle cranial fossa (Fig. 6).

The arteria ganglii vestibularis also permits the identification of Scarpa's ganglion in the course of the transtemporal approach. In contrast to the impression given by many artistic representations in anatomical textbooks, we found it very difficult, even under the operating microscope, to identify the vestibular ganglion from the main trunk and branches of the vestibular nerve if its blood supply is missing.

The present findings are summarized in Fig. 7. In general, two or more small arteries of nearly arteriolar size are seen to enter the internal auditory canal in man. These arteries never originate directly from the basilar trunk, but are branches of a larger cerebellar vessel (anterior inferior or accessory cerebellar artery). The arteries entering the internal auditory canal form an intricate arterial network, which can appropriately be called the *arterial system of the internal auditory meatus*. The labyrinthine artery or arteries belong to this system. The name of internal auditory artery should not be used, in order to avoid confusion with cerebellar vessels not primarily involved with the blood supply of the internal acoustic meatus and membranous labyrinth, as well as in consideration to the fact that more than one vessel is usually found to enter the porus acusticus internus in man.

Summary

The arterial system of the internal auditory canal in man has been investigated in 11 cadavers (22 temporal bones) by intravascular injection of a silicone rubber compound. With one exception, two or more small arteries of nearly arteriolar size have been seen to enter the porus acusticus internus of the specimens under investigation. The blood supply to the internal ear consisted of the single labyrinthine artery (mono-arterial type) in 9 cases, and of two labyrinthine arteries (bi-arterial type) in 11. The ramification pattern of the labyrinthine artery or arteries was similar to that observed by Siebenmann and by Konaschko. An extensive ramification of the labyrinthine artery or arteries was observed. These arterial branches, as well as the other vessels entering the internal auditory canal without reaching the internal ear, supply the structures lying in the meatus itself, particularly the cochlear and vestibular nerve. The largest arterial vessel not primarily concerned with the blood supply of the internal ear found in the internal meatus is an artery directed to the region of Scarpa's ganglion (arteria ganglii vestibularis). The reason for the existing confusion about the definition of the internal auditory artery is discussed. The name of the arterial system of the internal auditory meatus for the intricate arterial network found in the auditory canal is suggested. The labyrinthine artery or arteries belong to the system. The name of internal auditory artery should not be used, in order to avoid confusion with cerebellar vessels not primarily involved with the blood supply of the internal acoustic meatus and membranous labyrinth, as well as in consideration to the fact that more than one vessel is usually found to enter the porus acusticus internus in man.

References

Baker, A. B. & Iannone, A., *Neurology* (Minneap.), *9,* 391, 441 (1959).

Cavatorti, P., *Monit. Zool. Ital., 10,* 248 (1908).

Charachon, R. & Latarjet, A., *Compt. rend. Ass. Anat., 48,* 436 (1962).

Cushing, H., *Brain, 33,* 204 (1910).

Ferrari-Lelli, G., *Z. Anat. Entwicklungsgesch., 110,* 48 (1939).

Guerrier, Y. & Villaceque, F., *Compt. rend. Ass. Anat., 36,* 377 (1949).

Hansen, C. C., *Vascular anatomy of the temporal bone.* A preliminary report, in press (1967).

Konaschko, P. I., *Z. Anat. Entwicklungsgesch., 83,* 241 (1927).

Nabeya, D., *Acta Sch. Med. Univ. Kioto, 4,* 1 (1923).

Nager, G. T., *Ann. Otol., 63,* 51 (1954).

Nomina Anatomica. Prepared by the International Anatomical Nomenclature Committee appointed by the Fifth International Congress of Anatomists held at Oxford in 1950 and approved at the Sixth International Congress held in Paris in 1955, and including revisions approved at the Seventh and Eighth International Congresses of Anatomists held respectively in New York in 1960 and at Wiesbaden in 1965. Excerpta Medica Foundation (1966).

Siebenmann, F., *Die Blutgefässe im Labyrinthe des menschlichen Ohres,* Wiesbaden (1894).

Stopford, J. S. B., *J. Anat. Physiol., 50,* 131 (1916).

Transmeatal posterior fossa approach to acoustic neuroma

By Erik Fluur

Department of Otolaryngology, Karolinska Sjukhuset, Stockholm, Sweden

and Ladislau Steiner

Department of Neurosurgery, Karolinska Sjukhuset, Stockholm, Sweden

An acoustic tumour arises in the Schwann cells of the vestibular nerve, at the transition between the glial and fibrous portion, in the inner part of the internal auditory meatus. Consequently, in its initial stage, the tumour has an intratemporal localization. It is not until later, when it has extended into the posterior fossa, that it can be regarded as intracranial. Since it is situated in a region comprising the borderline between the field of activity of two specialities—i.e., otology and neurosurgery—it is not surprising that interest has recently been aroused in this tumour from the otosurgical point of view as well. One of the foremost reasons is, naturally, the improved methods of examination, which have permitted detection of tumours that are still confined to the internal auditory meatus.

In 1917, Cushing published his famous work on tumours of the acoustic nerve, and the suboccipital approach has subsequently been the classical method in removal of these tumours. Although, primarily, only subtotal intracapsular evacuation of the tumour was performed, Dandy (1925) later recommended total removal. Olivecrona has demonstrated that the 5-year survival rate is twice as high after total removal as after partial excision.

Unfortunately, the function of the facial nerve is often impaired after these operations. This applies particularly in total removal, when the nerve must be dissected free from the tumour before it can be removed. This procedure makes it difficult to keep the nerve intact. Various authors have stated that it remains undamaged in only 10–40% of cases. Olivecrona showed in his series that, even if the anatomical continuity of the nerve can be retained in about 40% of all cases, complete regeneration of its function cannot be anticipated in more than about 10%. The reason is that, during operation, the nerve is always traumatized to a varying degree, which implies that regeneration cannot be expected in 100%.

For many years there has, therefore, existed a great need of an improved surgical technique, precisely with the object of maintaining the function of the facial nerve in total removal of the tumour. This has, in fact, been stressed by several authors, among them Pool and Pava (1957). Concurrently with the advances in the possibilities of examination, new operative methods have been devised. Consequently, today, an acoustic tumour can be approached from three different directions:

1. Subtemporal extradural middle fossa (Kurze, 1958)
2. Translabyrinthine (Panse, 1904)
3. Transmeatal posterior fossa (Dandy, 1925)

The middle fossa and the translabyrinthine approach have subsequently been perfected by House (1964).

The subtemporal middle fossa approach can be used only in the presence of a small tumour, confined to the internal meatus. Unfortunately, tumours of this inappreciable size have hitherto been fairly rare. Among the advantages of the method are:

1. One need not enter the posterior fossa, which avoids the risk of damage to the cerebellum or brain stem.
2. The function of the facial nerve can usually be preserved.

The method has, however, drawbacks:

1. Limited field of exposure.
2. Interposition of the tumour between the posterior fossa vessels and the surgical field.
3. Difficulty of stopping bleeding in the medial part of the internal meatus.

The translabyrinthine method is used for a medium-sized tumour, which does not produce a rise in intracranial pressure. Even if operation is started by a translabyrinthine approach, the intervention nevertheless finally becomes purely intracranial. This is because one must, to provide access to the tumour, open the dura towards the posterior fossa, from the sigmoid sinus to the internal meatus. This small operative opening has the following advantages:

1. The cerebellum need not be retracted.
2. The function of the facial nerve can generally be saved.

This approach has, however, great drawbacks:

1. Limited field of action.
2. Total hearing loss before the tumour is visualized.
3. Increased risk of cerebrospinal fluid otorrhoea.
4. Great difficulty in dissecting the tumour capsule from the brain stem.

5. Major bleeding is difficult to control.

6. In about 40% of the tumours, only subtotal removal can be done.

The fact that the 5-year survival rate with complete removal of the tumour is twice that with subtotal removal makes neurosurgeons unwilling to accept the latter as a definite procedure, even if repeated removal can be carried out.

Consequently, in order to achieve the best results, and those safest for the patient, it seems most suitable for neurosurgeons and otologists to collaborate, using an operative method which both increases the possibility of total removal under reliable conditions, and permits the function of the facial nerve to be preserved. We have therefore, since 1964, used a method previously suggested by Dandy (1945) and Poppen (1960), i.e., a transmeatal posterior fossa approach. This technique has also been described by Rand and Kurze (1965) and Pool (1966). When the tumour has been exposed, the cerebellar hemisphere should be held in place by a self-retaining retractor, since a retractor held by an assistant may inadvertently shift and injure the cerebellum or the brain stem. The otologist then uses a dental drill to remove the posterior lip of the internal meatus as far as its bottom. The intracanalicular part of the tumour is removed, after which the facial and cochlear nerves can be traced in the central direction towards the tumour. It is easier to free the nerve from the tumour from this side than if it is sought on the brain stem side of the tumour, continuing in the peripheral direction. One of the drawbacks of the method is:

1. Cerebellar traction is necessary.

The advantages are, however, all the more numerous:

1. It is unnecessary to open the labyrinth, with its risk of meningitis from the middle ear.

2. No risk of postoperative cerebrospinal fluid otorrhoea.

3. Wide field of operation.

4. Direct visualization of the great vessels, and prompt control of bleeding.

5. Preservation of the facial nerve and total removal of tumour tissues in the internal meatus are possible.

The cochlear nerve can often be preserved as well. It is, however, our experience that even if one succeeds in doing this, it is hard to avoid damage to the internal auditory artery, which nourishes the tumour. This implies that the nutrition to the inner ear is lost and, concurrently with it, also the hearing.

Since only 5–10 tumours of the acoustic nerve are diagnosed annually at Karolinska Sjukhuset, it has not yet been possible to collect a large series. Total removal has been performed in altogether 12 cases. As a rule, the tumour was of the order of magnitude of 2–3 cm in diameter. In every case, the facial nerve was easy to identify in the internal auditory meatus. Nevertheless, in view of the localization of the tumour, we were unable to achieve adequate function postoperatively in four cases, even if the continuity of the nerve was preserved.

The neurosurgeon's dream is, naturally, to be able to operate on tumours that are confined to the internal meatus. Today, he has at his disposal two different approaches—the middle fossa approach and the transmeatal posterior fossa approach—both of which allow preservation of the function of the facial and cochlear nerves. The problem is to be able to diagnose the tumour already at its earliest stage. Our possibilities of establishing an early diagnosis have increased enormously in recent years. In fact, the only remaining difficulty is to get the patient to the physician as soon as possible.

References

Cushing, H., *Tumours of the nervus acusticus and the syndrome of the cerebellopontine angle,* W. B. Saunders Co., Philadelphia, Pa. (1917).

Dandy, W. E., *Surg. Gynec. Obstet., 41,* 129 (1925).

Dandy, W. E., *Surgery of the brain,* W. F. Prior Co., Inc., Hagerstown, Md., 671 (1945).

House, W. P., *Arch. Otolaryng.* (Chicago), *80,* 597 (1964).

Kurze, T., Unpublished data. Quoted from R. W. Rand and T. L. Kurze, 1965 (1958).

Olivecrona, H., *Läkartidningen, 65,* 1895 (1968).

Panse, R., *Arch. Ohrenheilk., 61,* 251 (1904).

Pool, J. L. & Pava, A. A., *The early diagnosis and treatment of acoustic nerve tumors,* Charles C. Thomas Publ., Springfield, Ill. (1957).

Pool, J. L., *J. Neurosurg., 24,* 483 (1966).

Poppen, J. L., *An atlas of neurosurgical techniques,* W. B. Saunders Co., Philadelphia, Pa. (1960).

Rand, R. W. & Kurze, T. L., *J. Neurol. Neurosurg. Psychiat., 28,* 311 (1965).

Exposure of the intra-petrous portion of the carotid artery

By Michael E. Glasscock, III

Otologic Medical Group, Los Angeles, California, U.S.A.

The intra-petrous portion of the carotid artery has to date been inaccessible to the neuro-vascular surgeon. This paper describes a technique for exposing the carotid artery within the temporal bone.

James T. Robertson, M.D. (Neurosurgeon, Memphis, Tennessee), was very instrumental in helping to develop this procedure. Our interest in this problem was stimulated by William F. House, M.D., who first mentioned the availability of the carotid artery through the middle fossa to us in 1965. Doctor Robertson and I did a number of cadaver dissections to work out the details of the technique for exposing the intra-petrous portion of the carotid.

Technique

The basic approach is that of the middle fossa route to the trigeminal ganglion. Refinements have been instituted in the form of the Zeiss operating microscope, House irrigation suction and the Jordan-Day otologic drill. The microscope provides excellent illumination and enough magnification to enable the surgeon to work in the confined space available to him.

The diamond burr of the otologic drill cuts the hard bone of the petrous apex but pushes the soft tissue of the vessel wall away without injury. The heat generated by the diamond stone is dissipated by the irrigation suction as it cleans the bone dust and blood from the wound. The diamond burr will become clogged with bone dust and cease to cut bone unless it is kept clear with the irrigation suction. This constant irrigation suction is essential when the patient is operated on in the supine position. Using these instruments, enough exposure is obtained to control backflow, incise the artery to remove clots or plaques and to suture the wall together. This entire procedure can be accomplished without destroying the function of the ear.

Routine prep and drape

The circulating nurse performs the standard half-head shave and prep on the involved side. Self-adhering plastic drapes are placed over the remaining hair. Once the patient is on the operating table the circulating nurse preps the skin, auricle and the plastic drape with zephiran chloride for ten minutes.

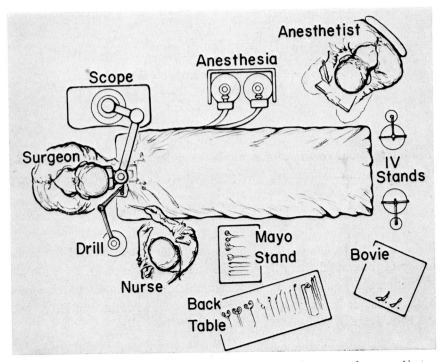

Fig. 1. The room arrangement has been designed to make maximum use of space and instrumentation.

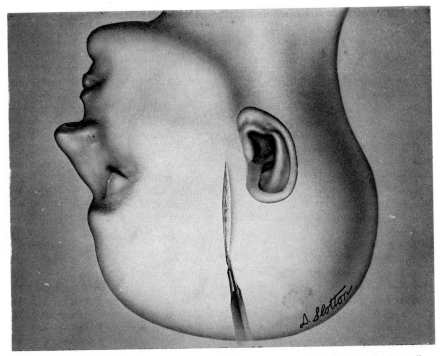

Fig. 2. The incision is basically that used for the classical approach to the trigeminal ganglion.

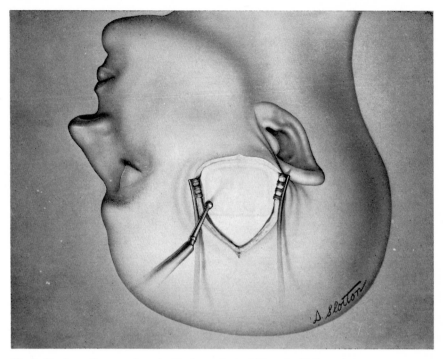

Fig. 3. The bone flap may be cut with the otologic drill or the Hall craniotome.

Room arrangement (Fig. 1)

The patient is supine with the surgeon seated at the head of the operating table.

Incision

A routine middle fossa craniotomy incision is made in the skin one finger's breadth anterior to the tragus of the ear (Fig. 2).

Craniotomy

The craniotomy will consist of a free-bone-flap being removed from the squamous portion of the temporal bone. This is a rectangular area approximately two-thirds in front of and one-third behind the external auditory canal (Fig. 3). The upper extent of the rectangle is at the level of the squamo-parietal suture line. It is important to keep the lines of the rectangle parallel to each other. The incision in the bone can be made with a cutting burr and irrigation suction or with the Hall craniotome. The Hall apparatus is by far the more rapid method. One must be very careful, however, to avoid a tear in the dura when using this instrument. Once all the edges of the bone flap have been clearly cut, it is removed revealing the underlying dura

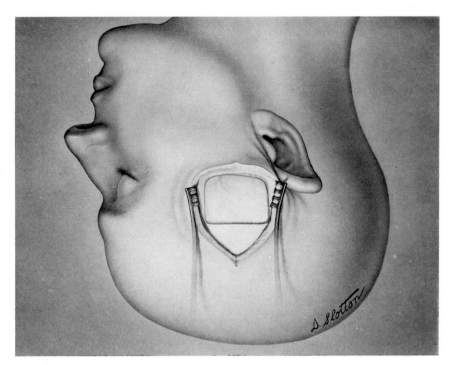

Fig. 4. Note the branch of the middle meningeal artery coursing through the dura.

(Fig. 4). The bone is then wrapped in a 4 × 4 sponge, soaked in saline and put aside until the end of the procedure.

Elevating the dura

Using the small House annulus elevator "gimmick" the dura is dissected away from the floor of the middle fossa. Once the dissection has been started the House-Urban self-retaining temporal lobe retractor is inserted between the edges of the craniotomy (Fig. 5). The blade of the retractor is placed into the wound and against the dura.

The first landmark is the middle meningeal artery as it enters the skull through the foramen spinosum. There is usually bleeding from the venous plexus that surrounds this artery. Once the artery has been isolated it is cauterized with the Bovie, ligated and the foramen spinosum is packed with cotton pledgets impregnated with bone wax.

The middle meningeal artery is the anterior limit of the dissection. Next the retractor blade is withdrawn slightly and attention is directed posteriorly where the second landmark is the arcuate eminence.

The dura is carefully elevated over the dome of the arcuate eminence and the blade of the retractor is advanced so that it fits over the lip of bone that corresponds to the superior petrosal sinus. The dura is then dissected free of

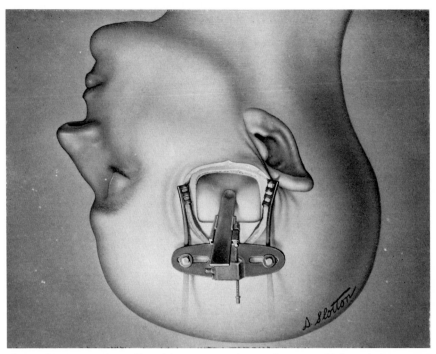

Fig. 5. The House-Urban self-retaining retractor elevates the temporal lobe and gives a good view of the floor of the middle fossa.

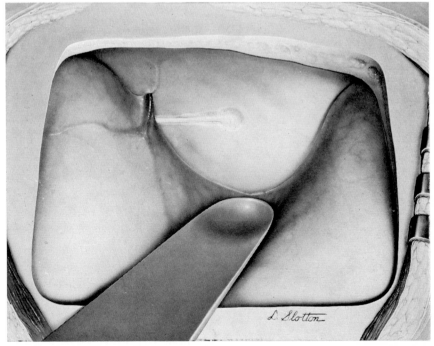

Fig. 6. A diamond burr has been used to expose the greater superficial petrosal nerve from the facial hiatus posteriorly to the geniculate ganglion.

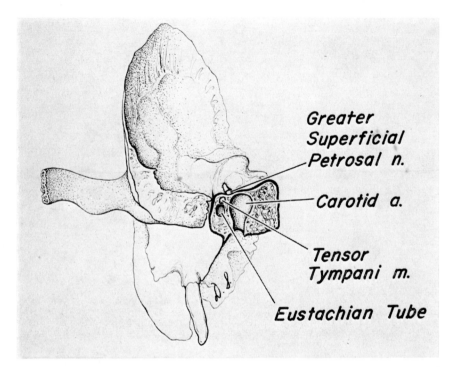

Fig. 7. Vertical cross section, right temporal bone, viewed from in front. Note relationship of carotid canal to greater superficial petrosal nerve, tensor tympani muscle, and eustachian tube.

the floor between the arcuate eminence and the middle meningeal artery. This step is very carefully performed because if the bony covering of the geniculate ganglion is dehiscent (fifteen percent) the ganglion may be injured. By approaching it from behind and stripping the dura away anteriorly, it is possible to find the third major landmark (the greater superficial petrosal nerve) without injury to the ganglion. Once the nerve has been located the retractor blade is moved slightly anteriorly so that it lies almost in line with the geniculate ganglion.

Exposure of the carotid artery

The greater superficial petrosal nerve is the landmark by which the geniculate ganglion and the facial nerve are identified (Fig. 6). The nerve is followed posteriorly to the geniculate by removing the bone with a diamond burr. Continuous irrigation suction protects the nerve from the heat of the diamond stone. Once the geniculate ganglion and facial nerve have been identified, the greater superficial petrosal nerve is severed just as it exits from the geniculate. The nerve is cut distally just before it passes under the trigeminal ganglion.

After the carotid is partially exposed in the floor of the middle fossa and when the greater superficial petrosal nerve is removed it can be seen to pulsate. The diamond stone is used to remove the bone from around the

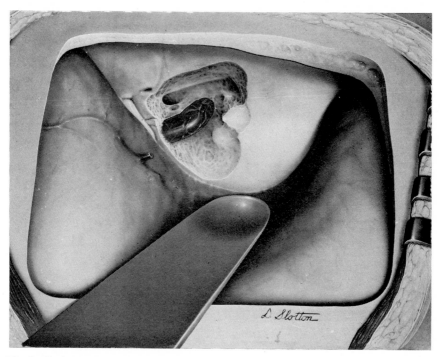

Fig. 8. The intrapetrous portion of the carotid artery has been widely exposed. Note the eustachian tube laterally and the cut ends of the greater superficial petrosal nerve.

artery. The most lateral dissection is performed first. This entails removing the belly of the tensor tympani muscle and the bony eustachian tube, both of which lie directly lateral to the carotid canal (Fig. 7). The inner table of the squamous portion of the temporal bone is removed next in order to obtain as much lateral exposure as possible. This lateral dissection is carried anteriorly to the cartilaginous portion of the eustachian tube and posteriorly to the middle ear. The medial dissection consists of removing the bone lying between the carotid artery, cochlea and internal auditory canal. When all the bone has been dissected free of the carotid artery it can be easily manipulated (Fig. 8). It is then possible to place a tie around the vessel or to open it to remove artheromatous plaques or propagating clots. If the artery is to be opened in the petrous segment, a second surgeon should have the carotid isolated in the neck with a clamp on the artery. It is possible to pass a probe directly through the artery into the neck from above. There is adequate exposure to suture the artery and to tie ligations.

Closure of the operative site entails removal of the Urban retractor blade allowing the temporal lobe to expand. The bone flap that was removed at the beginning of the procedure is replaced in its original position. The galea and skin are then closed in layers. A large absorbent bandage is applied.

Case report

(Surgeons—William F. House, Michael E. Glasscock, III, and William E. Hitselberger.) This 47-year-old housewife presented with a chief complaint of pulsating sound in her left ear for approximately thirty years. There had been intermittent bleeding and drainage from this left ear for several months, associated with headache and ear pain. The left ear contained a bulging red mass in the middle ear space that was pulsatile and extending into the external auditory canal. There was a total sensorineural hearing loss in the left ear. A paralysis of IX, X, XI, and XII was present. Polytome x-rays revealed a destructive lesion of the left jugulare bulb involving the carotid canal and the occipital bone to the foramen magnum and base of the clivis. A retrograde venogram indicated a complete block of the left jugular bulb. Bilateral carotid arteriograms showed that there was a great deal of crossed blood supply to the tumor. It was decided to ligate the carotid in the temporal bone simultaneously with the ligation in the neck to prevent the tumor from siphoning blood from the brain. On the polytome x-rays the carotid canal was obviously invaded by tumor so a total temporal bone resection was decided upon.

The first procedure consisted of a middle fossa exposure of the carotid artery within the temporal bone as described in the section on "Technique". Three ligatures were placed on the intrapetrous portion of the carotid artery just proximal to its exit into the cavernous sinus. At the same time a second surgeon was exposing the carotid artery in the neck. After the distal ligation in the temporal bone had been accomplished, the common and external carotids were ligated. The wound was then closed and the patient returned to the intensive care unit. She was closely observed for three days. On the fourth postoperative day she had not experienced hemiplegia and thus was returned to surgery where she had a subsequent total removal of her tumor. The carotid artery was severed and removed with the temporal bone. The facial nerve was sacrificed during surgery but IX, X, XI, and XII were spared. Her postoperative course was uneventful and she made a good recovery.

Discussion

We have used the exposure thus far only to ligate the artery or to remove the temporal bone from around it. At the present time indications for this operation are not clear-cut.

We have considered many possibilities; for instance, could this procedure be used to perform endarterectomies on the carotid artery within the temporal bone?

Artheromatous plaques are rare in the intrapetrous portion of the carotid but when present they are not readily controlled with current surgical techniques. The same holds true for propagating clots extending into this portion of the carotid from below. We certainly feel that endarterectomy is feasible, however, this has not been performed in a patient at the time of this writing.

Another possibility that comes to mind is to use a bypass graft to the carotid so that it could be sacrificed for carcinoma of the temporal bone. The five-year cure rate for carcinoma of the middle ear is very low. One reason for this is that the anterior wall of the middle ear is the carotid canal. This does not allow for adequate tumor margin, in many cases even with a total resection of the temporal bone. By being able to remove the carotid artery and the carotid canal in these cases, a much better cure rate should be possible.

As we learn more about the technical problems of the approach and of dealing with the artery in this area, the indications will undoubtedly expand.

Summary

A surgical procedure for the exposure of the carotid artery within the temporal bone has been presented. Endarterectomy, ligation and the possibility of bypass grafts have been discussed as indications for this approach. The surgical technique has been explained in detail.

General discussion

Ketcham to Lundberg

Did I understand correctly that when you reanastomose the transected facial nerve, or when you use a nerve graft to bridge an operative defect of the facial nerve, that functional results were poor? This is not the general experience when postoperative infection can be avoided, although it may take months for the resutured nerve to regenerate, and up to 8 to 12 months for the grafted nerve to function. Incidentally, nerve repair should be considered a semi-emergency procedure, as the successful regeneration is directly related to the interval between transection and repair.

Secondly, I failed to understand your recommendations concerning incomplete tumour removal. Are you suggesting that your results were satisfactory in spite of partial or subtotal tumour removal?

Lundberg to Ketcham

As I said in my lecture, hypoglosso-facial anastomosis was performed in 24 cases and accessory-facial in one. I prefer the former procedure, because I think the functional results are better and, not least, because of the painful hanging shoulder that is not seldom seen after severing the spinal accessory nerve. I cannot present the results of hypoglosso-facial anastomosis in figures, because I have not reviewed the cases in detail. There are some excellent results, a few failures and in the majority the results are fairly good.

By subtotal removal I mean radical extirpation, where a small fragment of tumour capsule firmly attached to the pons or the facial nerve is left behind, in order to save these structures from injury. (This definition differs from what other authors, e.g. Pool, mean by subtotal removal.) One question I tried to answer in my study was whether subtotal removal, in this sense, would be compromised by a high rate of recurrence. Since this does not seem to be the case, I think that subtotal removal is an eligible choice in selected cases, especially in elderly patients.

Ketcham to Fisch

My sincere compliments for a very comprehensive anatomical study presented in a most illustrative manner.

Wedenberg to Fisch and Fluur

Mr. Anderson spoke today about early audiologic diagnosis with help of the intra-aural reflexes. Instead of yesterday having this so-called "battery of audiologic tests" with a reliability of only about 50%, we today have presented one audiologic test with a remarkable sensitivity in the early diagnosis of acoustic neuromas.

My question: Using this sensitive test and our knowledge of the anatomy of the internal auditory artery, can it in the future be possible in early operation to protect the internal auditory artery, and in this way preserve the hearing? We heard from Drs. House and Hitselberger that this had been possible in a few cases.

In the case demonstrated by Dr. Fluur, he said that the hearing disappeared on the 3rd day. Do you not agree that if the internal auditory artery had been cut, the hearing loss would have occurred momentarily?

Fisch to Fluur

Beside the intracranial and the translabyrinthine operation, there is another way to explore the internal auditory meatus, and this is the approach through the middle cranial fossa. This transtemporal, extralabyrinthine approach allows inspecting the content of the internal meatus without taking any risk. We have performed this approach to date in 70 cases without a single complication. As shown in this short movie, the nerves lying in the meatus may be inspected without bleeding (the arteries present in the meatus are less than 200 microns in diameter). The nervous structures may be manipulated (in this case the vestibular ganglion) without producing a loss of hearing. The great advantage of the middle cranial fossa approach is to work mainly in the extradural space and to stay away from the arteria cerebelli anterior inferior, avoiding life-dangerous lesions of this vessel or of its main branches.

Lundberg to Fluur

I do not agree with Dr. House that the use of a dental drill intradurally means an increased risk of accidental damage to the nervous structures in the operative field, and I think that this opinion is supported by my results. As I mentioned in my paper, I have used the same procedure as Dr. Fluur since 1951 in altogether 53 cases, and I have not encountered any of the complications mentioned by Dr. House. I also wish to point out that unroofing of the porus has been used routinely by several neurosurgeons for many years. As far as I know, the procedure was first described by Dandy in 1925. Whether a drill or a chisel or a punch is used, it is an easy and safe procedure. I cannot see any reason for going through the temporal bone to expose the intrameatal portion of a neuroma.

Fluur to Wedenberg

I never said that we have cut the labyrinthine artery. If this had happened, the hearing would have disappeared momentarily, but the patient I have described had hearing for 3 days, and another explanation must be given. One explanation is bleeding through the lamina cribrosa into the internal ear, and clotting of the blood.

Fluur to Fisch

Dr. Fisch says that it is very easy to see the vessels in the internal meatus through the middle fossa approach. I would say that it naturally depends on the size of the tumour if you can see the vessels or not. The tumour is obtruding the canal, and therefore we can see a lot of oedema in the internal part of it. The possibility of seeing the vessels is naturally also depending on the amount of bleeding which blurs the view.

Fluur to House

To Dr. House I will say that during these 4 years that we have used this approach, we have found 2 cases of cysts. If we had used the translabyrinthine approach, we would have destroyed the whole internal ear, without finding any tumour at the end of the operation.

Portmann to Glasscock

I was very much impressed by the movie presented by Dr. Glasscock. If I understood his presentation, this patient had a big glomus jugulare tumour. I am not sure that it was so necessary to do a ligature of the carotid artery as a first stage of operation. Do you think it would not be better to perform directly the temporal bone resection and avoid this kind of injury?

Glasscock to Portmann

The glomus jugulare tumour was very extensive and had invaded the carotid canal. It was necessary to remove the entire temporal bone in order to remove the tumour. A preoperative carotid angiogram showed massive collateral circulation from the other side of the brain. We felt that it would be feasible to ligate the internal carotid without causing a hemiparalysis. The patient did tolerate this ligation and we were able to completely remove the tumour.

Chairman's summary of session II

G. Norlén

Mr. President, Ladies and Gentlemen. As Professor Olivecrona stated this morning, surgical treatment of the acoustic neuroma has been a hard problem for the neurosurgeon in the past, presenting with a high mortality and morbidity, especially with respect to the postoperative facial palsy. The tendency among the leading neurosurgeons today is radical removal, with saving the facial nerve if possible. Although the latter, as well as the operative mortality, are no doubt dependent mostly on the size of the tumour, I will also call attention to the age and sex of the patient in evaluating the prognosis of a surgical attack. Nowadays, neurosurgeons in different countries have presented series even of large tumours with an extremely low operative mortality and morbidity. I can mention a paper by Drs. Hullay and Tomits of Debrecen, Hungary, with a series of 50 radical removals with only one operative death and one late death, saving the facial nerve in 32 cases, with good or fair function in 80% of these cases. Unfortunately, the relation to the size of the tumour is not mentioned, but no doubt a large number of these lesions were large tumours. Dr. Drake, London, Canada, recently reported a series of 31 cases of total removal with four deaths, the facial nerve being saved in 16 cases. In six more cases, the nerve could be resutured in the posterior fossa, with four good results, and transplantation in four more cases with three good results. This means good functional recovery of facial nerve function in 63%. In his series, only two cases were considered as small tumours. Already in 1954, McKissock pointed out that small tumours could be removed safely with preserved facial function.

The House group in Los Angeles, U.S.A., has presented their translabyrinthine approach—so beautifully demonstrated here today—and no doubt the small and middle-sized tumours can be removed in this way with a low mortality, sparing the facial nerve. In the large tumours, House and Hitselberger had to rely on subtotal removal in a comparatively large per cent, but they consider it justified to reoperate later if necessary. This group has also demonstrated that earlier diagnosis of small acoustic neuromas is possible, and I think that we this morning had a good exposé of the otological and neuroradiological diagnostic possibilities.

Already Dandy removed the posterior lip of the internal auditory meatus, and even if he could see the facial nerve at this point, he did not save it. This technique has been used by us and Lundberg in order to remove the part of the tumour growing into the meatus, and from this point the nerve can easily be identified and followed to the brain stem. The difficulty with the facial nerve is not at the meatus, but at the tumour capsule closer to the brain stem. Just at the brain stem, it can be more clearly seen again. This technique has also been used by Dr. Kurze and Dr. Rand in Los Angeles, utilizing a microscope, and Dr. Fluur has today demonstrated his technique of this approach. As Olivecrona mentioned this morning, the operative deaths depend mainly on damage of the circulation to the pons.

As a neurosurgeon, it seems to me as if the translabyrinthine approach in the middle-sized and large tumours does not give a good view of the relation of the tumour to the brain stem and to the different structures in the cere-bello-pontine angle. The usual suboccipital approach will no doubt give a better view.

Is acoustic tumour an otologic disease or a neurosurgical disease? Well, the large tumours will always be a neurosurgical problem, the small and middle-sized tumours can be removed by the translabyrinthine route with excellent results, as Dr. House and his group have so nicely shown. However, the middle-sized tumour does not present a difficult problem to the experienced neurosurgeon, and this lesion can be removed by the usual suboccipital approach with a minimum of mortality and morbidity. I think that we need each other, the otologist, the neurosurgeon and the neuroradiologist, in order to improve the diagnostic methods, and I think that it has been shown today that improvement of the surgical results depends on earlier diagnosis. I think that we should give credit to Dr. House and his group, whose work has stimulated interest in earlier diagnosis, and contributed to improved surgical technique. Furthermore, the close working together of neurosurgeons and otologists will be of continuing advantage to the patient.

Considering the situation in Sweden, we will soon have 7 neurosurgical centres with about 20 so-called fully trained neurosurgeons. It seems to me rather unsatisfactory to scatter the sparse number of acoustic neuromas we have to deal with—amounting to about 35–40 per year—among 20 neuro-surgeons. It would be more absurd to disperse the material among the operat-ing otologists, of whom there might be 10 times as many as neurosurgeons.

The acoustic neuromas simply have to be concentrated to one or two centres, perhaps three. Otherwise there will be a conspicuous decline in the operative results.

In my opinion, the principal mission of the otologist is to improve his specialized diagnostic methods, in order to achieve early diagnosis when the lesion is still small or middle-sized. At this stage, the tumour can be removed by the translabyrinthine approach, and by the suboccipital route. The trans-labyrinthine approach has not improved the results compared with the results of the suboccipital approach as performed by the neurosurgeons today. For the large tumours, the conventional neurosurgical technique is also the most adequate, as demonstrated by Lundberg's results, but can undoubtedly be developed to further perfection by using operating microscopes, improved illumination and similar devices.

PITUITARY FUNCTION AND PITUITARY SURGERY

The anatomy of the pituitary gland

By Jan Wersäll

Department of Otolaryngology, Karolinska Sjukhuset, Stockholm, Sweden

General shape and embryological development

The pituitary gland in man is located in a deep recess in the sphenoid bone, the sella turcica. The gland is ovoid in shape, with a stalk which connects the gland with the hypothalamic region of the brain. The dura mater dips down to line the sella and thus envelops the pituitary gland as a tough capsule. A shelf of dura mater, the diaphragma sellae, extends over most of the top of the gland closely adapted to the sides of the pituitary stalk.

The gland measures about 1.5 cm in the transverse plane and about 1 cm in the sagittal plane, and is from 0.5 to 0.75 cm or more thick. It is naturally divided anatomically into three portions; the *pars anterior* (Fig. 1) which forms the main body of the gland, the thin extension upwards along the stalk from the pars anterior named the *pars tuberalis,* and the posterior part, the *pars nervosa*. The pars intermedius which is found to be fairly well developed in some animals is rudimentary in man. The pars anterior and tuberalis develop embryologically from a pouch-shaped protrusion from the roof of the oral fossa, the pouch of Rathke, which detaches from the ectoderm and forms a typical endocrine richly vascularized gland. The posterior part, the pars nervosa, is formed from a downward projection of epithelium of the neural tube, and retains its character of body of neuronal tissue.

Blood supply

Two main groups of vessels, the *superior* and *inferior hypophyseal arteries,* supply the gland. The *superior arteries* take their origin in the circle of Willis. The anterior group of these vessels enters the hypophyseal stalk in the anterior part of the upper end of the pars tuberalis. During their course downward through the stalk, these vessels send off branches, each of which ends in a cluster of tortuous capillaries. Similar branches and capillary clusters are formed by the posterior group of hypophyseal arteries. A large number of larger venous capillaries from the capillary arterial clusters fuse to form thicker veins in the hypophyseal stalk, and pass downward into the anterior lobe of the pituitary, where they empty into sinusoid canals formed between the cell cords of the pars anterior.

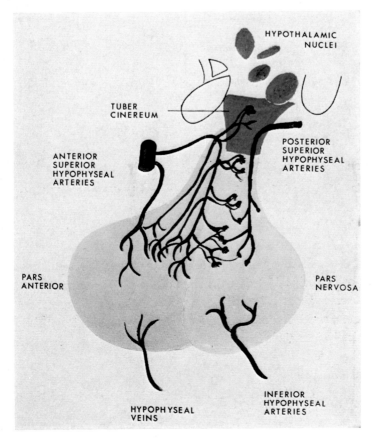

Fig. 1. Schematic drawing of the anatomy of the pituitary gland.

The blood supply to the pituitary through the superior hypophyseal arteries thus forms the blood supply for a portal venous system connecting the median eminence and the upper part of the hypophyseal stalk with the anterior lobe of the pituitary.

The pituitary gland is also supplied by arterial blood through two *inferior hypophyseal* arteries, which leave the inferior carotid arteries close to the posterior part of the cavernous sinus. Each inferior hypophyseal artery runs medially, and enters the capsule of the pituitary in its inferolateral aspect. Giving off numerous branches to the posterior lobe of the pituitary, the main branch passes forward, deeply penetrating the lateral part of the capsule from where arterioles penetrate the pars anterior, giving off an arterial supply even to this part of the gland. Communicating branches have been described to the superior portal system. It seems likely, however, that this is a not too important function of the inferior arteries, whose important function is to serve as the main source of arterial supply for the pituitary.

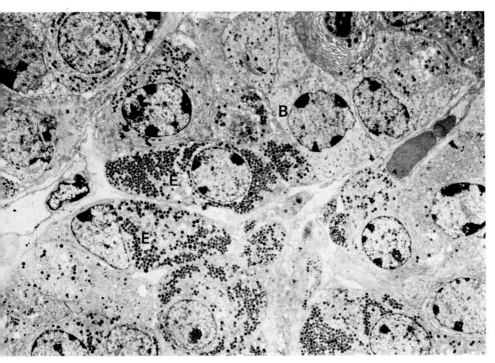

Fig. 2. Electron-micrographic survey of a section through the pituitary gland of a guinea-pig. E: Eosinophilic cell; B: Basophilic cell.

Microscopic structure of the anterior lobe of the pituitary

The cells of the anterior lobe of the pituitary form irregular branching cords supported by a framework of loose reticular fibers. The cords are separated by wide capillary spaces, supported by a somewhat more substantial layer of connective tissue. The capillary spaces are wider than ordinary capillaries, and lined by reticuloendothelial cells and are thus sinusoids rather than capillaries.

Staining of fixed specimens reveals a variation in the staining of various cells. Traditionally, the cells have been divided into chromophil cells which are fairly easily stained by ordinary staining methods, and chromophobes which "dislike" stain. The non-stained cells form clusters in the central part of the cell cords, whereas the most stained cells occupy the periphery of the cords.

Around 75 % of the cells stain intensely with acid stains, and are accordingly called acidophilic, whereas the remaining 25 % have a more or less basophilic cytoplasm.

The basophils tend to be more numerous toward the periphery of the gland.

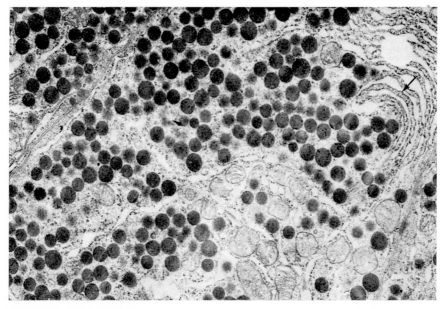

Fig. 3. Basophilic substance (arrow) and eosinophilic granules in an eosinophilic cell of the guinea-pig pituitary gland.

Extensive studies with different stains and hormone experiments have revealed the existence of various subtypes of basophil cells which have been related to the product of different hormones. The only clear relation between cell types and hormone production which seems to be valid for all animals studied is that the acidophil cells are related to growth hormone, whereas the majority of other hormones are related to basophil cells.

Electron-microscopic studies of the fine structure of the pituitary cells have revealed that the densely granulated acidophil cells contain granules of fairly constant size of around 3,000 Å to 3,500 Å (Figs. 2, 3), whereas some few acidophils have a larger variety of granules around 6,000 Å to 9,000 Å in diameter. The basophils have fewer granules which are around 1,000 Å in diameter (Fig. 2).

A combination of light and electron microscopy has shown that there is a large number of intermediate stages between nongranulated chromophobe cells and acidophil or basophil cells with varying degree of granulation. The basophilia of the cells depends to a great extent on the ribosome content of the cells, which in turn, is related to the activity of the cells. Thus cells might be highly basophilic with few granules of either the acidophil or baso-phil cell type or might contain little ribosomes or ergastoplasm and be filled with granules of either type.

Much work thus has to be done before we can identify a cell which produces a specific type of hormone, or can be characterized as to its physiological state.

Pars nervosa

The posterior part of the hypophysis is in intimate connection with the hypothalamic region of the brain. The core of the neurohypophysis contains the unmyelinated nerve fibres of the hypothalamo-hypophyseal tract, extending from cell bodies of the supraoptic and paraventricular nuclei of the hypothalamus. The nerve fibres are surrounded by glial cells, the so-called pituicytes. The nerve fibres form multiple nerve endings on the capillaries, which comprise a fairly dense network in the neurohypophysis. Of special interest are the neurosecretory granules which are formed in the cells of the supraoptic and paraventricular nuclei of the hypothalamus, transported along the nerve fibres, and stored in the nerve terminals. It is inferred from multiple experiments on the transport of secretion that the hormones of the posterior lobe are present in the neurosecretory granules, possibly bound to some carrier protein.

Roentgenological anatomy of the sphenoidal sinuses

By Gunnar Hammer

Department of Otolaryngology, Västra Frölunda Medical Centre,
Västra Frölunda, Sweden

and Claes Rådberg

Department of X-ray Diagnosis, Regionsjukhuset, Linköping, Sweden

The sphenoidal sinuses have been called the most variable bilateral cavities of the human body. Variations in their size will affect the boundaries of the pituitary gland, i.e., the anterior wall and floor of the sella turcica will possess a varying thickness and degree of protrusion into the sphenoidal sinuses. In planning and performing transsphenoidal pituitary surgery, the recognition of the individual topographic anatomy is of fundamental importance.

The body of the sphenoid develops from four symmetric nuclei. The various zones of fusion between the nuclei present a greater resistance to the pneumatization of the growing sinus than do the nuclei themselves. The bony septa found in the adult sinus are located at the sites of zones of fusion.

Embryologically and from a practical clinical standpoint, the sphenoidal sinuses are divided into three main types: a conchal, a presellar, and a sellar type (Fig. 1). The sellar type is by far the most common. Supernumerary sphenoidal sinuses are not seen.

Conchal type. The sphenoidal sinuses are very small and separated from the sella turcica by a cancellous bone wall approximately 10 mm thick (Fig. 2). This wall may, however, consist partly of sclerotic bone. The sphenoidal sinuses are situated well laterally, and are separated from each other by a thick bony septum.

Presellar type. In this type, the sella turcica is generally separated from the sphenoidal sinus by spongy bone, and the anterior wall of the sella turcica does not bulge into the sphenoidal sinuses (Fig. 3). The intersinusal septum generally runs in the sagittal plane, with no major deviations to either side. The pneumatization is not symmetrical, and one sphenoidal sinus is generally slightly larger than the other.

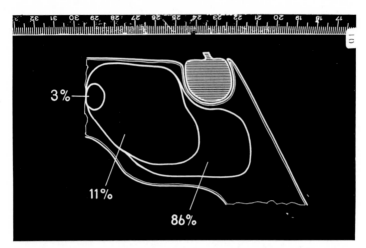

Fig. 1. Main types and frequencies of sphenoidal sinuses. Conchal type 3 %, presellar type 11 %, and sellar type 86 %.

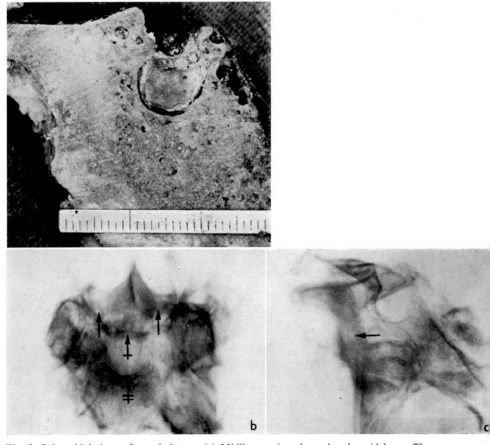

Fig. 2. Sphenoidal sinus of conchal type. (a) Midline section through sphenoid bone. The sphenoidal sinuses are situated lateral to this plane and are thus not seen in this section. (b) and (c) Axial and lateral roentgenograms of specimen. Sphenoidal sinuses (⇀), anterior wall of the sella turcica (↦), dorsum sellae (↦→).

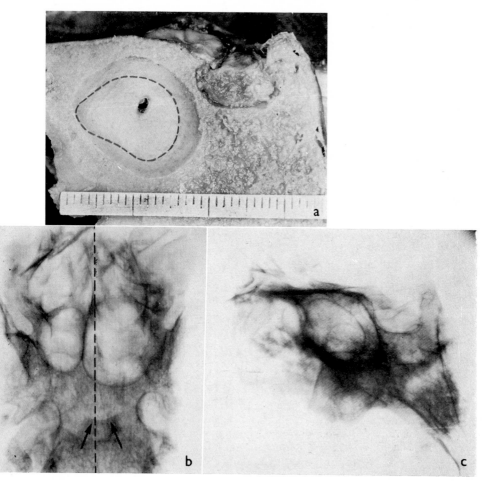

Fig. 3. Sphenoidal sinus of presellar type. (a) Midline section through sphenoid bone, right half as viewed laterally from inside. Right sphenoidal sinus marked by broken line. (b) Axial roentgenogram of specimen. Broken line indicates plane of section. Dorsum sellae (→). (c) Lateral roentgenogram of entire specimen. Anterior wall of sella turcica about three times as thick on the right side as on the left.

Sellar type. The anterior wall, and frequently the floor of the sella turcica, appear as a protrusion into the sphenoidal cells. As a rule, the anterior wall of the sella turcica is about 0.5 mm thick and does not contain spongy bone (Fig. 4). Cancellous bone is not infrequently found, however, in the floor. Both a presellar and a sellar type may be found in the same case.

Variations in the thickness of the anterior wall of surgical importance occur in the presellar type, as well as in cases with one sphenoidal sinus of presellar and the other of sellar type. The wall, as a rule, is thinnest on the sellar side (Fig. 5). It is usually possible, by comparing the appearance of the anterior wall in lateral and axial projections, to gain a fairly good idea

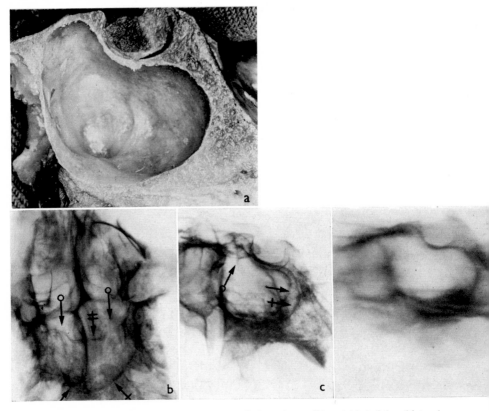

Fig. 4. Sphenoidal sinus of sellar type. (a) Right half of specimen. (b) and (c) Axial and lateral roentgenogram. Anterior wall of the sella (⊬→). Posterior wall of the spenoidal sinus on the left side (↦) and on the right (→). Carotid prominence (o→). (d) Tomogram through left sphenoidal sinus.

of the topography of the anterior wall, though tomography (preferably in a lateral projection) will provide more detailed information. Such an examination is usually necessary for correct estimation when the anterior wall is irregularly thickened, especially when it has a sloping course which prevents its demonstration in an axial projection, or when evaluation is complicated by the occurrence of septa having their attachments to the anterior wall, e.g. transverse and medial septa.

In addition to the intersinusal septum separating the two sphenoidal sinuses, others extending in different directions may be found. They may be classified as follows: transverse septum, medial septum, and lateral septa which are divided into frontal lateral and sagittal lateral (Fig. 6). The posterior part of the intersinusal septum often deviates more or less to the sides, and is accordingly often attached laterally to the anterior wall of the sella, or sometimes as far laterally as in the carotid prominence, i.e., in the most anterior portion of the carotid groove. This variant is found in 20%.

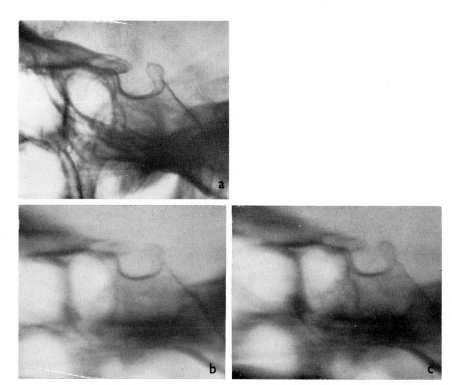

Fig. 5. Varying thickness of anterior wall of sella turcica. (a) Lateral roentgenogram. (b) and (c) Lateral tomograms through the right and left parts of sella. Right part of anterior wall is considerably thicker than the left part.

A transverse septum is generally confined to one sinus. The surgical approach should preferably be through the contralateral sinus, since this septum impedes orientation. The transverse septum or crest is of surgical significance in so far as it has its attachment in the anterior wall and causes local thickening (Fig. 7).

The other septa are of minor importance. However, a frontal lateral septum may confuse orientation during surgery.

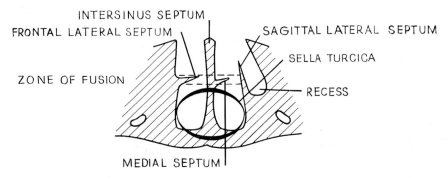

Fig. 6. Schematic representation of horizontal section through sphenoid bone, showing varying types of septa in the sphenoidal sinuses.

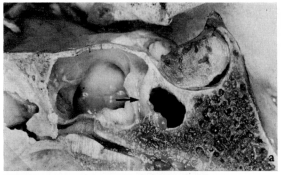
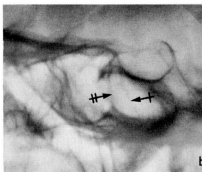

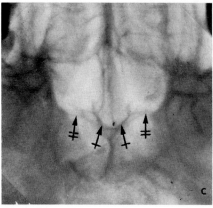

Fig. 7. Transverse septum. (a) A transverse septum (→) extends to the floor of the sphenoidal sinus from the upper part of the anterior wall of the sella. (b) and (c) The medial portion (↦) of the transverse septum is more curved than the lateral portion (⊬).

In some cases, the tuberculum sellae is situated relatively far below the roof of the sphenoidal sinus. On piercing the anterior wall of the sella turcica, an operator unaware of the true anatomy may easily go too high, and enter the intracranial cavity above the diaphragma sellae into the region of the cisterna chiasmatica and the optic chiasma (Fig. 8).

By X-ray examination, sometimes including tomography, all anatomic variants of the sphenoidal sinuses can be analyzed before surgery.

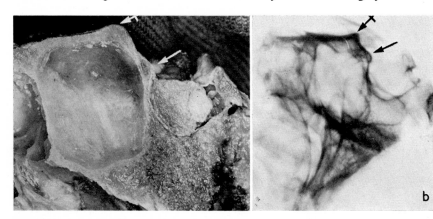

Fig. 8. (a) and (b) Tuberculum sellae (→) situated considerably below the roof of the sphenoidal sinuses. Sphenoidal limbus (↦).

Transsphenoidal hypophysectomy

By John Angell James

Litfield House, Clifton Down, Bristol, England

The situation of the hypophysis in the party wall between the cranial cavity and the upper respiratory passages has tantalized the interest of both neurosurgeons and rhinologists for many decades. Nature seems to have intended to protect this vital gland from any influence that could interfere with it by placing it in the centre of the skull and surrounding it with large vascular spaces to maintain a constant temperature and perfect metabolic conditions.

Following the early attempts to operate on hypophyseal tumours by the transsphenoidal route which brought to light the risks of the three major complications of cerebrospinal rhinorrhoea, meningitis and intractible haemorrhage the balance swung greatly in favour of the transcranial approach. The great impetus given to hypophyseal surgery following the introduction of Cortisone which opened the way to major hormone surgery and the application of the binocular microscope to rhinologic surgery has completely reversed this trend. The advantages and disadvantages of the two routes may be summarized as follows:

Advantages

Transcranial	*Transsphenoidal*
Route of access is aseptic.	Short, almost imperceptible scar.
The hypophyseal stalk and diaphragm are clearly visible and the stalk can be removed if desired.	Short operation with minimal shock and with haemorrhage easily controllable.
No cerebrospinal fluid rhinorrhoea.	Very slight postoperative discomfort and morbidity.
Suprasellar extension of tumour is freely accessible.	Direct view with binocular operating microscope.
	Suprasellar extensions of tumours are presented into the empty sella by intracranial pressure.
	Precise partial hypophysectomy is feasible leaving the stalk and the upper part of the gland intact.

Disadvantages

Transcranial	Transsphenoidal
Operation of considerable magnitude requiring an osteoplastic flap.	Nasal sepsis is an absolute contraindication.
Damage to ocular and olfactory nerves. Morbidity and mortality from shock oedema and haemorrhage.	C.S.F. leak and meningitis are now very rare.
It is impossible to see into the full depth of the sella.	Ocular and olfactory nerve damage is very rare.
Meticulous removal of all deep fragments of the gland cannot be controlled by observation under the operating microscope.	Lack of pneumatisation of the sphenoidal sinuses in 3% of patients greatly increases the difficulty of exact localisation of the gland and the avascular window in the dura enclosing the gland.

The transsphenoidal approach

There are four main routes of access to the hypophysis by the transsphenoidal approach:

1. Trans-ethmoidal (Chiari, 1912)
2. Trans-antral (Hamberger, 1961)
3. Osteoplastic nasal (Macbeth, 1961)
4. Transseptal (Cushing, 1912)
5. Transpalatal

Each of these routes has its own minor advantage or disadvantage compared with the others and any surgeon operating on the hypophysis should be prepared to adopt the route that best suits his skill and experience and the particular anatomy of the individual patient. The individual anatomical development of the sella, the sphenoidal bone, its air sinuses and the venous sinuses determines the relative ease or difficulty with which the transsphenoidal operation can be performed.

1. Trans-ethmoidal

The trans-ethmoidal approach is the shortest from the surface and if advantage is taken of the nasal fossae for the passage of the instruments an unrestricted view is obtained of the anterior wall and cavities of the sphenoidal sinuses and finally into the sella for the removal of the gland.

If the nasal septum is deviated this should be resected but need only add a few minutes to the length of the operation and in practice this procedure is not often required.

2. Trans-antral and transpalatal

The trans-antral and transpalatal routes have the advantage of exposing a slightly more upward view into the sella and thus the diaphragm and any suprasellar extension of a tumour is more easily visualised. However they have the disadvantage of an incision in the mouth which cannot be rendered completely aseptic and it is more difficult to obtain the full advantage of the binocular operating microscope.

3. *Osteoplastic nasal*

The osteoplastic nasal route provides very good access and a clear indication of the midline but has the disadvantages of the magnitude of the wound and the instruments are used in the direct line of vision.

4. *Transseptal*

The transseptal route suffers from the disadvantages of longer distance and restricted field of vision.

Whichever of these routes is employed it is important that the operator should have wide experience of nasal and sinus surgery and of the use of the operating microscope if he is to exploit all the advantages of these approaches.

My own choice of route has been in practically every case the transethmosphenoidal combined with the transnasal or the transseptal.

The latest technique of performing this operation is as follows:

Access

A curved incision is made over the lateral aspect of the nose anterior to the lachrymal sac and internal tarsal ligament. The orbital periosteum is very carefully elevated carrying with it the trochlea of the superior oblique muscle, the attachment of the internal tarsal ligament and the lachrymal sac. The elevation is carried posteriorly to the anterior ethmoidal artery which is coagulated with diathermy. The ethmoidal labyrinth is then opened and the cell walls excised right up to the fovea ethmoidales and the cribriform plate. A window is cut in the posterior third of the nasal septum to show the anterior surface of the left sphenoidal sinus. The window is enlarged downwards to the floor of the nose. The anterior portion of the lamina papyracea of the ethmoid is excised only so far as is necessary to obtain an uninterrupted view of the anterior surfaces of the sphenoidal sinuses. The rostrum of the sphenoid is then removed with the anterior walls of both sphenoidal sinuses. The mucous membrane is stripped down from the posterior surface of the sphenoidal sinus to expose the bony covering of the sella. The motor driven surgical drill is then employed to drill through the usually thin layer of bone covering the dura over the anterior surface of the hypophysis. The dura is freed from the posterior surface of the bone and the bony window enlarged as widely as possible until the margin of the cavernous sinuses laterally, the circular sinus above and the inferior intercavernous sinus below are exposed.

Exposure of gland

The surgical diathermy needle is now employed to make a cruciate incision. Since it is very difficult always to be certain of the exact distance to which the cavernous sinuses encroach on this window the needle is pressed firmly against the dura which is tented inwards and then the current switched on to burn through. This will seal any shallow extension of a cavernous sinus and avoid troublesome bleeding at the edge. A series of adjacent needle punctures are made in this way to complete a cruciate incision.

Dissection of gland

With special dissectors the gland is then dissected from its capsule laterally and then inferiorly and superiorly and finally the stalk is torn through.

Removal of gland

The gland is then seized with the gland forceps. These have been designed with special non-kick action so that there is a minimal rise of the jaws as the forceps are closed. Any small remnants of gland are then carefully removed with dissectors, curettes and forceps until the whole cavity is perfectly clear and the diaphragm can be seen bowing downwards.

Closure of dura

A circular patch of fascia lata cut from the lateral aspect of the thigh is then placed over the diaphragm to close the operculum. It is held in place with an angled dissector and the cavity of the sella beneath is packed tightly with muscle from the vastus externus until the patch is firmly held in place and the whole sella is tightly packed. If there is a good sheet of mucous membrane available from the posterior sinus wall this can be replaced to cover over the muscle directly but if this does not make a good seal an additional disc of fascia lata is then placed over the muscle and the opening in the bone and the mucous membrane returned over that.

The cavity of the sphenoidal sinus and part of the adjacent ethmoidal sinuses are then packed with absorbable gauze impregnated with sulphonamides and proflavine or antibiotics. The gauze is threaded with a nylon thread to facilitate removal which is performed on the 8th day after operation.

Table 1.

Total operations 394

Mammary carcinoma	338	Acromegaly	4
Mammary carcinoma, male	2	Chromophobe adenoma	4
Diabetic retinopathy	22	Granulosa cell tumour of the	
Prostatic carcinoma	14	ovary	1
Melanoma	7	Cushing's syndrome	1
		Ovarian carcinoma	1

Post-operative complications

51 Cerebrospinal leak (1 only in last year)
    5 were repacked with fascia and muscle and all ceased.
11 Meningitis
    5 fatal (4 in 1 month in an influenza epidemic in 1963)
 2 Ocular palsy
    (1 of these developed an arteriovenous aneurysm)

Post-operative mortality 7.6%

5 Cortisone crises	7 Hepatic metastases
1 Inhaled vomit	8 Pulmonary metastases
1 Coronary thrombosis	3 Cerebral metastases
1 Perforated gastric ulcer	1 Pericardial metastases
2 Intestinal haemorrhage	1 Hypofribrinogenaemia

Results

In 8 years I have performed 394 hypophysectomy operations. The majority have been performed for hormone ablation for advanced metastatic mammary cancer. The overall results of the total number is shown in the accompanying Table 1. Very significant developments have taken place in the technique employed during these years and as a result of the improved technique the results in the last 100 cases are of particular significance (Table 2).

Table 2.

Complications in last 100 cases

Cerebrospinal leak	1 (Duration 3 days)
Ocular palsy	0
Meningitis	0

Results in the last 100 cases

Directly attributable to the operation:
  1 Cortisone crisis   1%
Attributable to the disease:
  2 Pulmonary metastases
  2 Pulmonary embolism
  1 Intestinal metastases with   7%
    haemorrhage
  1 Abdominal perforation
  1 Hepatic metastases

Post-operative mortality —   Total 8%

The most important detail in technique that has completely altered the number of complications is the fascia muscle fascia sandwich method of sealing off the subarachnoid space. The remarkable efficiency of this technique may be illustrated by a particular patient who had a chromophobe adenoma of considerable size and who had been treated by partial transseptal removal and a heavy course of radiotherapy. She developed a cerebrospinal rhinorrhoea for which my neurosurgical colleagues operated closing the leak with compressed muscle. This was not successful and the patient developed meningitis which required intensive treatment with antibiotics. By the trans-ethmoidal approach we were able to see the leak, remove the tumour completely leaving a sizeable remnant of gland, and seal off the leak by the sandwich technique with complete success. The patient has had a perfect result and although she takes a small dose of Cortisone she is not entirely Cortisone dependent except under stress.

Surgery for diabetics

There is considerable difference of opinion as to the value of hypophysectomy for diabetic retinopathy.

In our series there have been some good and some disappointing results. Our criteria for selection of patients for this operation is summarized as follows:

1. There should be a predominantly haemorrhagic retinopathy which is obviously threatening vision.
2. That neither retinitis proliferans nor extensive retinal degeneration should effect both eyes severely.
3. That renal failure is absent.
4. That the patient is sufficiently intelligent to understand the implications of pituitary removal and to co-operate fully in taking replacement therapy.

A series of partial hypophysectomies for diabetic retinopathy has also been performed. The series is too small to be conclusive but some success was achieved and some hypophyseal function was retained. It seems that a total hypophysectomy is more likely to have the maximum beneficial effect on the retinopathy.

Because the rhinologic surgeon specialises in sinus and microsurgery he will in the future continue to have an important technical role in the team of specialists concerned with the management of the hypophysis.

References

Chiari, O., *Wien. Klin. Wschr., 25,* 5 (1912).

Cushing, H., *The pituitary body and its disorders,* Lippincott, Philadelphia (1912).

Hamberger, C.-A., Hammer, G., Norlén, G. & Sjögren, B., *Arch. Otolaryng.* (Chicago), *74,* 22 (1961).

Macbeth, R. G., *J. Laryng., 75,* 1 (1961).

Transsphenoidal approach to the pituitary—Movie

By Kurt Burian

Department of Otolaryngology, Filialstation der Universitätsklinik, Wien, Austria

Since the use of the surgical microscope and consequent improvement of microsurgical technique, the transsphenoidal approach to be base of the skull has become more frequent. The main indications are: tumours of the hypophysis, hypophysectomy for metastasizing cancer, for diabetic retinopathy and, finally to close cerebrospinal fistulas. Although the transsphenoidal approach becomes more frequent (better results due to better lighting and more subtle preparation), it should not rival the transcranial approach but complement it to improve results.

To judge between the usefulness of either technique, it is necessary to appreciate the individual limitations. The transsphenoidal approach is not suited for tumours which extend far above the sella. On the other hand, it is often not possible to remove the origin of a tumour within the sella with the necessary radicality by transcranial operation. The high rate of relapses after transcranial operations and the necessity of postoperative X-ray treatment confirm this. These facts lead to the conclusion that it is possible to improve the results with a combination of both methods. In co-operation with the neurosurgical clinic of the University of Vienna, we have utilized two-stage procedures for more than five years in suitable cases, and obtained much better results than before, in spite of the fact that no postoperative X-ray treament has been administered. The movie will elucidate the indications for the transsphenoidal and for the two-stage procedure. The transsphenoidal approach is mainly indicated for removal of purely endosellar tumours. Suprasellar tumours with a wide sella aperture can be approached either transcranially, transsphenoidally or, if necessary, in two sessions combined: transcranially and transsphenoidally.

In cases of suprasellar tumours with narrow sella aperture, the transcranial approach is preferred; should tumour removal be incomplete, a secondary transsphenoidal extirpation of intrasellar tumour residues is indicated. For tumours extending into the posterior region, a transsphenoidal tumour resection and decompression should precede the transcranial tumour extirpation.

Of 80 operations performed up to this day, 60 cases have been analyzed

Table 1.

Surgical approach	Number of cases	Rhinorrhea	Meningitis	Mortality	
				up to 2 weeks postop.	following 2nd postop. week
Primary transsphenoidal	40	1 case (3 weeks)	—	1 case: Meningeoma and malig. argentaffinoma	1 case: Endocrine derailment (5th postop. week)
				1 case: Brain-damage due to penicillin	
				1 case: Aspiration of mucus, endocrine imbalance	
Transsphenoidal following transcranial procedure	20	1 case (4 weeks)	1 case (4th week postop.)	1 case: Transsphenoidal decompression following transcranial procedure	—
Total	60	2	1	4	1

in the following tables. The follow-up covers periods of 6 months to more than 5 years. In 40 of these cases, the transsphenoidal technique was the primary and only method of operation; in the remaining 20 cases, a two-stage procedure or transsphenoidal reoperation was performed because of relapse after one or two transcranial operations.

The complications observed are shown in Table 1. Liquorrhoea, dreaded by the neurosurgeon, occurred only twice and stopped without surgical intervention. Meningitis developed in a patient in the fourth postoperative week, although there was no cerebrospinal fistula postoperatively. It quickly subsided on treatment with antibiotics.

Among the 60 cases, 4 deaths occurred during the first 2 postoperative weeks, but only two of them can, however, be counted as surgical fatalities. In one case there was brain damage due to penicillin; in this case the sella had been packed with muscle tissue soaked in penicillin. A severe epileptic state developed, in the course of which a haemorrhage into the tumour side occurred, causing the death of the patient. In the second case, of acromegaly combined with diabetes, a severe metabolic disturbance developed, with loss of consciousness and aspiration of mucous 12 hours after the operation.

Table 2.

Surgical approach	Postoperative observation (years)					
	$\frac{1}{2}$–1 yr.	1–2 yr.	2–3 yr.	3–4 yr.	4–6 yr.	Total
Primary trans-sphenoidal	7	6	5	3	3	24
Recurrences	–	—	–	–	–	—
Transsphenoidal following transcranial procedure	7	10	6	9	–	32
Recurrences	–	—	–	–	–	—

The two remaining deaths are not due to the transsphenoidal operation. In one case the preoperative diagnosis was insufficient. Besides the hypophyseal tumour, the patient also suffered from a malignant argentaffinoma with hepatic metastases and a meningeoma in the tentorial fissure; the operation was, therefore, not indicated.

In the second case, because of rapidly increasing cerebral pressure, we had to open the sella from below 24 hours after a transcranial operation. The decompression was, however, insufficient and the patient died several hours later.

A late fatality occurred during the fifth week after operation in a patient with acromegaly and diabetes. He did not follow instructions to undergo a blood-sugar level determination, and died in diabetic coma.

Table 2 shows the results. It should be noted that in the group where two-stage operations were performed, no relapses have occurred so far. This is despite the fact that in those cases relapses after the first transcranial operation occurred within a much shorter time than the period of observation that has passed since the transsphenoidal reoperation.

General discussion

Notter to Angell James

As far as I remember, observation on fishes are published which have shown certain relations of a third lobe between the adeno- and neurohypophysis and the melanophoric system. This may have been the theoretical reason for hypophysectomy in man. The results were, however, negative with the exception of a few cases reported with good response of the tumour or its metastases. We ourselves have not tried hypophysectomy in melanomas.

Palva to Angell James

I should like to ask Dr. Angell James how often he finds it necessary to use the X-ray apparatus as an aid in localization of the hypophysis, particularly in cases of a small sphenoid sinus and dense bone. Secondly, does he find it necessary to ligate or coagulate the anterior ethmoid artery often, while working through the ethmoid labyrinth?

Luft to Angell James and Burian

I would like to ask the two last speakers whether they have operated on non-tumourous pituitary glands. If so, have you tested pituitary function after the operation in order to find out whether there are any remnants of the pituitary? Also, have you made serial sectioning of the tissues of the sella after operation in patients who died at short or long intervals after the surgical intervention?

Furthermore, I would like to discuss the advantage of leaving normal pituitary tissue when removing tumourous one. The replacement therapy after complete removal of the pituitary is simple and standardized. Therefore, I think that it is advisable to remove all pituitary tissue in instances where you cannot be absolutely certain that you have not left any small parts of the tumour.

I have not discussed the possibility of combining removal of the pituitary with postoperative radiotherapy. This may be of great advantage in some instances.

C.-A. Hamberger to Angell James

During the first years, we had hypophysectomized patients together with general otolaryngeal cases, but nowadays we isolate these cases for about 10 days. We never have infectious complications.

Olivecrona to Angell James and Burian

Do you use a binocular microscope during the whole operation?

Angell James to Palva

In answer to Dr. Palva, I use X-ray localization in cases with conchal type pneumatization 3 % and in most of those with the presellar type 11 %. The anterior ethmoidal artery is always coagulated, as it reduces the bleeding in the nose.

Angell James to Luft

When using high magnification, it is possible to differentiate between tumour and normal gland tissue with certainty in the case of chromophobe tumours, and usually in the chromophil tumours. However, in case of any doubt, the whole gland is removed to ensure that there is no recurrence of the tumour.

Angell James to C.-A. Hamberger

The complete isolation of hypophysectomy patients has not been possible, owing to lack of facilities. This has made it more than ever important to ensure in every case that the dura is closed with fascia, as muscle alone is not an absolute barrier to the passage of bacteria from the nose in the post-operative period.

Angell James to Olivecrona

I use a head light and loupe for the earlier nasal stages of the operation, and transfer to the binocular microscope when the posterior wall of the sphenoidal sinus is drilled.

The wound is closed completely without drainage. The fascia patch is held in place with an absorbable gauze pack in the sphenoidal sinus, which will be partly softened, and can be painlessly removed in one week.

Escher to Burian

Did you have no complications, filling the empty sella with gelatin? After liquefication, gel-foam may be a nest for infection. According to the experience of Riskaer and Angell James, the whole packing with muscle and covering with fascia may be safer.

Burian to Escher

In our first 20 cases, we implanted only muscle tissue into the sella. Later on, we have seen that there is no difference in the postoperative course using spongostan or muscle tissue. The one case of meningitis we observed happened in a patient where muscle tissue was implanted. Therefore, we prefer spongostan in cases without cerebrospinal leakage.

Burian to Luft

I agree with Dr. Angell James that it is easily possible to differentiate between normal and pathological tissue. Therefore, we should try to save the normal gland tissue. Even if it is possible to replace hypophyseal function, I prefer to save a rest function if it is possible.

Burian to Olivecrona and C.-A. Hamberger

We use the head light till we open the sella. The preparation into the sella is done under the microscope. The film is photographed through the microscope, to demonstrate to the neurosurgeon that there is much better lighting and view with the help of the microscope.

Preoperative evaluation of pituitary function

By Rolf Luft

Department of Endocrinology, Karolinska Sjukhuset, Stockholm, Sweden

In the 1940's, before the cortisone era, the surgical endocrinology of the pituitary was a rather underdeveloped field. The laboratory procedures available for the diagnosis of endocrine insufficiencies were few and inaccurate. It was noticed by neurosurgeons and endocrinologists that patients with non-hormone producing tumours of the hypophysis, in general, could be divided into two groups: 1. those with normal appearance and normal secondary hair growth, and 2. those with pale dry skin, some increase in body weight and reduced or absent secondary hair growth. The appearance of the latter group was very characteristic, and it was termed "chromophobe", since most of the patients with this syndrome happened to have chromophobe adenomas of the hypophysis.

Not until the late 1940's was it established that the group of "chromophobe" patients had adrenocortical insufficiency in addition to hypogonadism and hypothyroidism, i.e., that they had panhypopituitarism. It then also became understandable why this group of subjects constituted such a poor surgical risk.

Today, the situation in the area of surgical endocrinology is completely different. Our diagnostic procedures are well established, and hormones are available for the replacement of most of those not produced in sufficient amounts.

The surgical endocrinology of the hypophysis deals with two main subjects:

A. preoperative evaluation of pituitary function, and
B. preoperative substitution therapy

Preoperative evaluation of pituitary function

The evaluation comprises direct tests of the secretion of pituitary hormones and procedures for evaluation of the functional status of peripheral endocrine glands. The purpose is to decide which pituitary functions have to be replaced before operation and also afterwards.

1. *Hypothalamic—pituitary—adrenocortical function*. A series of tests are used regularly for this purpose:

   a) cortisol in plasma, diurnal variation of cortisol in plasma
   b) excretion of 17-ketogenic steroids
   c) ACTH infusion test
   d) metopyrone test
   e) vasopressin test

These different procedures evaluate, at different levels, the capacity of the pituitary to produce ACTH.

a) Measures the actual concentration of cortisol in plasma, and also the diurnal variation in cortisol concentration. This changes rhythmically, and mirrors similar fluctuations in ACTH production. It is dependent on an intact pituitary gland.

b) Measures the amount of cortisol metabolites in 24-hour urine.

c) Tests the capacity of the adrenal cortex to respond to ACTH. While this response is absent in primary adrenocortical failure or Addison's disease, it may be present, although delayed and sluggish, in adrenocortical failure due to insufficient ACTH secretion.

d) Vasopressin acts as a direct stimulator of ACTH secretion, and thereby increases cortisol concentration in plasma. This function also depends on an intact pituitary gland. This test has limited diagnostic value.

e) Gives a measure of the capacity of the pituitary to increase ACTH production when cortisol secretion is blocked by metopyrone. This capacity is usually lacking in pituitary insufficiency.

2. *Thyroid function*. The functional state of the thyroid gland is evaluated by PBI and free thyroxine in plasma and the T_3-resin test. In addition, by administration of TSH, we measure the capacity of the thyroid gland to respond to its pituitary stimulator. This is lacking in primary thyroid insufficiency, and mostly delayed and sluggish in thyroid insufficiency secondary to pituitary failure.

3. *Gonadal functions*. While, e.g., adrenocortical or even thyroid function may be intact in patients with tumours of the pituitary region, some degree of gonadal insufficiency is almost always present in such instances. However, these functions do not have to be replaced before operation, and usually are not evaluated before the final replacement therapy.

4. *Direct measurement of pituitary hormones*. It should be emphasized that, in the near future, we shall have available methods for direct measurement

of all pituitary hormones in blood and, probably, also in urine. This is made possible by the introduction by Berson and Yalow of radioimmunological assay methods for polypeptide hormones. At present, all these hormones have actually been measured, but all the antibodies to the hormones necessary for the procedure are, as yet, not generally available.

In this connexion, the insulin test should be emphasized. By giving intravenously 0.05–0.1 IU of insulin per kg body weight, a hypoglycaemic state is reached, which induces an increased secretion of HGH, ACTH (and cortisol) and catecholamines. It therefore serves as a good screening test for several endocrine functions.

Preoperative substitution therapy

The evaluation of pituitary function before surgical intervention on the gland tells us if hormonal replacement is necessary. As a general rule, it may be said that no such substitution therapy is necessary when adrenocortical function is intact. When adrenocortical insufficiency is present, the patient—who then, as a rule, also has panhypopituitarism—needs replacement therapy.

The ideal situation for the internist in instances of panhypopituitarism is when enough time is available for as complete removal of the signs of panhypopituitarism as possible. We then prefer the following regime:

1. cortisone acetate 25 mg $\times$ 2 daily
2. thyroxine 0.1–0.2 mg daily
3. one injection of long-acting androgens (in males)

The administration of cortisone and thyroxine is continued till the day of operation, preferably for a couple of weeks. When necessary, the operation may be performed without replacement therapy during the days before surgery.

In all instances with adrenocortical insufficiency, replacement is given in the morning of the day of operation with cortisone acetate 100 mg i.m., and 100 mg of a cortisol derivative in 500 ml of saline-glucose administered during the whole duration of the operation. It is followed during the rest of the day of operation by 50 mg of cortisone given every 4 hours.

Postoperative treatment of the hypophysectomized patient

By Björn Sjögren

Department of Medicine IV, Sahlgrenska Sjukhuset, Göteborg, Sweden

From an endocrinologist's point of view, the postoperative management of the hypophysectomized patient does not present too many problems. During the first postoperative days, we are mainly concerned about the dose of cortisone and the possibility of polyuria. We have given cortisone acetate by the intramuscular route in a dose of 100 mg before the operation and another 100 mg in the afternoon after surgery. During the following 2 days, 75 and 50 mg, respectively of cortisone acetate have been given twice daily. Depending on the general condition of the patient and especially on the presence of fever, the dose is rapidly decreased to 25 mg of cortisone acetate orally twice daily. It is most important, however, to increase the dose of cortisone in case of complications with fever.

In most cases, the general condition of the patient has been very favourable after surgery. Fever has occurred only for a few days (less than 38°C) and most often the patients have been able to take water after 24 hours.

Polyuria appears in many cases and may be impressive. Its occurrence depends on the degree of trauma to the pituitary stalk and the height of its section. Polyuria is often rapidly decreasing in severity, but may persist for prolonged periods. It is important to follow the urinary flow carefully until the patient is able to drink freely. At that time he is able to select the adequate amount of water spontaneously. During the first days, the urinary volume is measured every 4–6 hours. Glucose is administered intravenously and adjusted to match urinary flow and expected insensible loss of water. The adequacy of water administration is checked by repeated measurements of plasma sodium concentration or plasma osmolality. Antidiuretic hormone is given after the appearance of polyuria as Pitressin tannate®, a long-acting preparation. One ml is given i.m. each or every other day according to the need. Alternately, the hormone can be administered as a spray (Vasopressin®).

Difficulties with respect to water balance may arise in case of complications leading to decreased consciousness of the patient. As he can no longer react to thirst, water has to be given only with the guide of plasma sodium or osmolality, which must be determined several times a day.

Patients with diabetes mellitus should receive 1/3–1/2 of their usual daily dose of insulin subcutaneously before surgery. A glucose drip is given before the operation, and continued until the patient can take food adequately. Insulin is given in repeated, small doses as rapid acting insulin according to the blood sugar level. After successful hypophysectomy, the daily dose of insulin most often can be reduced to 1/3–1/2 of the previous dose. Furthermore, the tendency to ketosis disappears.

After a few weeks, the completeness of the hypophysectomy is checked according to the methods already discussed by Professor Luft. In the case of pituitary insufficiency, cortisone acetate is given in two daily doses of 12.5 mg each. There is no need for a mineralocorticoid, as the secretion of aldosterone is adequate and independent of pituitary function. It is extremely important to instruct the patient carefully how to increase the administration of cortisone in case of "stress" (fever and surgery!).

Sodium thyroxine is given in a dose of 0.2–0.3 mg daily. It is of some importance to note that cold intolerance and dryness of skin cannot always be interpreted as signs of inadequate replacement of thyroxine, as these symptoms often persist in the face of full replacement. Moreover, the basal metabolic rate often continues to be lower than before operation in case of pituitary insufficiency.

Testosterone is given to male patients as a long-acting preparation, 250 mg every 3–4 weeks. Estrogen replacement is desirable in female patients unless contraindications exist (mammary cancer!). We have used ethinylestradiol in a daily dose of 0.1 mg in periods of 3 weeks. Alternately, a combined estrogen-gestagen preparation can be given in a cyclic fashion. In some women, the administration of a small dose of an androgenic steroid is helpful with respect to decreased sexual drive.

Providing that the basic disease of the patient is controlled, the hypophysectomized patient most often is in good condition and few symptoms occur, which can be explained by the absence of the pituitary. There is a tendency to increase in weight, which can be controlled, however, by dietary restrictions. Some patients complain of persisting tiredness, and it is difficult to know whether it can be explained by the endocrine situation. As has already been noted, some patients complain of dryness of the skin and intolerance to cold. In our experience, the muscular development of the hypophysectomized patient does not change if he continues an active life. Moreover, we have not observed development of osteoporosis in our cases.

Pituitary ablation or destruction in diabetes mellitus

By Rolf Luft

Department of Endocrinology, Karolinska Sjukhuset, Stockholm, Sweden

The classical observation by Houssay and Biasotti in 1930 demonstrated that ablation of the pituitary gland could ameliorate the metabolic defects in animals deprived of the pancreas. Over the years, several observations in experimental diabetes were added which demonstrated the significance of the pituitary—and mainly the so-called growth hormone produced by the gland —for the "Houssay phenomenon". When Luft and Ikkos in 1960 showed that human growth hormone (HGH) could induce diabetes in humans, the cycle of experimental evidence seemed to be completed, which gave to growth hormone the role of a prominent diabetogenic substance.

We may say that, up to this day, the rationale for the removal of the pituitary in patients with diabetic vascular disease is based only on the early findings in experimental diabetes, to which was later added the experience from studies with HGH in man.

The early results of hypophysectomy in patients with diabetic retinopathy, reported by Luft et al. (1953, 1955) seemed encouraging. Later reports by a number of authors gave conflicting evidence of the significance of the procedure in diabetic patients. Furthermore, it has been stressed by us and others that the surgical risks, and later risks mainly of fatal hypoglycaemia, might be of such magnitude that possible therapeutic gains by the procedure might be negligible. In the following, some viewpoints on hypophysectomy in diabetic retinopathy will be presented.

Criteria for selection of patients

The following rather rigid criteria have been adhered to since about 1958 in the selection of diabetic patients for hypophysectomy (see also Ray et al., 1968):

1. *Age limit of 40 years.* Older diabetic patients tolerated the operation less well. Also, in general, they were in a more advanced stage of disseminated vascular disease.

2. *Useful vision remaining in one or both eyes.* It was taken as a general criterion that the remaining vision should be sufficient for work in the patient's profession and for reading ordinary print in a newspaper. Hypophysectomy provides no benefit for patients with gravely impaired vision.

3. *Progression of retinopathy.* Only those patients are selected in whom progression of the retinopathy is identified during a period of months. This excludes patients in whom resorption of retinal haemorrhage with resultant improvement of vision occurs spontaneously.

4. *Absence of retinitis proliferans.* Over the years, we have found that vision is little benefitted by hypophysectomy in the presence of retinitis proliferans. Changes like exudates, microaneurysms and neovascularization most often were greatly improved.

5. *Adequate renal function.* We are, in general, not willing to submit to operation patients with increased creatinine concentration in serum, decreased glomerular filtration rate (less than 60 ml per min), albuminuria of major degree and hypertension. Chronic urinary tract infection also contraindicates hypophysectomy.

6. *Reasonable intelligence and willingness to cooperate.* In principle, the management of the patient after hypophysectomy is not difficult. Over the years, we have learnt that, in order to avoid fatal hypoglycaemia, the patient must be intelligent enough to follow the regimen outlined for him, especially regarding insulin dosage and need for increased doses of cortisone under certain conditions.

Techniques for pituitary destruction or ablation in diabetic patients

Most of the techniques used over the years for pituitary destruction or ablation, mainly in metastatic breast cancer, have also been used in patients with diabetic retinopathy. It may be said that, as a rule, any of these techniques will fulfil its purpose in patients with diabetes, provided that the surgeons and those handling the postoperative care of the patient are familiar with the special problems related to the diabetic state. The main such circumstances are:

1. *The vascular disease.* Vulnerability of the small blood vessels is a common sign in diabetic vascular disease. This demonstrates itself in minute haemorrhages on the brain surface when this is touched during operation, and increased tendency to cerebral oedema after the operation.

2. The effect of *sudden alteration of the hormonal state* after removal of the pituitary. This requires extra carefulness in the management of the hypophysectomized diabetic patient.

These facts should be considered when choosing among the available procedures. The transcranial approach for hypophysectomy—as the one used by us in the 1950's and, e.g., Ray—would therefore seem to be less suitable, and the transantral procedures to be preferred. The methods using implantation of radioactive material in the intact pituitary or external irradiation with protons or alpha particles also have several advantages.

Complications of hypophysectomy in diabetic patients

These may be immediate ones and such appearing at a later stage. The *immediate ones* are those connected with the procedure as such, partly such related to any surgical intervention applied to a diabetic patient.

The major *late complication* is fatal hypoglycaemia. This is the main cause of fatal outcome in these patients not related to the vascular disease as such. It is also one of the reasons why there has been some hesitation among many colleagues to suggest hypophysectomy in diabetic patients. The hypoglycaemia can be avoided by careful replacement therapy, especially under conditions of increased need for cortisone. However, experience has shown that it is almost a prerequisite for the prevention of hypoglycaemic attacks that the patient is reasonably intelligent and is willing to cooperate with the physicians taking care of him.

Results

We have no new personal results demonstrating what can be achieved by hypophysectomy in diabetic retinopathy and other parts of the late diabetic syndrome. Therefore, we prefer to illustrate this with reports by two other groups.

1. Ray and coworkers (1968) reported that of 47 evaluated hypophysectomized diabetic patients, 31 showed regression of the retinopathy, in 6 it was arrested and in 10 unimproved. Thus beneficial results were obtained in 79%. There were 4 deaths in the first 18 patients (unselected group), none in the next 38 patients (selected group).

2. Lundbaek and his group from Aarhus, Denmark, reported in 1967 at the International Diabetes Congress in Stockholm on the first controlled study on the effect of hypophysectomy in diabetic retinopathy. There was a significant difference between the hypophysectomized group and the group of matched diabetic controls, from 5 years to 6 months after the first group had been operated on.

With the above criteria for the selection of patients and these results in mind, we may today consider hypophysectomy a safe and worthwhile procedure in the treatment of diabetic retinopathy in a selected group of patients.

References

Houssay, B. A. & Biasotti, A., *Rev. Soc. Argent. Biol., 6*, 251 (1930).

Ikkos, D. & Luft, R., *Lancet, 2,* 897 (1960).

Luft, R. & Cerasi, E., *Diabetologia, 4,* 1 (1968).

Luft, R. & Olivecrona, H., *J. Neurosurg., 10,* 301 (1953).

Luft, R., Olivecrona, H., Ikkos, D., Kornerup, T. & Ljunggren, H., *Brit. Med. J., 2,* 752 (1955).

Luft, R., Olivecrona, H. & Sjögren, B., *Nord. Med., 47,* 351 (1952).

Ray, B., Pazianos, A. G., Greenberg, E., Peretz, W. L. & McLean, J. M., *JAMA, 203,* 79, 85 (1968).

Pituitary ablation in acromegaly

By Björn Sjögren

Department of Medicine IV, Sahlgrenska Sjukhuset, Göteborg, Sweden

Surgical treatment of acromegaly is by no means a recent development. Sixty years ago, Stumme and Cushing independently described cases in which partial hypophysectomy had led to considerable improvement. Cushing also predicted that *partial hypophysectomy* would become the method of choice in the treatment of acromegaly.

Before the cortisone era, complete hypophysectomy was obviously impossible. Victims of acromegaly were operated on only in cases presenting with suprasellar extension of the tumour, and the operation was only palliative. The effect of surgery on the non-neurological manifestations of acromegaly has generally been disappointing. Today, also, most patients with acromegaly are not operated on in the absence of neurological symptoms. Pituitary irradiation has generally been thought to arrest progression of the disease. Recent experiences with measurements of plasma growth hormone, however, raise serious doubts as to the efficacy of such treatment.

As yet, the follow-up of cases submitted to more radical treatment of eosinophilic tumours has been too brief for conclusions concerning its effectiveness. The present material comprises 1 male and 8 female patients, who were reinvestigated 10 years after transsphenoidal hypophysectomy (performed by Professor C.-A. Hamberger and Professor G. Norlén).

At the time of surgery the length of the case history ranged from 2 to 18 years (Table 1). Two patients, only, had small suprasellar extensions of the pituitary tumours (M. J. and E. Z.). B. A. presented with severe headache, excessive perspiration, soft tissue growth, muscular weakness and insulin-requiring diabetes. Severe headache was a main complaint also in cases R. H., D. S. and E. L. In all cases except B. A., the disease was developing rather slowly with moderate metabolic symptoms.

In 4 cases, the acromegaly had progressed in spite of earlier, conventional X-ray treatment (Table 1). All patients had noted progressive body changes, including enlargement of hands and feet, as well as growth of lips, nose and tongue. At examination, all subjects showed clear-cut acromegalic features. Severe disfigurement was not, however, present. Cases G. L. and E. Z. presented with fairly slight tissue swelling.

Table 1.

Patient	Born		Case history years	Age at operation years	Time of postop. observation years	X-ray treatment
B. A.	♂	18	2	38	12½	—
L. N.	♀	22	4	33	12½	—
A. G.	♀	17	8	40	11	+
R. H.	♀	20	5	37	10½	—
D. S.	♀	12	7	46	10½	—
E. L.	♀	13	18	44	10½	+
M. J.	♀	11	11	47	9½	+
G. L.	♀	09	5	51	8½	+
E. Z.	♀	25	5	36	7	—

All patients were reinvestigated in 1968. The time of postoperative observation ranged from 7 to 12.5 years (mean 10 years). On the whole, the results are favourable. All subjects are living an active life and most of them are free of symptoms. Progression of acromegalic features has not been observed. Three subjects complain of some headache and of moderate tiredness (cases A. G., R. H. and D. S.). Moderate sweating persists in case D. S.

Objective improvement of acromegalic changes are most clearly evident in cases B. A., E. L. and G. L. As a matter of fact, it is difficult to see that these subjects have been victims of acromegaly. Tissue swelling is minimal or absent also in cases A. G. and D. S., but these patients still look somewhat acromegalic. Cases R. H. and E. Z. also have somewhat coarse features which are, however, less pronounced than before surgery. There is probably no improvement of the acromegalic features of patients L. N. and M. J., who nevertheless are completely free of symptoms.

Postoperatively, pituitary insufficiency was demonstrated in 6 cases (Table 2). In cases L. N., R. H. and M. J., thyroid and adrenal function is normal. The most gratifying improvement occurred in cases B. A., A. G., E. L. and G. L., in whom pituitary insufficiency developed. Case B. A. has been free of glycosuria after surgery and his blood sugar is normal. In spite of having developed pituitary insufficiency, case D. S. still shows some symptoms compatible with acromegaly.

The body weight did not change much after operation in the present series of patients. A few subjects increased somewhat in weight, while others lost a few kg. One subject (M. J.) showed evidence of osteoporosis before operation, but the radiological appearance of the skeleton has not changed afterwards. Osteoporosis has not developed in any patient.

Detailed laboratory studies, including measurements of body composition

Table 2.

Patient	Normal activity	Symptoms	Pituitary insuff.	Acromegalic face
B. A.	+	—	+	no-improved
L. N.	+	—	–	yes-unchanged
A. G.	(+)	a, b	+	yes-improved
R. H.	+	a, b	–	(yes)-improved
D. S.	(+)	a, b, c	+	yes-improved
E. L.	+	d	+	no-improved
M. J.	+	–	–	yes-unchanged
G. L.	+	–	+	no-improved
E. Z.	+	–	+	(yes)-improved?

a = moderate headache.   b = tiredness.   c = perspiration.   d = nervousness.

and plasma growth hormone, will be presented in a forthcoming publication.

It is concluded that in the present series of 9 cases of acromegaly with an average postoperative follow-up of 10 years, the result is good with respect to general health and activity in all patients. Definite progression of acromegalic features has not been observed. Significant improvement in soft tissue swelling has occurred in 6 cases also showing pituitary insufficiency. These results are better than could be anticipated after conventional radiological treatment.

The main objection of hypophysectomy in acromegaly arises from the knowledge that the disease follows a fairly benign course in many cases. The operative risks must be shown to be minimal before hypophysectomy will become widely used in slowly developing cases without pronounced subjective or metabolic symptoms. Furthermore, pituitary insufficiency follows radical surgery.

Remission in dependence of the hormonal elimination in hypophysectomy of breast cancer

By Franz Escher

Department of Otolaryngology, University Hospital, Berne, Switzerland

Under the influence of Luft and Olivecrona, we started in June 1955 with hypophysectomy in patients affected with cancer of the breast in advanced stages.

As a disciple of F. R. Nager, whose Semon lecture in 1939 "The Paranasal Approach to Intersellar Tumors" gave a lucid survey of 30 years' activity, I chose the same way.

I suppose that the technique is known. The first period was marked by the overcoming of technical difficulties.

a) closure of the open sella with transplantation of muscle, fascia, galea against rhinorrhoea and meningitis.

b) stabilization of the blood circulation by steroids, which were not yet generally used in 1955.

c) wide exposure of the sella and wide opening of the capsule, in order to judge the whole contents of the sella.

d) use of binocular magnifiers or microscope for the control of eventual remains of the pituitary.

The problems a–c were soon resolved. The problem of pituitary remains will be discussed later.

In the next period, we concentrated our activity on the aim for better results.

e) differentiation of the prognosis.

f) better choice of the patients for hypophysectomy.

For this goal, we had constant contacts with the different groups, especially with those of Vienna, Stockholm, Copenhagen and London. This co-operation was dealt with in our book "Hypophysectomy" (1965) and the symposium M. Dargent (1966).

My actual report is based on my own experience. I cannot give you a tremendous number of cases from our small centre, but it is sufficient to allow some remarks and conclusions. All these patients are exactly followed by our endocrinological service, and furthermore I know and knew each patient personally and not only as a case. What a number of tragedies! Overlooking these 13 years of experience, I have a very ambivalent feeling. I ask myself if—besides more security and perfection of the technique—we have really made great progress. I feel that my report will not bring essentially new facts. But I am happy to have the occasion of putting a number of questions for the discussion. I think that one of the most important aims of this symposium is to clear up unelucidated problems.

Remarks on remission

The American Joint Committee on endocrine ablative procedures in disseminated cancer of the breast has fixed the conception of remission, namely:

6 months' regression in persistent focus and
no appearence of metastasis in other regions.

The world statistics of remissions lie between 32 and 40%. In our own progressive analysis of the cases, we are just in these limits ±3 round about 35%, in dependence of good and bad series. Instead of a statistical calculation, I tried to make a graphic in the chronological representation of the cases (Fig. 1). This was an impressive surprise even for myself. Considering that in Berne we perform 7 to 8 hypophysectomies a year, you may imagine

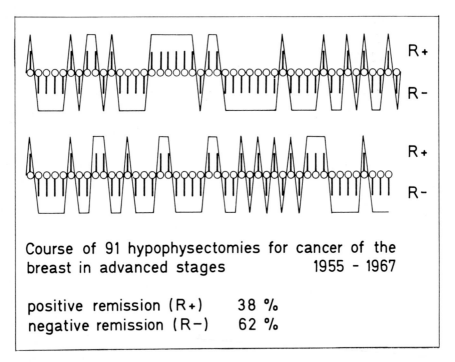

Course of 91 hypophysectomies for cancer of the
breast in advanced stages   1955 - 1967

positive remission (R+)   38 %
negative remission (R−)   62 %

Fig. 1

Average survival

remission positive (R+)
19.2 months
remission negative (R-)
5.7 months

Fig. 2

how discouraging a bad series is and how stimulating a good one is. When a doctor starts a surgical or another method and has bad results for over a year, he probably will be definitely disappointed. On the other hand, a good series will prematurely convince him of the superiority of the chosen method. A graphic like this is like a temperature card with chills of hope and deception. This hazardous medical activity is by that time a real psychological burden for a physician, the more this therapy finally is a palliative one, even in remission cases (Fig. 2). These considerations lead to the fundamental question: "How can we get better results"?

a) Selection of the cases

    1. refinement of the selection corresponding to empiric facts.

    2. Value of preoperative tests for the selection.

b) Importance of the radicality of the operation.

a. 1. Comparing the different statistics, the following facts are generally admitted:

As a rule, the results are rather poorer in young women. The incidence of remission increases 5 years after the menopause. More important than the age seems the velocity of the course of the illness. A long free interval extending to the appearance of the first metastatic lesion has a definite prognostic value. When the interval is short, few remissions are observed; as it increases, so does the incidence of remission.

This rule—mentioned by Dargent—may occasionally be broken. We observed cases with a long free interval, followed by a high-speed evolution once the metastasis appeared. Surveying the years, I get the impression that each case of breast cancer which has not been cured by the primary therapy has more or less a predestinated individual course which can be influenced only partially.

A further important prognostic factor is the response to the oophorectomy. In patients who failed to respond, a worse result will be expected in hypophysectomy. Having in mind these general considerations, I would like to pose the following questions to the symposium:

— Do you still consider hypophysectomy to be indicated even if a patient had no response to oophorectomy?

— Do you believe that we should renounce hypophysectomy in a case with high-speed evolution of metastasis? It is preferable in this situation to try first chemotherapy with antimitotic substances?

— After a successful oophorectomy, should we start first a hormonal therapy once the remission after the castration has passed? Or is this the best moment to undertake hypophysectomy?

This question is important because everybody knows that therapy with androgens often has severe side-effects, and therapy with oestrogens and cortisone is not strictly defined.

— In addition to these questions, we have to consider the almost miraculous relief of pain and frequently spectacular improvement of general symptoms. Do you still believe that a hypophysectomy is indicated for that subjective reason, even in a bad case?

a. 2. According to the investigations of biological factors by Atkins (discriminant factors), the remissions are more frequent when the level of etiocholanolone is elevated in relation to the 17-hydroxysteroids. Have you personal experience of this test, should we use them as a routine, or have you other biological tests for a more precise indication?

b) The importance of the radicality of the operation.

In all publications, great stress is given to the radicality of hypophysectomy. Already Olivecrona mentioned this important fact. He emphasized the special felt polishing burr and the use of Zenker's solution to destroy the remains of the hypophysis on the inner wall of the capsule. B. Ray used the same procedure. Furthermore, the use of optic magnifiers or the microscope was introduced. Theoretically, it seems easy to accomplish the radicality, practically it is much more difficult. Even with a developed technique and an excellent exposure, you may sometimes have difficulties in achieving an absolutely dry sella, free from any bleeding, a prerequisite for a certain inspection. In other cases, you may be sure that the sella is empty, but nevertheless after months you will find some positive endocrinological functions again. A repeated admission of operated patients to hospital to plot the whole hormonal constellation is not possible in any case.

I would like to demonstrate a graphic of 32 hypophysectomies with a complete postoperative hormonal investigation (Fig. 3). The most impressive fact is the variety of the postoperative hormonal constellation. Only in two cases we still have all hormones existing. These are therefore really incomplete

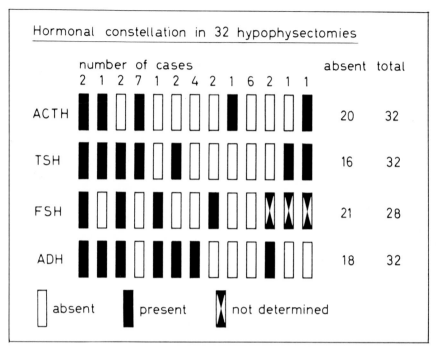

Fig. 3

hypophysectomies. In all the other cases, almost one hormone is lacking. Very important is the total absence of FSH in $3/4$ of this series.

What is now the relation between the totality of the elimination and the remission? If we consider the graphic of the variability of the postoperative hormonal constellation, it is not so clear to establish a norm. An approximative rule is helpful, if you separate the cases which need a hormonal substitution from those without it. This schema seems to prove clearly that the group with substitution has a higher rate of remission (Fig. 4).

In spite of these facts, a number of unelucidated questions are still present.

● How many remains are necessary to entertain an endocrinological function? This question is of great importance, not only for the surgical ablation, but especially for the elimination with radioactive substances, today mainly with yttrium. With a high radioactive charge for total destruction, the percentage of severe side-effects—rhinorrhoea—increases (15–30%). Riechert says in his new book that an elimination of 80% is sufficient. Is this opinion really acceptable?

● Do you suppose that a regeneration of specific hypophysic cells from small remains is possible? In postmortem histological controls of the contents of the sella, we sometimes found nests of hypophysic cells, in cases which

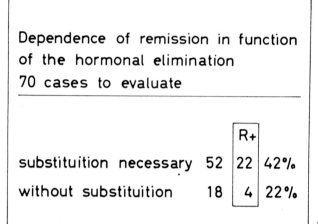

Fig. 4

apparently had an exact hypophysectomy. Or may other possibilities of compensation occur? I am extremely interested in Moberger's paper concerning the pharyngeal hypophysis.

Finally, I would like to discuss two observations. The longest survival of 6 $^1/_2$ years was observed in a woman with a bad prognosis: pulmonary lymphangiosis, carcinomatous pleurisy with respiratory insufficiency. And precisely this hypophysectomy was incomplete.

• In one patient with bone metastasis, I was forced to stop the operation before opening the capsule. I had the intention of removing the hypophysis in a second stage. But the patient refused a second operation, because after this "pseudohypophysectomy" she immediately had been free from pain and had a remission of 8 months.

All these contradictory and to a certain extent illogical facts create an insecurity which is hard to tolerate, especially from the point of view of medical ethics.

In conclusion, I feel uncomfortable bringing up all these questions instead of new scientific results. I thank you for helping me in the following discussion.

References

Escher, F. et al., Advances in Oto-Rhino-Laryngology, XII. Hypophysectomy, S. Karger AG, Basel (1965).

Dargent, M., Major endocrine surgery for treatment of cancer of the breast, Colloque int. Lyon. SIMEP Editions, Lyon (1967).

Mundinger, F. & Riechert, T., Hypophysentumoren, Hypophysektomie, Georg Thieme Verlag, Stuttgart (1967).

Hypophysectomy in mammary carcinoma

By Theodore R. Miller

Pack Medical Group, New York, N.Y., U.S.A.

The breast is the most common site of primary carcinoma in women, accounting for about 22 per cent of all malignant tumors. Shimpkin (1963) of the National Cancer Institute, has stated that during an anticipated life span of 72 years, carcinoma of the breast will develop in one out of every 18 women, an incidence of 5.5 per cent. Extrapolating on the basis of the present United States population, about fifty thousand new cases of mammary cancer will appear each year, and more than 60 per cent of these patients will have metastases in spite of the best current modes of treatment. Metastases will bring death to 80% of those in whom mammary cancer is found in the lymph nodes at all levels of the axilla.

Therapy for carcinoma of the breast is based on the knowledge that the organ is normally dependent upon endocrine control, and that the lesion is to some degree dependent on the hormone produced by the host for a variable period of time before becoming autonomous. The dependent tumor cells retain characteristics of the normal cells from which they arise, and the tumor cells function like those of the tissue of origin. Carcinoma of the breast is, at first, rarely autonomous or intrinsically self perpetuating. It usually is sustained and propagated by endocrines functioning at normal or subnormal levels.

Choice of therapy

The selection of the type of therapy for the patient with advanced carcinoma of the breast depends upon the patient's functional endocrine status, which can be described in three basic groups of women: (1) premenopausal, those actively menstruating; (2) menopausal, those in the menopause, either natural or induced, up to ten years after its occurrence, including the occasional woman who, though well past the menopause, shows evidence of active estrogen production in her vaginal smear; (3) postmenopausal, those past the menopause ten or more years, including the rare patient who shows no estrogenic activity regardless of her age.

Hormonal therapy. In women ten years or more past the menopause, that is, group 3, the addition of exogenous estrogenic hormone is a most satisfactory primary treatment. It is to be noted that the older the patient is at the onset of treatment, the more likely is the regression of the tumor. The value of androgens is well established in the primary treatment of the meno-pausal patient with metastatic disease in the bone, or secondarily for the patient with recrudescent osseous disease after failure of response to oophor-ectomy, adrenalectomy, or estrogen therapy. While estrogenic therapy is valuable only in the postmenopausal patient, since it causes progression of the disease in the premenopausal group, androgens prove of value in both groups. In the American Medical Association Subcommittee's report (1960) on 580 patients treated with androgens for disseminated mammary car-cinoma, objective responses were obtained in only 21.4 per cent.

Objective improvement with corticosteroid therapy is generally less fre-quent and of shorter duration than that following other types of hormonal therapy. Sherlock and Hartmann (1962) in a retrospective analysis of 204 patients who died of carcinoma of the breast, observed that patients given additive adrenal steroid therapy showed a significant increase in metastases. This may well be due to the dosage schedules used, since small doses of cortisone tend to stimulate the growth of many forms of cancer without suppressing adrenal function and concomitant production of estrogen.

Progesterone has been reported (Landau *et al.,* 1962) to be effective in the therapy of mammary carcinoma. This is particularly true after other hor-monal substances have produced a response and then failed. While the exhibition of various hormonal substances singly or in combinations at various ages of patients with advanced mammary cancer has been partially successful in producing objective as well as subjective improvement, it does not appear to be as complete nor as long-lasting as ablation of the ovaries, adrenals, or hypophysis.

Ablative therapy. In 1896, Sir George Beatson (1896) first reported that inoperable mammary carcinoma in women could be induced to regress by excision of the ovaries. In the first group, or premenopausal patient, it re-mains the best primary method of treating advanced carcinoma of the breast. Surgical castration is preferable to roentgen castration, since it is more likely to be complete, has an insignificant mortality rate, and offers an objective remission in about 44 per cent of premenopausal patients, lasting an average of about 14 months. The response is thought to be due to the removal of the endogenous estrogenic hormone.

In reviewing many reports, it is obvious that ablative therapy, carried out at the time of first recurrence of mammary cancer, is of more benefit than if done after other forms of therapy have been exhausted. It is unfortunate that because hormonal therapy, radiation therapy, and chemotherapy are capable of producing a partial regression, ablative therapy is all too often deferred until a more advanced stage of the disease, limiting its effectiveness.

Oophorectomy is the ablative therapy of choice for the group 1 patient. Further response after failure can be had by sequential adrenalectomy and hypophysectomy. Combined bilateral oophorectomy-adrenalectomy is the best primary method of treatment in patients in group 2, as shown by Huggins (1952) while hypophysectomy offers the best palliation for patients in group 3. In case of recurrence, sequentially performed oophorectomy, adrenalectomy, and hypophysectomy will produce a regression of metastatic mammary cancer in a fairly high percentage of cases, provided the original oophorectomy has been of value.

It seems paradoxical that the *addition* of estrogen in group 3 patients produces regression, while the *removal* of estrogenic hormone in the group 1 patients produces regression of advanced mammary cancer, yet the evidence is indisputable.

Advantages of hypophysectomy

Luft, Olivecrona and Sjögren (1952) introduced hypophysectomy as a therapeutic measure for advanced mammary cancer. Since that time, the pendulum of opinion has been swinging to and fro as to which of the three ablative procedures is best. Oophorectomy-adrenalectomy appears to be of benefit by virtue of the removal of the endogenous estrogenic hormone and its stimulating effect upon the hypophysis as well as on the tumor. Hypophysectomy is superior because it attacks the problem directly, stopping the production of estrogen by the abolition of gonadotropic and adrenotropic hormones, and removing the source of mammotropic and growth hormones.

At the International Conference on Major Surgery in the Treatment of Breast Cancer in Lyon, 16 authors reported on 865 surgical removals and 2,182 radiation hypophyseal destructions, and concluded that hypophysectomy was superior to adrenalectomy-oophorectomy. Their end results showed figures varying from 33 to 50 per cent regressions to as high as 70 per cent in the surgical removal of the pituitary in patients of 65 years of age and over.

Howard Dunbar (1967), in reporting results of hypophysectomy at the Cornell-New York Hospital Medical Center, stated that 41 per cent of patients showed a remission when done in the first five years after menopause; 51 per cent from 6 to 10 years after menopause; and 70 per cent in the age group after 65. In patients who had previously responded to castration, 91 per cent were reported to have responded to hypophysectomy. However, only 6 per cent of those patients who had not responded to castration responded to hypophysectomy.

The advantages of hypophysectomy over adrenalectomy-oophorectomy are as follows:

1. While ovariectomy is not necessary with hypophysectomy, as it is with adrenalectomy, in many cases combined bilateral oophorectomy and adrenalectomy can be done through a transabdominal approach, allowing abdominal exploration for metastases and exploration of possible ectopic adrenal glands.

2. Besides having the same effect on estrogen productivity as do oophorectomy-adrenalectomy, hypophysectomy eliminates the growth hormone and prolactin which probably affect the growth of cancer.

3. Some patients in whom remission has followed oophorectomy and adrenalectomy have another remission after hypophysectomy. While this is rare and may represent inadequate or incomplete adrenal surgical techniques, it is sufficiently frequent to warrant the surgical procedure if good response has been noted after bilateral oophorectomy-adrenalectomy.

4. Although fluid and electrolyte balance is easier to manage after adrenalectomy-oophorectomy than after hypophysectomy, only about 10 per cent of our patients have developed fluid and electrolyte problems that require special measures. Most patients after adrenalectomy require 50 to 75 mg of cortisone daily, whereas following hypophysectomy only 35 to 50 mg are required. The occasional patient who develops severe diabetes insipidus and hyponatremia can be controlled by salt-retaining corticosteroids such as Dexamethisone, varying the daily intake of salt, and the use of pitrissin in oil or as snuff.

5. While oophorectomy-adrenalectomy or hypophysectomy will induce complete regression of mammary cancer for varying lengths of time, the administration of small doses of estrogen will reactivate tumor growth after oophorectomy-adrenalectomy, but after hypophysectomy the tumor is unchanged by the administration of estrogen. It has been shown (Pearson *et al.*, 1954) that bovine growth hormone, estrogen, and progesterone or combinations of these hormones, with or without replacement therapy with cortisone or thyroxin, fail to reactivate tumor growth after hypophysectomy. This would indicate that hypophysectomy is superior to either of the other forms of ablative therapy.

Selection of cases

The difficulty lies in selecting the patient who is suitable for hypophysectomy. The following conditions can be used in predicting good results of hypophysectomy, although occasional remissions have been observed in patients in whom none of these criteria were present: (1) a prolonged interval, usually more than three years, between the mastectomy and the manifestation of metastatic involvement; (2) previous response to oophorectomy and androgen therapy; (3) evidence of estrogenic activity as shown in a menopausal type of smear; (4) well differentiated mammary cancer; (5) the age group between 40 and 65 years.

Surgical technique of hypophysectomy

Many different approaches to the hypophysis have been described in the literature. The neurosurgical approach through a transfrontal craniotomy has the advantage of avoiding contamination of the dural sac, but is a major surgical endeavor and is accompanied by many possible complications. The various approaches through the nose, maxillary antrum, or middle wall of the orbit have their devotees. We have found, however, that the approach through the maxillary antrum and the sphenoidal sinus, described by Hamberger *et al.* (1961) is the most satisfactory. The main complication is the possibility of rhinorrhea with its concomitant risk of meningitis. This can be prevented by the use of a plug of muscle in the sella turcica, supplemented by a skin graft placed over the posterior wall of the sphenoidal sinus. This approach is simple and it should now be possible to study the effect of hormonal ablation on breast cancer in its earlier phases.

Suggestions for further approaches to the problem

The question of whether or not hypophysectomy or other ablative therapy should be used as the primary treatment for this disease can best be answered by noting the fact that localized cancer of the breast can be cured by excision. This has been proved by the high rates of cure that follow radical mastectomy for disease confined to the breast (Welch, 1966). As a corollary, cancer can also be cured in many instances when metastasis is confined to nodes that can be excised. Even those cases in which the interpectoral or Rotter's node is involved can be cured by the extirpative approach. Patients with widespread metastatic disease and untreated breast cancer have been shown to have a regression of the local disease as well as the distant metastasis following ablative endocrine therapy. However, no complete cure such as follows radical mastectomy has been reported.

I have attempted removal of the adrenals, ovaries, and pituitary glands in two operative seances several times, with resulting disappearance of the tumor, but it is too early to determine whether or not this more complete excision of the endocrine system is of any more value than hypophysectomy alone.

While it is essential that hypophysectomy be total to produce longlasting suppression of hormone-dependent mammary cancer, I have observed that partial ablation of the pituitary will produce shorter-lived or temporary regression and relief. Selective anterior hypophysectomy has been used in the treatment of diabetic retinopathy (Hardy and Ciric, 1968). From a study of the specimens in our series, removed by the transantrosphenoidal approach, it would seem feasible to remove the anterior lobe in its entirety without disturbing the posterior lobe, thus avoiding the distressing consequence of diabetes insipidus.

Patients in whom nodes at all levels of the axilla are involved have an 80 per cent chance of recurrence and/or metastasis, and should form an interesting group for the study of the prophylactic value of hypophysectomy.

Continued study to develop the ability to predict which patients have hormone-dependent tumors should lead to improved therapeutic management. It is unfortunate that experience with ablative endocrine treatment of patients with breast cancer has, for the most part, been confined to the late phases of the disease. Hypophysectomy at the time of the first recurrence should yield a longer period of remission than the usual measures, such as use of hormones, radiation therapy, chemotherapy, and bilateral oophorectomy with adrenalectomy. An important unanswered question is whether breast cancer in its earliest phases is more dependent upon the endocrine environment than in its later phases. Transantrosphenoidal hypophysectomy offers a simple means of accomplishing optimum endocrine alteration and should permit an approach to this potentially rewarding possibility.

References

Beatson, G. T., *Lancet, 2,* 104, 162 (1896).

Dunbar, H. S., *Hypophysectomy for advanced breast cancer.* International conference of Lyon: Major endocrine surgery for the treatment of cancer of the breast in advanced stages. SIMEP Editions, Lyon, 105 (1967).

Hamberger, C.-A., Hammer, G., Norlén, G. & Sjögren, B., *Arch. Otolaryng.* (Chicago), *74,* 22 (1961).

Hardy, J. & Ciric, I. S., *JAMA, 203,* 73 (1968).

Huggins, C. B. & Dao, T., *Ann. Surg., 136,* 595 (1952).

Landau, R. L., Ehrlich, E. N. & Huggins, C., *JAMA, 182,* 632 (1962).

Luft, R., Olivecrona, H. & Sjögren, B., *Nord. Med., 47,* 351 (1952).

Pearson, O. H., West, C. D., Hollander, V. P. & Treves, N., *JAMA, 154,* 234 (1954).

Sherlock, P. & Hartmann, W. H., *JAMA, 181,* 313 (1962).

Shimpkin, M. B., *JAMA, 183,* 358 (1963).

Subcommittee on breast and genital cancer of the AMA council on drugs. JAMA, 172, 1271 (1960).

Welch, C. E., *Surgery, 59,* 908 (1966).

General discussion

Ketcham to Luft

I gather that your prime indication for recommending hypophysectomy is progressive deterioration of vision as a result of diabetic retinopathy. Yet you are so highly selective in your criteria for recommending surgery such as that they must have vision, fairly good renal function, etc. This suggests to me that the results may be less than ideal. I ask if hypophysectomy in diabetics should be more often considered; are you really enthused about this form of treatment?

Bateman to Luft

We have operated on 24 cases of diabetic retinopathy in the period 1959–61. These cases were unselected according to Dr. Luft's criteria, and it appeared that the elderly cases in the series were rendered more vulnerable to their diabetic vascular disorders by the operation. Has this sort of experience led Dr. Luft to fix his age limit at 40 years?

Angell James to Luft

Partial hypophysectomy for diabetic retinopathy has been performed in 5 cases. The first was not intentional and had a very good result with striking improvement. In these cases the improvement has been in the haemorrhagic element and not in the other manifestations.

Luft to Ketcham

Dr. Ketcham asked me whether I am enthusiastic about hypophysectomy in diabetic retinopathy. The simplest reply would be that I am in favour of hypophysectomy in a group of diabetics selected along the lines described in my slide.

Luft to Bateman

Since several years we have not touched patients where amaurosis was expected to appear within one year. The prognosis is too poor in this group. We know today, mainly thanks to the work of Ashton, that the changes in the vessels in the eye grounds are very marked and advanced even when the findings in the ophthalmoscope are moderate. This is another reason why we stick to the strict criteria for the selection of patients outlined in my slide.

Arslan to Sjögren

Ultrasonic hypophysectomy, which was performed in our Department in 95 cases (1965–1968), has the advantage of not definitely destroying the pituitary, but of suppressing its hormonal function. This is very important in Cushing's disease, in which the aetiology is "hyperfunction" of the gland. In cases of diabetic retinopathy, the results were the same as in surgical hypophysectomy.

Notter to Escher

In our opinion, better tumour regression occurs after total than after partial depression of pituitary activity. In our material, the difference in the survival between these two groups is significant. This could also be shown in 5 of our first partially hypophysectomized patients who had a second and longer tumour regression following total hypophysectomy.

In a series of 13 hypophysectomized patients, no difference existed between the hormonal state of the patient and tumour regression, but a clear-cut correlation between histological and biological malignancy of the tumour and tumour regression, respectively, survival of the patient.

Recovery of hypophyseal cell function after temporal suppression by interstitial irradiation is possible, and clearly demonstrable by recovery of hormonal excretion several months after implantation.

To the question about the most suitable time for hypophysectomy in breast cancer patients: we believe that it should be done in a relatively early stage of tumour dissemination, when the patient still has sufficient resistance and general condition to react to the hormonal operation. This is no longer the case when he has extended liver, brain and bone metastases.

Selection of the patients is necessary and may be done according to their reaction to oophorectomy, irradiation of the ovaries, cortisone medication or special patterns of hormonal excretion.

Angell James to Escher

In our group of 331 hypophysectomy operations for metastatic breast cancer, the best results were obtained in the age group 60–69 years, in the patients with osseous metastases, in those with high urinary gonadotropin and in those with a long interval between the primary operation and the appearance of metastases. In 8 patients who had had previous adrenalectomy, oophorectomy, there was a further remission in 3.

Every effort should be made to ensure a total hypophysectomy, though a microscopically perfect removal is impossible. From animal studies, pituitary regeneration is possible, and it may well be that this can occur also in the human.

Luft to Escher

Professor Escher raised a number of important questions that were really to the point. Unfortunately, most of these cannot be adequately answered to-day. At least I cannot do so, but I could always add a number of equally important questions to the list of Professor Escher's.

When we say today that we do not know exactly the place of hypophys-ectomy in the treatment of breast cancer, the same argument can be applied to any of the methods for endocrine treatment of tumours. There has been a tendency to extrapolate from the experience gained in experimental breast cancer in inbred strains of mice to breast cancer in humans. We have no idea if these two types of breast cancer have anything in common. For instance, whether the synergism of lactogenic hormone and oestrogens for the development of experimental breast cancer also is valid for the disease in women, or whether viruses ("Bittner factor") also play a role when breast cancer develops in a woman. We have to await answers to such and other problems before being able to understand why hypophysectomy is successful in 30–40 % of unselected patients with metastatic breast cancers.

Professor Escher also raised the question about the significance of the radicality of hypophysectomy for its effect on breast cancer. I believe that most workers in the field are of the opinion that as complete a hypophys-ectomy as possible gives better results than subtotal removal of the gland. We know that grossly incomplete pituitary ablation sometimes does the job. However, to my mind, there can be no doubt that we must aim at com-plete removal. Only then can we come to a conclusion as regards the place of hypophysectomy in the treatment of metastatic breast cancer. May I remind the surgeons that even when you do your best to empty the sella turcica completely, you sometimes—and not so seldom—end up with sub-total hypophysectomy.

The interesting question why incomplete hypophysectomies sometimes are followed by remission cannot be adequately answered. One tentative explana-tion is that breast cancers may have different degrees of hormone sensitivity, and that those with the greatest sensitivity may react already to less extensive alterations of the hormonal milieu of the body.

The results obtained with hypophysectomy in unselected groups of pa-tients with metastatic breast cancer are generally quoted at about 35 % worth-while remissions. It should be emphasized that the number of remissions is much higher if you work with groups of patients who had previously re-sponded well to other forms of endocrine therapy, such as oophorectomy in menopausal women and oestrogen treatment in the postmenopausal ones. The schedule should therefore be to start with the latter procedures, and later add hypophysectomy only to those that proved to be hormone-sensitive.

As Professor Escher mentioned, it has been found that patients reacting well to hypophysectomy had increased amounts of etiocholanolone in the urine. I think that he refers to the work by Bulbrook and coworkers. What they actually showed was that these patients demonstrated an increased discrimination index in which etiocholanolone was involved. Although these results are interesting, they have not been generally accepted as prognostic signs. Nor is it generally accepted that determination of the excretion of any hormone in the urine can be used for the selection of patients for hypophysectomy.

Professor Escher's longest survival was 6 years. We had a patient with breast cancer with widespread metastases to the bones, in terrible pain, who survived hypophysectomy for 10 years and who had a remission lasting for about 7 years. These instances are rare, however.

When we introduced hypophysectomy in metastatic breast cancer, our aim was to remove by one single step the production of all hormones possibly involved in the development and/or progression of breast cancer. Today we know of at least one alternative method which, when used as a primary therapeutic procedure, gives approximately the same number of remissions as hypophysectomy: the combination of oophorectomy and cortisone administration of Nissen-Meyer of Oslo. Future research will perhaps tell us the role played by oestrogens and each of the pituitary hormones discussed for the progression of breast cancer in man. Until then, our endocrine therapeutic measures must be considered as empirical.

Ketcham to Luft

We here in this room are primarily interested in the anatomical area of the head and neck, and I believe that we are correctly left with the impression that hypophysectomy may play a very favourable role in the control of metastatic breast cancer symptoms. It has been said this morning that it is the ablative treatment of choice. May I remind you that last month at a meeting of urologists, they left their meeting having been told that adrenalectomy gave much more favourable palative results. So just as with melanoma and thyroid tumors we have a bizzare behaving tumor, most unpredictable and often with long-term survival of 10 to 20 years before metastatic disease causes death. It is for this reason that we know so little about breast cancer and must be careful in being too dogmatic in our recommendations. It is a sad state of affairs indeed that the cancer which causes death in women in greater numbers than any other cause continues to be so poorly understood. It will remain so until all of us are willing to place our patients into controlled long-term collaborative study protocols, which may then eventually give us some answers which will be scientifically and statistically reliable.

H. C. Andersen

I should like to report a controlled clinical trial concerning the effect of hypophysectomy on diabetic retinopathy. The trial was carried out under the leadership of Knud Lundbæk and started 6 years ago and stopped $1^{1}/_{2}$ years ago. The patients were selected according to criteria mentioned by Professor Luft, and candidates for operation were chosen at random. A total of 30 patients belongs to the trial and it turned out that the operated and the control group were completely identical concerning sex distribution, average age (31 years) and average effective vision (57%). We have followed these two groups every third month, presenting an observation time ranging from $6^{1}/_{2}$ to $1^{1}/_{2}$ years. The last follow-up examination has shown that the average effective vision in the operated group has dropped from the preoperative level of 57% to 49%, but in the control group it dropped from 57% to 32%. In the control group we have seen 5 cases of the very unpleasant condition of haemorrhagic glaucoma, which did not occur in the operated group.

One patient died of postoperative meningitis and in the same group one died elsewhere from incorrectly treated hypoglycaemia.

It is our intention to continue with the follow-up examination as long as patients and members of the group are still alive.

Ketcham to Escher

I believe that these collaborative studies which are presently few and far between will require large numbers of patients entered into the study, due to the long life history of breast cancer. Most important is the need to have physicians agree to enter these patients in a study, and then carry out the specific treatment which the study calls for under the circumstances of the patients' disease.

Escher to Ketcham

I would refer to the Dargent Symposium in Lyon 1966. Both groups: urologists and hypophysectomy surgeons were present. The results of adrenalectomy + hypophysectomy are about the same. But the next question is, which intervention is more dangerous, adrenalectomy or hypophysectomy? Here I am sure that adrenalectomy is the severer intervention, and furthermore for the destruction of the hypophysis you have the choice of different methods.

C.-A. Hamberger

Dr. Ketcham earlier mentioned malignant melanomas and Dr. Angell James also mentioned that in his paper. Does anyone have experience of treatment with endocrine surgery in such cases? We have hypophysectomized 5 cases without improvement. We have also tried hypophysectomy in a few cases of prostatic cancer. In these we have seen a good remission.

Ketcham to C.-A. Hamberger

Malignant melanoma is not ordinarily recognized as a hormonally dependent tumor. Yet at times it has behaved as such, and for this reason I advise against pregnancy in any woman who has had melanoma. I have not performed nor recommended adrenalectomy or hypophysectomy for melanoma but others have, and I am not sure that any favourable success has been obtained.

Miller to C.-A. Hamberger

In answer to Dr. Hamberger, we have done hypophysectomies on 12 cases of malignant melanoma with widespread metastases, on the theory that the removal of the melanin-stimulating hormone might influence the course of the disease. There have been several reports in the literature that irradiation of the hypophysis in similar cases had produced regression of the metastases.

Unfortunately, there was no response in any of our cases.

We have noted almost uniform symptomatic relief in prostatic cancer with metastases. Adrenalectomy appears to have little or no effect in this disease.

Angell James

Seven cases of malignant melanoma have been operated on. In 3 there was a response. In 1 it persisted for 6 months with considerable regression of the skin tumours. In general, the response is short and may be dangerous. In the first case, death was due to haemorrhage from shrinking cerebral metastases, 3 weeks after hypophysectomy. Seventeen patients with metastases from prostatic carcinoma have been operated on, with response in 40%.

Chairman's summary of session III

G. Bateman

There has been discussion about whether total hypophysectomy should be aimed at or whether it was adequate to aim at partial surgical hypophysectomy in certain diseases or even in all diseases. As Dr. Luft has pointed out we do not at present know the results of total hypophysectomy in many diseases and until we have some figures about the results of total hypophysectomy we shall only add confusion to confusion by introducing deliberate partial hypophysectomy.

As chairman I would urge the members of the symposium to aim at total hypophysectomy in all cases. I say "aim" because autopsies of the post-operative pituitary fossa always show that pituitary cells are still present on histological examination and often there are macroscopic nodules of pituitary tissue still present in the fossa when the surgeon thinks he has done a total operation. It may be that some new technical trick will enable us to perform total hypophysectomy of normal pituitaries when the object of operation is hormone ablation. As regards surgical hypophysectomy for pituitary tumours with an expanded sella turcica, I am convinced that we should aim at total hypophysectomy and I am also convinced that we seldom, if ever, achieve total removal. Fortunately, the surgical mortality in these cases is almost non-existent so that we cannot check our surgical achievement in the post mortem room. We shall have to wait for the remnants to proliferate and once more produce symptoms before the incompleteness of the operation is demonstrated.

There has been a suggestion made that gelatin sponge or some other extraneous material should be used for filling the pituitary fossa after hypophysectomy. I am convinced that autogenous material, e.g. muscle, should be used for this purpose. I do not think it is important whether fascia and muscle or muscle alone is used, but I do regard it as important that autogenous material should be used.

I am glad that the organizer of this symposium has chosen his participants in such a way that we have not had to spend the morning arguing the relative merits of surgical ablation of the pituitary and destruction of the pituitary by the implantation of irradiated material such as Yttrium 90. We have been trying to elucidate problems of more basic importance than this. Escher's questions need answering and many of them are still unanswerable. Luft has suggested some answers and some methods by which further answers can be arrived at. I am grateful to him for taking on his shoulders this part of the chairman's responsibility. The fact that this gathering cannot supply the answers shows the validity of the questions and their penetration to the core of our problems.

Finally I thank, on behalf of the participants, Professor Hamberger and his colleagues for calling together so many doctors interested and active in this field of surgical and scientific advance.

Changes of the sella turcica in pituitary tumours

By Tore Laurén

Department of X-ray Diagnosis, Kronprinsessan Lovisa's Children's Hospital, Stockholm, Sweden

At roentgen examination without contrast medium, the following findings may be expected in cases of pituitary tumours; alteration of the sellar shape, increased volume and destruction of the sella or adjacent parts of the sphenoid bone.

Eosinophilic adenomas expand the sella in a balloon-shaped way, and chromophobe adenomas give a cup-shaped type of expansion and are more liable to erode the dorsum and extend outside the sella. These findings are fairly reliable, but there are many cases with intermediate shape and, as has been described by Greitz and Ross, the findings may be reversed. In basophilic and mixed adenomas, sellar changes are absent or atypical.

The volume of the sella is perhaps not as important to evaluate as its shape. To assess the volume accurately, it is of course necessary to measure not only the length and depth but also the width, which is visualized in the standard p.a. skull projection in almost all cases. A well developed sphenoid sinus facilitates the visualization, and in some cases with a small sinus tomography is necessary. A number of authors have assessed normal sellar volume, for instance Di Chiro and Nelson, who made an elaborate radiographic and volumetric study in cadavers. The normal variation was found to be wide, and assessment of the volume is therefore of limited diagnostic value in the individual case.

A careful study of the sellar floor is important in searching for bone destruction. Fig. 1 demonstrates the p.a. projections of the sellar floors, drawn directly from the skull films of 50 patients without history of endocrine disorders. It is obvious that a moderate lateral inclination is not pathologic, which is in agreement with earlier observations. In the most marked cases, a corresponding asymmetry of the sphenoid sinus was found. It is also evident that there is a considerable variation in width. The diagnostic consequences of these variations in the shape of the floor are illustrated in Fig. 2. It demonstrates that the sellar floor may appear with one, two or even three contours in the lateral projection. It is also obvious that the sella may appear normal in the lateral projection in cases of small bone destructions. Figs. 3

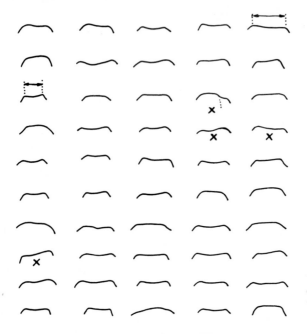

Fig. 1. P.a. projections of the sellar floor in 50 normal cases. Note lateral inclination (X) and difference in width (↔).

and 4 demonstrate that these concepts of the anatomy of the sellar floor are of practical importance.

In a survey like this of sellar radiology, it seems important to stress the following points: The sella should be studied in both frontal and lateral projections, and bone destruction with tumour extension into the sphenoid sinus should be carefully looked for. In most cases the sella and the adjacent

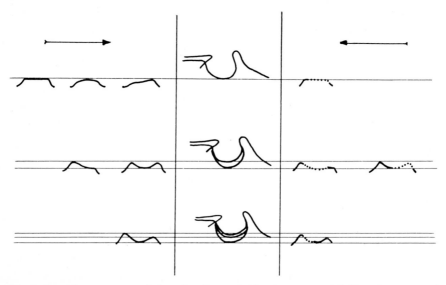

Fig. 2. Lateral appearances of the sellar floor resulting from normal (left) and constructed pathologic cases (right). The fine lines indicate the beam of X-rays.

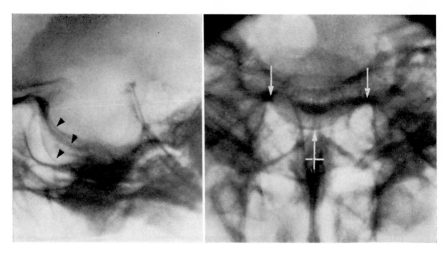

Fig. 3. Eosinophilic adenoma. Lateral projection (left) with the sellar floor represented by three contours (▼). P.a. projection (right) with lateral margins (→) and centre (↦) of the sellar floor.

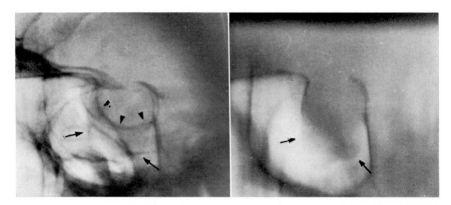

Fig. 4. Eosinophilic adenoma with destruction of the floor. In the lateral projection (left) the floor looks intact (▼), but a tumour (→) is bulging down into the sphenoid sinus. In the tomogram (right), the tumour is more clearly visualized and the bone destruction is evident.

skull base can be studied in plain films, but occasionally tomography is necessary. In some cases of doubtful enlargement of the sella, assessment of the volume is helpful.

Of course, sellar radiography is just a detail in the roentgen examination in cases of pituitary tumours. A complete skull examination with special projections of the optic foramina should always be performed. Pneumo-encephalography with special attention to the chiasmatic and interpeduncular cisterns and the floor of the third ventricle must be performed in almost all cases, because suprasellar growth may be present without demonstrable sellar changes. Usually, the extrasellar extension occurs into the suprasellar region, but in rare cases a tumour may extend into the anterior, posterior or middle cranial fossa. In the last-mentioned case, carotid angiography may be useful to visualize lateral displacement of the internal carotid artery. Besides, the vascular pattern may sometimes give information about the nature of the tumour, as has been described by Ross and Westberg. Phlebography of the cavernous sinus may occasionally give information about the lateral border of the pituitary.

References

Camp, J. D., *Radiology, 53*, 666 (1949).

Di Chiro, G. & Nelson, K. B., *Amer. J. Roentgen., 87*, 989 (1962).

Krueger, E. G. & Unger, S. M., *Amer. J. Roentgen., 98*, 617 (1966).

Lindgren, E., *Röntgenologie Bd. II, Handbuch der Neurochirurgie,* Springer Verlag, Berlin (1954).

Oon, C. L., *Brit. J. Radiol., 36*, 294 (1963).

Ross, R. J. & Greitz, T., *Radiology, 86*, 892 (1966).

Taveras, J. M. & Wood, E. H., *Diagnostic Neuroradiology,* Williams and Wilkins, Baltimore (1964).

Westberg, G. & Ross, R. J., *Acta Radiol.* [Diagn.] (Stockholm), *6*, 475 (1967).

Pituitary tumour pathology

By Jan Wågermark

Department of Pathology, Danderyds Sjukhus, Danderyd, Sweden

Classification

Traditionally, the pituitary cells are divided into three main classes: the *chromophobes,* the *acidophils* and the *basophils.* Tumours arising in the gland are also traditionally classified in the same manner, according to their dominating cell type.

Light microscopy

The tumours are not encapsulated and are not sharply demarcated from the surrounding tissue. They are thus difficult to separate from areas of focal hyperplasia, which are very common in the organ. This applies especially to the basophil adenomas, which never reach any prominent size.

The acidophil adenomas are larger, but most often limited to the sella. They may show degenerative changes, such as bleeding and fibrosis, but seldom cyst formation. The chromophobe adenomas grow very large, have a tendency to erode the surrounding bone walls and often show supracellular vegetations. Their central parts degenerate, and cyst formation is a common finding.

Histologically, subdivisions of each main type can be done according to the arrangement of cells and the amount of stroma. Thus, diffuse and sinusoidal types (according to some authors also a papillary type) can be recognized. This separation is, however, without any practical and clinical significance, being merely a morphological pecularity.

Malignancy

Regarding the malignancy of pituitary tumours, some authors have denied the existence of this state. However, few but well documented cases with distant metastases are described in literature. On the other hand, especially the chromophobe adenomas show "local malignancy" and destroy the surrounding tissues. The more aggressive adenomas show more prominent cellular atypia, and they also have a tendency to recur.

Electron microscopy

What information can now be added in the diagnostic work on pituitary adenomas from the knowledge obtained in research work recently? One matter that has interested workers in the field is if the morphologist can confirm secretory activity in cases of hormone overproduction. This is best studied in cases with acromegalia caused by acidophilic adenomas. We have been able to investigate this problem ourselves, and I can exemplify by personal findings.

Material

Our material consists of 15 patients with acromegalia, investigated at the endocrinologic clinic at Karolinska Sjukhuset and operated on at the ear, nose and throat department of the same hospital, where transsphenoidal hypophysectomy was performed. At operation, material was taken for electron microscopy and the activity of the cells was studied.

Cellular activity

Signs of activity in these protein-synthesizing cells are a prominent Golgi apparatus, well-developed endoplasmic reticulum and richness of mito-

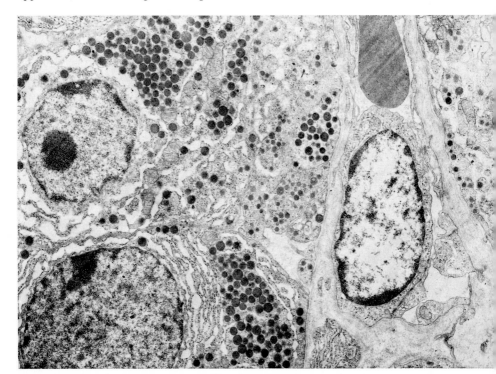

Fig. 1. Actively hormone-producing acidophil adenoma. The cell in the lower left corner is typical, with its well developed endoplasmic reticulum and the peripherally located granules. × 3000.

Table 1. *Comparison between "clinical activity", growth hormone concentration in the blood plasma and activity as estimated in the electron micrograph. Fifteen cases of acromegaly.*

Case	Clin. activity	HGH (mμg/ml plasma)	Electron micr.activity
1	+ + +	160	active
2	+ + +	50	moderately active
3	+ + +	50	active
4	+ + +	47	inactive (regr.)
5	+ + +	96	active
6	+	17	inactive (regr.)
7	+ + +	270	very active
8	+	20	moderately active
9	+	15	regressive changes
10	+ + +	42	active
11	+	30	regressive changes
12	+ +	28	moderately active
13	+ +	24	moderately active
14	+ + +	75	inactive
15	+(+)	26	moderately active

chondria. Secretory granules are few and peripherally located (Fig. 1). From these criteria, the last column in Table 1 is constructed. It will be compared with the clinical evaluation of the acromegalic activity, which now can be confirmed by estimations of the plasma content of growth hormone.

Correlation between morphology and function

As can be seen, there is generally a good correlation between morphology and function in *eosinophilic adenomas*. We have no cases with a morphologically active picture which is not associated with a clinically active disease. However, the reverse is true for some cases. The explanation might be that the investigated tumour tissue came from necrotic and degenerated areas not representative of the hormone-producing parts. Thus, with the electron microscope, the secretory activity can be evaluated with accuracy.

Chromophobe adenomas

We have also been able to study cases with *chromophobe adenomas*. Ultramorphologists working with normal pituitary glands can recognize a special cell type for every one of the hormones produced in the organ. However, as the main difference between the cell types is the characteristics of the granulation, it is not possible to determine of the cell population of these adenomas is composed of only one type of tropic cells. Most of the work is also done on animals, and little is known about the ultrastructure of the normal human pituitary gland.

We have made a preliminary investigation of 15 chromophobe adenomas.

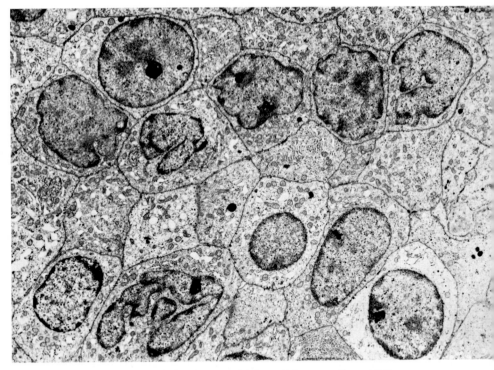

Fig. 2. "Empty" type of chromophobe adenoma with few cellular organelles. × 2000.

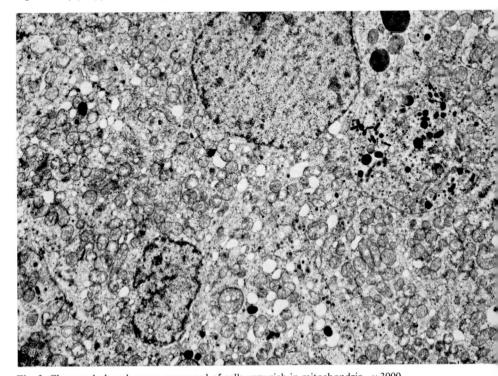

Fig. 3. Chromophobe adenoma composed of cells very rich in mitochondria. × 3000.

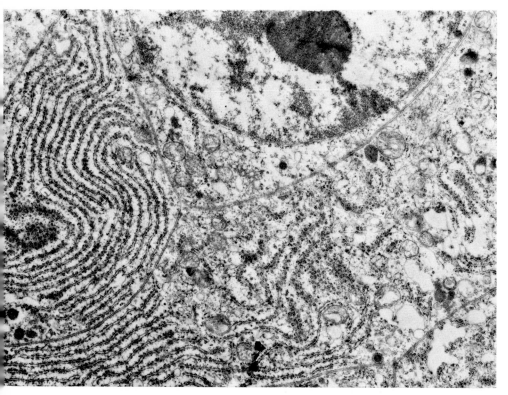

Fig. 4. Detail of cells of the third type of chromophobe adenoma, showing a characteristic endoplasmic reticulum. ×4000.

We then observed some different morphological patterns: The majority (9 of 15) are "empty", *i.e.,* are composed of densely packed cells with very few cellular organelles, including secretory granules (Fig. 2). Others are rich in mitochondria, showing high metabolic activity (Fig. 3). A third type shows, in addition to mitochondria, a characteristic endoplasmic reticulum (which is ultrastructural evidence of protein production) (Fig. 4). Up to now, however, we have not been able to correlate these ultramorphological subtypes with any characteristics in the clinical picture, nor with any laboratory data on the patients. But we hope that by extending to other methods—mainly the fluorescent antibody technique—we will be able to identify the tumour nature better and hereby also perhaps give some clues to the aetiology.

Ultrasonic selective hypophysectomy for advanced prostate or breast cancer and for pituitary diseases (Cushing's syndrome, acromegaly, diabetic retinopathy, etc.)

By Michele Arslan

Department of Otolaryngology, University Hospital, Padova, Italy

Surgical applications of ultrasound which have appeared to be very useful are the following: (1) Treatment of advanced, hydropic labyrinthosis (Ménière's disease), (2) Hypophysectomy, (3) Removal of larynx papilloma by direct application of the probe (through direct laryngoscopy) to the papilloma, and (4) Treatment of facial hemispasm, through direct application of the probe to the surgically exposed nerve trunk (Arslan, 1952, 1961, 1967).

The advantages, offered by this type of ultrasonic irradiation through a surgical approach, may be summarized as follows:

1. The possibility of destroying "at a distance" deep-lying organs or structures, without causing severe anatomical or functional damage to the surrounding tissues, thus greatly reducing surgical risks. The actual surgical part of the operation is thus limited to the production of a pathway to the target organ.

2. It is possible to produce selective lesions, both as regards the type of cell destroyed and the extent of the size and degree of destruction.

3. Harmlessness of ultrasound irradiation on the tissues immediately surrounding the target organ.

4. It is possible to repeat the ultrasound irradiation, possibly varying some of its characteristics, if the results of the first irradiation have proved insufficient. Irradiation may be repeated painlessly, as the access pathway produced at the time of the first irradiation remains patent.

Hypophysectomy is indicated at present in the following diseases: advanced cancer of the breast and prostate with bone metastases, diabetic retinitis, malignant exophthalmus, Cushing's syndrome, and acromegaly.

Different methods of destroying the function of the pituitary gland are currently used: (1) surgical excision of the gland through one of three approaches, *i.e.*, transfrontal, trans-ethmoidal, or transseptal, (2) implantation in the pituitary fossa of radioactive elements, (3) teleradiation of the pituitary, with X-rays or with alfa particles, protons, and accelerated neutrons, and (4) stereotactic cryohypophysectomy. These methods may be associated, in a certain percentage of cases, with complications such as intrasellar bleeding, cerebrospinal fluid rhinorrhoea, meningeal infection, damage to the optic chiasma or the hypothalamus, and oculomotor nerve palsy.

For some diseases, complete hypophysectomy with the resultant complete functional suppression of the pituitary, and the need for substitutive hormonal therapy, can represent a therapeutic mistake. In cases of pituitary "hyperfunction", such as in Cushing's syndrome, total excision of the gland is unnecessary, since its inhibition to a varying extent is sufficient to achieve a stable improvement of the clinical picture.

Experimental investigations

Research was first carried out on dogs. The histological and hormonal effects produced by the direct ultrasonic irradiation of the pituitary applied with variable intensity and duration were studied (Arslan and Ricci, 1967). The hypophysis of the dog was approached via the transpalatal route. In this method the soft palate was incised under general anaesthesia and the soft tissues of the rhinopharynx detached. A 5–6 mm hole was then drilled in the bone anterior to the spheno-occipital synchondrosis and after removal of all bone fragments the dural layers covering the hypophysis were completely exposed. A rod, similar to that used for ultrasonic irradiation of the human pituitary, was applied to the dural capsule through the bone opening. After irradiation the cavity was filled with antibiotic powder and the palate sutured.

Numerous experiments have been done with the new Siatem ultrasonic generator (Fig. 1) on groups of 5 dogs, one animal in each group being a control. The results of some of these experiments are reported as follows:

Group 1: Dogs subjected to irradiation of 2–5 W/cm^2 for 20 minutes.

Group 2: Dogs irradiated with 2–5 W/cm^2 for 40 minutes.

Group 3: Dogs irradiated with 15 W/cm^2 for 10 minutes or with 45 W/cm^2 for the same length of time.

Results

The animals showed a definite fall in the urinary 17-ketosteroids. In no case were appreciable histological lesions of the suprasellar endocranial region seen. A direct relation between the severity of cellular lesion and the intensity and length of time of irradiation, or both, was observed. We therefore believe that a selectivity of the protoplasmic effect of ultrasound, as re-

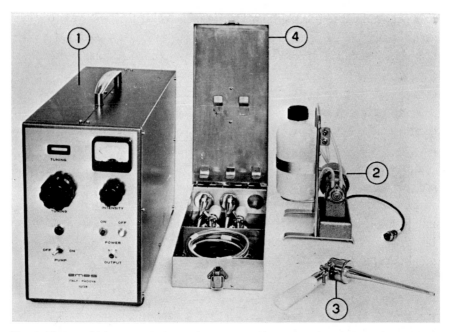

Fig. 1. The new high-powered ultrasonic generator Siatem for hypophysectomy, Ménière's disease, laryngeal papilloma, etc. 1. Generator. 2. Pump for continuous water circulation. 3. Ultrasonic probe. 4. Container of different probes.

corded by Fry (1958), can achieve in some cases a normalization of pathological hormonal secretory processes.

The effect of ultrasonic irradiation of the hypophysis is to produce cellular lesions with the damage very evident in the cytoplasm and less marked or absent in the nucleus. The cytoplasm of the basophil cells seems to be the most sensitive of the pituitary cells to the effect of ultrasound. This observation is confirmed by reduction of the 17-ketosteroids in irradiated animals. It is also noted that the effect of ultrasound on the hypophyseal parenchyma is irregular, resulting in areas with very severe lesions adjacent to areas in which the tissue seems to be less damaged. Everywhere, however, diffuse hyperaemia and sometimes small interstitial haemorrhages can be observed. In no case were lesions of the suprasellar endocranial region seen.

Clinical applications

This method of removing pituitary function by ultrasound at high intensity has the advantage of eliminating the complications which may be associated with surgical hypophysectomy, radioactive implantation of the pituitary, or of cryohypophysectomy. In fact, the application of ultrasound to the pituitary does not open, or perforate through, the capsule of the pituitary and there-

fore does not cause intracapsular bleeding. It avoids the possibility of trans-
sellar intracranial infection and it can be repeated several times without
danger. Finally, if low intensity ultrasound is used, it does not completely
abolish pituitary function but can bring about a "selective", *i.e.*, differential
cytolysis in the different types of cells that make up the pituitary tissue.

As to what concerns surgical technique, the trans-ethmoidal approach requires the demolition of bone walls, or of the ethmoid or the turbinate, and
leaves external face scars.

From another point of view, there is no doubt that the postoperative
complications which may be associated with surgical hypophysectomy or
with radioactive implantation may arise, directly or indirectly, either from a
narrow and deep operative field, with poor illumination or from excessive
bleeding due to the greater removal of bone by the trans-ethmoidal or transnasal approach.

The new principles upon which we have based our technique are essentially as follows: (1) The transseptal approach is used so that destruction of
nasal or sinus bones is not necessary and an external face scar is avoided,
(2) Increased visibility of the sella is achieved by means of two expedients:
a) a short incision at the base of the columella in order to remove the
columella from the operative field, and b) the use of the Zeiss operating
microscope, (3) Opening of the sella is done by using a drill with a curved
handle and with the help of operative microscopy. This allows an extremely
delicate action, which avoids damage to even the smallest vein of the capsule, (4) The ultrasonic probe is pressed firmly against the capsule which is
neither cut nor transfixed.

The surgical steps we employ consist of the following:

a) general anaesthesia with induced hypotension;

b) V incision of the nasal columella;

c) vertical incision of the septum at the level of the anterior margin of
the quadrangular cartilage (Fig. 2);

d) submucous resection of the middle part of the septum: this is mobilized
and lifted to the side of one of the two nasal fossae, so as to unify extensively
the two nasal fossae now forming a single cavity;

e) the anterior wall of the sphenoid sinuses is removed to create a wide
route of access to the sphenoidal sinuses;

f) very wide opening into the sphenoidal sinuses;

g) exact localization of the region corresponding to the sella turcica by
X-ray pictures taken during operation;

h) removal with a drill, under microscopic control (Zeiss operating microscope), of the postero-superior wall of the sphenoid sinuses;

i) the capsular sheath of the pituitary is freed as much as possible;

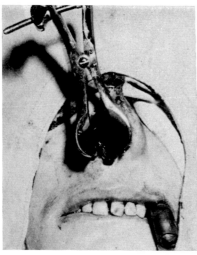

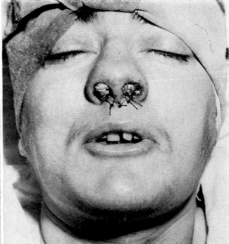

Fig. 2. Transcolumellar approach.   Fig. 3. Postoperative clcsure.

j) application of the irradiating probe, firmly held on the capsule of the hypophysis (Fig. 4);

k) cooling of the irradiator by circulating physiological saline at room temperature;

l) irradiation with ultrasound beam having the following characteristics: frequency 3 Mhz; intensity from 30 to 40 W/cm^2 ultrasound (average value); duration of irradiation 20 minutes or more;

m) replacement of the anterior septum in its primitive median position;

n) accurate suturing of the columellar incision;

o) loose packing of the operative cavity (posterior packing is useless) (Figs. 2 and 3).

After an interval of a month or more, the irradiation may be repeated in a completely bloodless way, by introducing the probe through one nasal fossa, with X-ray control.

Complications

The complications are summarized in the Tables 1 and 2.

Clinical effects of ultrasonic hypophysectomy

1. *Advanced cancer of the breast or prostate*

Fortyfive patients were treated with this method in our Department. General conditions improved very much and pain due to metastasis was rapidly lessened or disappeared altogether in all the patients.

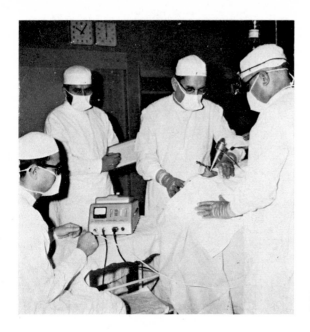

Fig. 4. Ultrasonic irradiation of the pituitary gland.

Hormonal tests showed pituitary inhibition as measured by doing 17-KS and 17-OHCS (hydroxycorticosteroid) determinations before and after the ultrasonic intervention. Inhibition was achieved on a second ultrasonic irradiation in 8 cases.

It must above all be stressed that there was in all our cases a total absence of surgical complications. The only complication we observe is a polyuria which decreases in some weeks with the use of posterior pituitary hormone.

Table 1. *Complications of the ultrasonic selective hypophysectomy. I.*

1964–1968 (1st June) Number of cases: 45

	Advanced breast cancer 33 cases	Advanced prostate cancer 12 cases
Post-operative death (0–4 weeks)	0	1 (*)
Cerebrospinal fluid rhinorrhoea	0	0
Cerebral haemorrhage	0	0
Cerebral thrombosis	0	0
Diabetes insipidus	1	0
Transient polyuria	29	8
Anosmia	0	0
Oculomotor palsy	0	0
Visual field defects	0	0
Mental changes	0	0

(*) *Man aged 60. Cause of death: cardiac arrest at 10th day after operation. Post-mortem examination revealed neither pituitary nor endocranial lesions.*

Table 2. *Complications of the ultrasonic selective hypophysectomy. II.*
1964–1968 (1 st June), *Number of cases: 45*

	Cushing's Disease 18 cases	Acromegaly 15 cases	Diabetic Retinopathy 12 cases
Post-operative death (0–4 weeks)	2 (*)	1	0
Cerebrospinal fluid rhinorrhoea	0	0	1
			(duration: 12 days)
Cerebral haemorrhage	0	0	0
Cerebral thrombosis	0	0	0
Diabetes insipidus	2	0	0
Transient polyuria	12	7	5
Anosmia	0	0	0
Oculomotor palsy	0	0	1
			(recovery after 2 months)
Visual field defects	0	0	0
Mental changes	0	0	0

(*) Case 1 Woman aged 63. Very severe progressively worsening Cushing's syndrome with sclerosis of myocardium. Cause of death: cardiac arrest at 7th day after the operation. Case 2 Man aged 60. Advanced prostate cancer with bone metastases. Cause of death: cardiac arrest at 10th day after operation.
Post-mortem examination in both cases revealed neither pituitary nor endocranial lesions.

In not even one case did we observe either cerebrospinal fluid rhinorrhoea, meningeal infection or nervous troubles.

Reduction of bone metastasis was observed in nearly all patients: in some the metastasis seemed to have completely disappeared. In some patients, 6 months or later after the intervention, the metastases reappeared in extension and number (Table 3).

2. Cushing's syndrome

Cushing's syndrome is a complex disease, characterized by adiposis, predominantly of the trunk with reddish skin, "full moon" face, bone fragility, hypertricosis, increase of blood pressure, hyperglycaemia, troubles of the metabolism of calcium and phosphorus, and frequent trophic lesions of the muscles (manifesting themselves through asthenia).

Eighteen patients were operated upon by ultrasonic hypophysectomy.

Table 3. *Response to the ultrasonic selective hypophysectomy (1964–1967).*

Number evaluated	Total	Regression	Static	Remission (R + S)	Pro-gression	Number still alive
1. Advanced breast cancer	33	15	9	24	9	23
2. Advanced prostate cancer	11	5	2	7	4	6

Postoperative course and clinical and hormonal effects on these patients can be summarized as follows:

a) *Postoperative course.* In 16 cases it was very good. All the patients could stand up 4–6 days after intervention. In no case was there meningeal symptoms, visual trouble, cerebrospinal fluid rhinorrhoea, etc.

In all cases a considerable increase of the diuresis was noted on the days immediately after the intervention; after 30 to 40 days, however, the urinary secretion returned to normal. The plasmatic rate of antidiuretic hormone (ADH), at first very much reduced, later became normal.

This would seem to indicate that the ultrasonic irradiation determines a reversible inhibition in the posterior pituitary.

b) *Actual clinical conditions.* After the operation the characteristic clinical symptoms of Cushing's syndrome decreased or disappeared. In particular, the disappearance of the full moon face was noticed; loss in weight oscillated between 10 and 20 kg; roughness of skin and facial rubor as well as hypertricosis were lessened. In the majority of cases, the blood pressure was considerably lower in the days following the intervention, and afterwards it was stabilized on 160/100 mm Hg. In some cases menstruation reappeared, normal and regular.

c) *Variations in the hormonal picture.* The postoperative variations in the rate of the urinary corticoids of four patients, 6 months after intervention, were measured.

Both the 17-KS and the 17-OHCS which were considerably increased before intervention, following it diminished so as to come back to normal limits.

The normalization of urinary corticoids is highly important, as it indicates clearly that the ultrasonic energy acts at the level of the hypophysary cells secreting the adrenocorticotrope hormone (ACTH), thus striking the fundamental factors of Cushing's syndrome.

In some cases the hypophysary gonadotropines have been measured: parallel to the normalization of the gonadotropine rate, menstruations which were absent pre-operatively reappeared and were normal as to rhythm, quantity and duration.

In some cases, in which there was a slight "prediabetic" condition, with slight increase of the basal glycaemia and diminished tolerance for glucose, the ultrasonic irradiation of the hypophysis practically corrected this metabolic alteration, bringing the glycaemic values down to normal. This appears as an extremely important datum, as it gives us the basis for planning, in the future, a possible new treatment for severe diabetic conditions.

Studies are now being carried out in the Department of Endocrinology of our University Hospital (Dr. Crepaldi *et al.*) on the variations both of the

Table 4. *Response to the ultrasonic selective hypophysectomy* (1965–1967).

Number evaluated	Total	Marked improvement No.	%	Light improvement No.	%	Static No.	%	Impairment No.	%
3. Cushing's disease	16	11	72	4	23	1	5	None	—
4. Acromegaly	14	9	—	3	—	2	–	None	—
5. Diabetic retinopathy	12	5	—	4	—	3	–	None	—

plasmatic cortisol rate and of the notesterified fat acids (NEFA) in 24 hours; it is known that disappearance of the nictemeral rhythm of the cortisol is actually considered as pathognomonic for Cushing's syndrome. Our observations up to now clearly indicate that in our patients this rhythm of the plasmatic cortisol that previously had disappeared for the disease was brought, after the operation, again to normal.

These first observations on the development of Cushing's syndrome after direct ultrasonic irradiation of the pituitary, seems to indicate that the effect of the ultrasonic energy is not of destruction but of correction, as regards the function of this gland. Naturally, the concept of "normalization" of the pituitary function is brought forward as a hypothesis for future researches. In this regard we would like to stress that if necessary a second, and even a third irradiation, is extremely easy to repeat, without any new surgical procedure, as approach to the sella remains open forever.

However, we can affirm that the results obtained up to now are highly satisfactory, both for the clinical improvement of the patients, and for the absence of any postoperative complications (Table 4).

3. *Acromegaly*

Fifteen patients were operated upon. One case died a week after operation: autopsy showed the presence of a tumor (adenoma) which was expanded at the suprasellar level and was not preoperatively recognized. By other cases, after the operation, there was a clear reduction of the hyperplasia of the face tissues, of the hands and the feet and of other clinical troubles. Variations of ACTH and of blood cortisol were observed. Variations of NEFA mobilization were observed too (Table 4).

4. *Diabetic retinopathy*

It is well known that diabetic retinopathy represents today a severe disease, and even a social clinical problem.

The diabetic retinopathy consists essentially of the following eye lesions: microaneurysms, haemorrhagic lesions, soft exudates in the vitreous body and, in the more advanced stages, neoformation of vessels.

Twelve patients were operated upon. Only two transitory complications

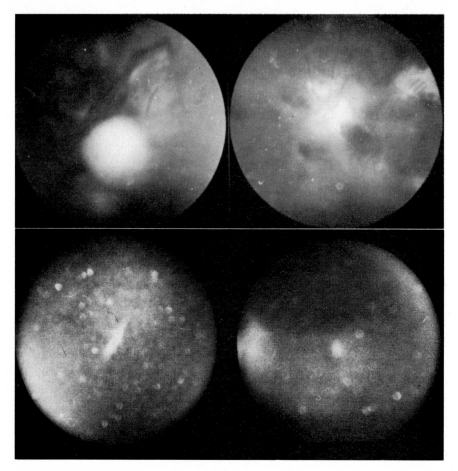

Fig. 5. Photographs of retina in 2 cases of diabetic retinopathy treated by ultrasonic hypophysectomy (on the left side: before the treatment).

were observed in two patients (Table 2). Following ultrasonic hypophysectomy, we have observed a partial resorption of the exudates of the vitreous body, with a moderate amelioration of vision (Fig. 5). As the patients had insulin-deprived primary diabetes, there were no appreciable variations in the basal glycaemia; on the contrary, the sensitivity to insulin was clearly increased, and the diabetes now balanced with a dose of insulin corresponding to less than half the dose which was necessary before the intervention.

This fact indicates that ultrasonic irradiation induces a diminished secretion of anti-insulin hormones, as happens, in Cushing's syndrome and acromegaly, for ACTH and the somatotropic hormone.

Summary

Results obtained with a new method of selective cellular inhibition of the hypophysis by means of a beam of ultrasonic waves of 30–40 W/cm² (average value) and 3 Mhz frequency are described. The method has been improved with a new surgical technique and used in a group of patients with advanced breast and prostate cancer, Cushing's syndrome, acromegaly and diabetic retinopathy. The clinical and hormonal improvement obtained with the operation was the same as those obtained with surgical hypophysectomy or intrasellar implantation of isotopes. Inhibition of the hypophysis with ultrasound does not require any incision or transfixion of the dura mater of the sella. This procedure has the great advantage of giving rise to no postoperative complications whatsoever.

References

Arslan, M., *Vint. Congr. Otorhinolaryng.*, Amsterdam, 429 (1953).

Arslan, M., *Minerva Otorinolaring., 15,* 1 (1965).

Arslan, M., *J. Laryng., 80,* 1 (1966).

Arslan, M., *Ann. Otol., 75,* 798 (1966).

Arslan, M., *Acta Otolaryng.* (Stockholm), *63,* 252 (1967).

Arslan, M. & Ricci, V., *Proc. Roy. Soc. Med., 61,* 7 (1968).

Arslan, M., Sala, O. & Molinari, G. A., *Acta Otolaryng.* (Stockholm), *56,* 154 (1963).

Cushing, H., *The pituitary body and its disorders,* Philadelphia & London (1912).

Fanucchin, F., Minetti, L. & Polvani, F., *Considerazioni metodologiche e ricerche sperimentali sulla possibilità della applicazione clinica dell'irradiazione ultrasonora ipofisaria.* Scritti Medici in onore del Prof. L. Villa. Milano, 315 (1957).

Frazier, C. H., *Ann. Surg., 57,* 145 (1913).

Fry, W. J., *Advances Biol. Med. Phys., 6,* 281 (1958).

Gordon, D., *Ultrasound as a diagnostic and surgical tool,* Edinburgh & London (1964).

Lawrence, J. H., Tobias, C. A., Born, J. L., Gottschalk, A., Linfoot, J. A. & Kling, R. P., *JAMA, 186,* 236 (1963).

Luft, R. & Olivecrona, H., *Cancer, 8,* 261 (1955).

Macbeth, R. G., *J. Laryng., 75,* 70 (1961).

Molinari, G. & Crepaldi, G., in press.

Molinatti, G. M., Camanni, F. & Tedeschi, M., *J. Clin. Endocr., 19,* 1144 (1959).

Rand, R. W., Dashea, M., Paglia, D. E., Conway, L. W. & Solomon, D. H., *JAMA, 189,* 87 (1964).

Rasmussen, H., *Acta Otolaryng.* (Stockholm), *52,* 519 (1960).

General discussion

Hammer to Laurén

Dr. Laurén's last slide showed a radiopaque structure in the posterior part of the sphenoidal sinus after transsphenoidal hypophysectomy. In an investigation with light, X-ray and fluorescence microscopy after tetracycline administration, we have shown this structure to consist of two different tissues: a dense organic matrix and newly formed compact bone. Postoperatively, the remineralization activity in the rebuilt area decreases gradually, being very minute after a year.

Wersäll to Wågermark

This morning we saw a beautiful slide demonstrating the localization of ACTH-producing cells as shown in Professor Arslan's laboratory. Could Dr. Wågermark comment on the possibility of demonstrating with some degree of specificity the localization of the various pituitary hormones in cells of varying type?

Wågermark to Wersäll

It is difficult to get pure preparations of pituitary hormone. Thus, it is hard to get specific antibodies. We have tried with fluorescent anti-growth hormone and found this to concentrate in eosinophilic cells.

Angell James to Arslan

Does Professor Arslan use cooling and, if so, by what means? What dosage does he use in the human being, since in the dog it required 40 watts cm² to cause necrosis? It seemed from the film that only 2.5 watts cm² was used in the human operation. In our experience in the rat, an intensity of 20 watts cm² is required to cause even partial necrosis. At this intensity the temperature rises 15°C in the gland even when continuous cooling is employed on the surface.

Bateman to Arslan

Will Professor Arslan explain the difference between polyuria and diabetes insipidus when he used these terms in his table of complications?

Grahne to Arslan

I should like to mention another method for doing hypophysectomy with a very minor surgical risk. That is the use of a cryogenic probe. We have used this method until now in 12 cases of advanced breast cancer. Through the septal approach we put the probe in the hypophysis, using $-60°C$. We cannot achieve a total destruction of the gland in all cases, but our experience of this kind of hypophysectomy is good, and above all the surgical risk is a very minor one.

Arslan to Angell James

In all our experiments, great care was taken to avoid any thermic action on the living pituitary submitted to ultrasonic irradiation. The new Siatem U.S. generator functions with circulating water constantly cooling the tip of the irradiator; by this technical arrangement, the thermic action is completely avoided.

Arslan to Bateman

The diagnosis of "diabetes insipidus" was made by endocrinologists, who routinely investigate our patients submitted to ultrasonic hypophysectomy.

Stereotaxic treatment of craniopharyngiomas

By Erik-Olof Backlund

Department of Neurosurgery, Karolinska Sjukhuset, Stockholm, Sweden

The mortality reported after attempts at radical surgical removal of cranio-pharyngiomas has usually been very high. In some surgical units where extraordinary interest and work have been devoted to this problem, it has been possible to reduce the mortality at primary operations, especially in children (Matson, 1964). In a few cases, when the tumour is mainly intrasel-lar, the transsphenoidal route can be used (Hamberger *et al.,* 1960). Never-theless, many experienced neurosurgeons agree with Olivecrona when he states that: "major surgical operations of craniopharyngiomas have probably lost most of their importance" (Olivecrona, 1967, Hamlin, 1968). Irradiation alone has been used with encouraging results (Kramer *et al.,* 1961, 1968). Nevertheless, there is considerable risk of radiation damage to the optic nerves and the adjacent structures. Thus, a new method in the management of these tumours is desirable, particularly in older patients and cases of recurrence.

In many craniopharyngiomas, the clinical manifestations are caused by a solitary, expanding cyst. The mere evacuation of such a cyst may be benefi-cial. However, recurrences are common after such treatment. In 1951, Lek-sell and Lidén in one case injected radioactive isotope directly into the cyst cavity to destroy its lining (Leksell and Lidén, 1952). Similar cases have since been described by other authors (Klar, 1953, Wycis *et al.,* 1954, Campbell and Hudson, 1960, Overton and Sheffel, 1963, Volkov *et al.,* 1963, Bond *et al.,* 1965).

Since 1960, the trial of this approach has been resumed at the Department of Neurosurgery, Karolinska Sjukhuset (Leksell *et al.,* 1967). The following tentative program has been formulated.

1. Diagnostic puncture of the tumour

Using the standard stereotaxic technique (Leksell, 1949, 1966), the tumour is punctured through a burr-hole. To avoid damage to the vessels of the circle of Willis, the coordinates of the anterior communicating artery are deter-

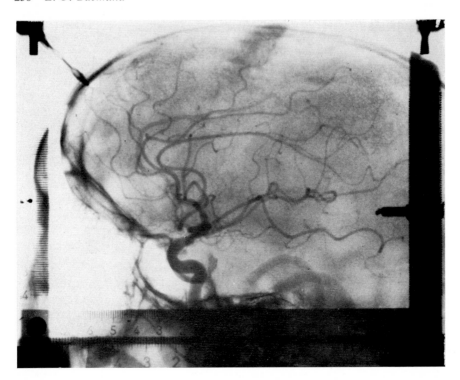

Fig. 1

mined after angiography (Fig. 1). This puncture shows whether the lesion is solid or cystic and, if the latter, the volume of the cyst. In the cystic cases, this diagnostic puncture often causes improvement in the clinical condition.

2. Therapeutic procedure

a) *Cystic lesions*

With the same stereotaxic technique, a heavy dose of beta-emitting isotope is injected into the cyst. If a pure beta emitter is used, the half-value depth of the radiation is about 1 mm.

^{32}P in the form of bismuth phosphate suspension is a useful compound because of its radio-opacity, but gives a very uneven dose distribution. Colloidal yttrium has proved to be superior to the phosphorus compound. As the Bremsstrahlung is sufficient for making a scintigram of the head, it is possible to demonstrate the distribution of the isotope postoperatively (Fig. 2).

b) *Solid lesions*

If at the diagnostic puncture the tumour is found to be predominantly solid, the choice of therapy is more difficult. We have attempted treatment by

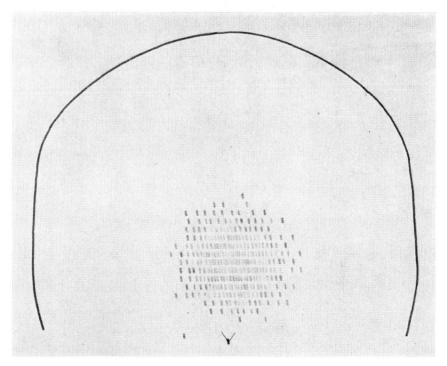

Fig. 2

stereotaxic radiosurgery in order to deliver a sufficient dose of radiation to the tumour without damage to the surrounding structures.

The technique has been developed primarily for thalamotomy in Parkinsonism and pain (Leksell, 1968). The radiolesion is produced by intense cross-firing of the target by a large number of narrow beams of gamma radiation. The radiosurgical apparatus consists of a hemispherical metal body with 179 beam sources of radioactive cobalt, and a movable operating table, to which a collimator helmet is attached. The beams are sharply focused on to the centre of the hemisphere. According to the coordinate determination, the patient's head is fixed to the helmet, and when the operating table is moved into the radiation unit, the tumour target will be placed in the beam focus.

The dose fall-off is extremely steep. A dose of 20 krads given to ordinary brain tissue in pain surgery (Leksell, 1968) has induced necrosis in a sharply demarcated area, shaped like a disc, with a maximum radius of 10 mm (Fig. 3).

Present series

The present series consists of 14 patients. Two of them had solid tumours and were treated radiosurgically. The 12 remaining patients with cystic

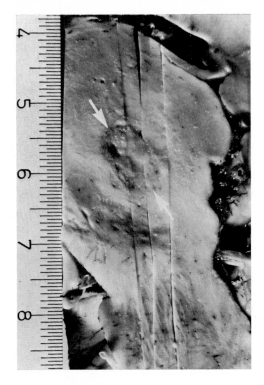

Fig. 3

tumours have been treated with isotope. One of these had two separate cysts which were treated at different times.

In the first six cystic cases, ^{32}P was used and the inside of the cyst wall received a heavy dose of about 200 krads. The next six cysts were treated with colloidal yttrium. With this compound, a dose of 20 krads to the cyst wall seems to be enough to induce shrinkage of the cyst. It should be mentioned that three patients received two injections of isotope because of re-accumulation of cyst fluid after the first injection. It was thought that the initial dose had been too small.

Table 1.

Symptoms and signs before treatment	Symptoms and signs after treatment			
	Impairment	No change	Improvement	Comments
Visual acuity disturbed in 9 cases	1		8	
Visual fields disturbed in 9 cases	3		6	
Headache in 5 cases	1		4	
Pathological *X-ray findings* in all 11 cases			7	Not yet controlled in the last 4 cases

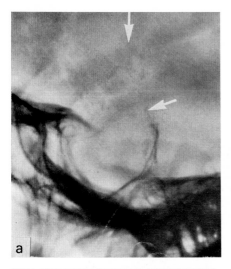

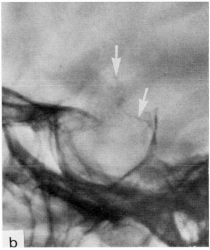

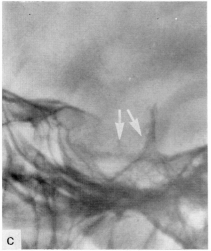

Fig. 4. In this case, the plain skull films showed scanty suprasellar calcification (a). An encephalogram revealed a rounded, apparently cystic tumour. The cyst was treated with ^{90}Y. Since then, the calcification has sunk gradually (pictures b and c), almost to the floor of the sella, probably indicating collapse of the cyst. Picture (c) was taken 10 months after the treatment.

Results

In the *cystic* group, there was one fatal case, a girl with a very large tumour and high intracranial pressure, who did not respond to the puncture and died in another hospital 3 months later. All the remaining cystic cases are well and had improvement of symptoms. The average observation time in the isotope group is 3 years and 1 month. The effect of the treatment on the most frequent symptoms and signs can be seen in Table 1. The radiological changes have often been dramatic (Fig. 4). In this isotope group, no serious complications or side-effects have been encountered.

Finally, a brief description is given of the two *solid* craniopharyngiomas treated with radiosurgery. The first occurred in an 18-year-old boy who had

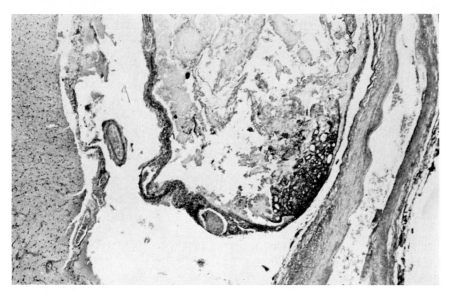

Fig. 5. A part of the tumour is seen between the brain stem and the basilar artery. The tumour is necrotic except for a thin crescent of vital craniopharyngioma tissue which can be seen close to the vessel.

a calcified tumour mass extending into the interpeduncular cistern, displacing the brain stem backwards. A Pudenz shunt had been inserted 6 months previously. Unfortunately, 4 months after a course of 2000 rads, he died as a result of obstruction to the shunt. This was confirmed at autopsy. There was almost complete destruction of the tumour, with only a thin crescent of surviving craniopharyngioma tissue. The surrounding brain substance was reported to be completely normal (Fig. 5).

In the other case, investigation showed a rounded tumour, extending backwards from the sella. At the diagnostic puncture, the tumour was felt to be very tough, and two small silver rods were inserted as indicators. A radio-surgical lesion was made in the centre of the tumour with a dose of 5000 rads. The position of the silver rods has been checked regularly since. One of the indicators has moved towards the site of the lesion, indicating shrinkage of the tumour (Fig. 6).

Conclusion

Intracystic injection of a heavy dose of beta-emitting radioisotope has proved to be a safe and effective treatment for craniopharyngioma cyst. In the management of predominantly solid tumours, particularly in older patients or those with recurrent lesions, the radiosurgical technique with precise, stereotaxically directed narrow gamma beams may offer a new solution to an old problem. Time will show the long-term merits of this technique.

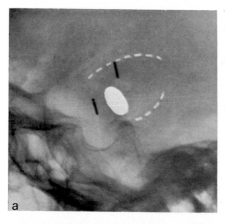

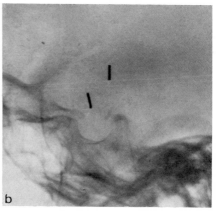

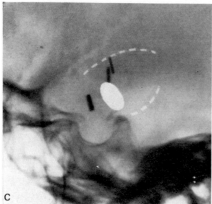

Fig. 6. In (a) the dotted lines represent the tumour surface as seen in the air study. The size and position of the radiosurgical lesion are indicated on the film by the white oval between the two silver indicators. (b) Eight weeks after the treatment, the posterior indicator is located closer to the site of the lesion. This can be seen more easily in (c), where the pictures (a) and (b) are superimposed.

References

Bond, W. H., Richards, S. & Turner, E., *J. Neurol. Neurosurg. Psychiat., 28,* 30 (1965).

Campbell, J. B. & Hudson, F. M., *Surg. Gynec. Obstet., 3,* 183 (1960).

Hamberger, C.-A., Hammer, G., Norlén, G. & Sjögren, B., *Acta Otolaryng.* (Stockholm), *52,* 285 (1960).

Hamlin, H., *Personal communication* (1968).

Klar, E., *Langenbeck Arch. Klin. Chir., 276,* 117 (1953).

Kramer, S., McKissock, W. & Concannon, J. P., *J. Neurosurg., 17,* 217 (1961).

Kramer, S., Southard, M. & Mansfield, C. M., *Amer. J. Roentgen., 103,* 44 (1968).

Leksell, L., *Acta Chir. Scand., 99,* 229 (1949).

Leksell, L. & Lidén, K., *A therapeutic trial with radioactive isotopes in cystic brain tumor.* Radioisotope techniques Vol. 1: Medical and physiological applications. H. M. Stationary Office, London (1952).

Leksell, L., *Some principal and technical aspects of stereotaxic surgery.* In Pain. Ed. by Knighton and Dumke. Little, Brown & Co, Cambridge (Mass.) (1966).

Leksell, L., Backlund, E.-O. & Johansson, L., *Acta Chir. Scand., 133,* 345 (1967).

Leksell, L., *Cerebral radiosurgery. I. Gammathalmotomy in two cases of intractable pain. Acta Chir. Scand.,* in press.

Matson, D. D., *Clin. Neurosurg., 10,* 116 (1964).

Olivecrona, H., *The craniopharyngiomas.* In Handbuch der Neurochirurgie, IV/4. Springer Verlag, Heidelberg (1967).

Overton, M. & Sheffel, D., *J. Neurosurg., 20,* 707 (1963).

Volkov, A. A., Vaskin, I. S., Zobina, M. D. & Muratkhodzhaev, M. K., *Med. Radiol.* (Moskva), *8,* 23 (1963).

Wycis, H., Robbins, R., Spiegel-Adolf, M., Meszaros, J. & Spiegel, E., *Confin. Neurol., 14,* 193 (1954).

Interstitial irradiation of the hypophysis

By Gustaf Notter

Department of Radiotherapy, Regionsjukhuset, Örebro, Sweden

Interstitial irradiation of the hypophysis is a relatively simple and rapid method to decrease and destroy the hormonal activity of the gland, and it is practically without operative mortality. For these reasons, it is often preferred to major surgical procedures.

However, the normal hypophysis is very radioresistant, and tolerates much higher doses than its surroundings. With ^{90}Y and ^{198}Au implants, pituitary necrosis does not develop until after radiation doses of 70–100 krad (Greening, 1957, Notter, 1959), while hypothalamus, optic chiasm and cranial nerves tolerate only 5000 rad.

A study of the hypophyseal topography shows that, usually, the distance from the periphery of the gland to the optic chiasm and the carotid artery is about 5 mm, and to the cranial nerves 10–15 mm. Accurate implantation of pure beta-emitters with localized radiation effect is therefore required if the hypophysis is to be irradiated intensively, without damage to the surrounding tissue, or if selective destruction of the adeno- or neurohypophysis is to be achieved.

Concerning irradiation of the more radiosensitive and voluminous pituitary adenomas, a lower but more extended dose distribution from gamma sources such as ^{198}Au or ^{192}Ir is preferable.

Two techniques of isotope implantation can be distinguished. The first is the stereotactic one suggested by Talairach (1956), in which the hypophysis is implanted centrally with multiple short pellets. This produces a relatively large source in the centre of the gland, and increases the dose to the periphery. Overdosage to the optic nerves can be avoided by implantation of inactive pellets near the diaphragm (Juret and Hayem, 1960). However, adequate irradiation to the lateral parts still remains difficult, due to the oval shape of the hypophysis.

In the non-stereotactic technique, which is used by most operators, the isotopes are inserted centrally in each half of the hypophysis under fluoroscopic control. This provides a better dose distribution to the lateral parts of the gland. However, if the cylinders are not implanted accurately 3–4 mm from the midline, remnants of pituitary tissue will survive.

The best dose distribution is achieved by a combination of the two techniques, with implantation of 30 small spheres in each half of the gland (Notter, 1959). With this technique, total histological destruction was achieved in 80%, but cerebrospinal rhinorrhoea occurred in 30%. To improve our results, we followed the suggestions of Mullan and Harper (1963), using a ^{90}Sr-^{90}Y needle.

We produced two identical ^{90}Sr applicators, containing 95 mCi, with an active length of 4.5 mm. The source was placed in the top of a needle with 1 mm outer diameter. The dose rate at 4 mm distance from the surface of the needle was 800 rad/min, and 40 krad could be delivered simultaneously to both sides of the hypophysis within 50 min.

However, the active length of 4.5 mm was too short to effect total destruction of the gland when the source was placed centrally on both sides. Histological examination of some hypophyses showed remnants of surviving tissue in the anterior and posterior part of the gland. Two applications were therefore necessary on both sides, one in the anterior and another in the posterior part of the gland. By this means, total hypophysectomy was achieved in all accurately implanted cases.

To shorten the operative time, a new applicator with adjustable length from 1–14 mm, containing 500 mCi ^{90}Sr, was constructed. The source can be covered by a shutter of 0.5 mm steel, which absorbs 93% of the primary radiation. This applicator delivers 40 krad in 4 mm distance within 25–35 min, depending on the length of the source.

During the last two years, we have irradiated 27 patients with the ^{90}Sr applicator with good clinical results, and without complications (Notter et al., 1968).

The complications after interstitial irradiation of the hypophysis are usually of two types: radiation damage to the cranial nerves, and cerebrospinal leakage. The first complication can be avoided completely by accurate implantation. The second one cannot be predicted. In most instances, it can be prevented by screw implantation in the front wall of the sella (Forrest, 1958), or better by paraffin injection (Hayem and Juret, 1962). We have used both techniques, but now prefer the intrasellar injection of 0.1 ml of a paraffin-Y_2O_3 mixture under fluoroscopy through a special, electrically heated cannula. This prevented cerebrospinal leakage in our last 25 patients and stopped it in three earlier operated cases (Notter and Melander, 1968). Compared to the permanent implantation of ^{90}Y or ^{198}Au seeds, the use of a ^{90}Sr applicator offers several advantages:

The applicator can be used for many years, because of the long half-life of 28 years, which means decreased costs per irradiation.

The dosimetry is easier and more accurate.

The implantation is easier and more reliable; moreover, fractionated and postoperative irradiations can be performed safely.

The radiation dose can be reduced significantly, because of the high dose rate. According to Harper's and our own experience, 40 krad given in 30–60 min correspond to 70–100 krad given with ^{90}Y.

The use of a ^{90}Sr applicator seems, for these reasons, to be the method of choice for interstitial irradiation of the hypophysis, and we wish to recommend this technique to all who are interested in this form of radiation therapy.

Also, if gamma radiation is required, the applicator can be used, because the ^{90}Sr-^{90}Y source can easily be changed to a ^{192}Ir source.

References

Forrest, A., Blair, D. & Valentine, J., *Lancet, 2,* 192 (1958).

Greening, W., *Proc. Roy. Soc. Med., 50,* 867 (1957).

Hayem, M. & Juret, P., *Presse Med., 70,* 1582 (1962).

Harper, P. V., Strandjord, N., Moseley, R. & Lathrop, A., *Nuclearmedizin,* suppl. 3, *29,* 447 (1964).

Juret, P. & Hayem, M., *Presse Med., 68,* 1044 (1960).

Mullan, S., Harper, M., Tani, E., Vailati, G. & Lathrop, K., *J. Neurosurg., 20,* 940 (1963).

Notter, G., *Acta Radiol.* (Stockholm), suppl. 184 (1959).

Notter, G. & Melander, O., *Acta Radiol.* (Stockholm), *6,* 491 (1967).

Talairach, J., Aboulker, J., Tournoux, P. & David, M., *Neurochirurgie, 2,* 3 (1956).

Holmér, A., Bärring, N., Melander, O., Notter, G. & Widell, C., *Fortschr. Roentgenstr., 106,* 574 (1967).

Pharyngeal hypophysis following hypophysectomy

By Gunnar Moberger

Department of Radiopathology, Karolinska Sjukhuset, Stockholm, Sweden

As far back as in 1838, Rathke presented evidence that the adeno-hypophysis was embryonically derived from the nasopharyngeal mucosa. He also showed that, in the adult organism, remnants of this epithelial deviation exist in the form of a strand of cells along the so-called canalis craniopharyngeus, commonly known as Rathke's pouch. Because of the minute dimensions of this strand, which is macroscopically invisible, it requires a special technique to be demonstrated. The strand follows the dorsal margin of the vomer, passes through the posterior portion of the sphenoid bone, and enters the sella turcica from below (Fig. 1).

By means of serial sectioning of the soft tissue in the roof of the nasopharynx, some remnants can always be found. A negative finding is likely to be due to a faulty technique. In 20 autopsy specimens with normal hypophysis, we were able to demonstrate a pharyngeal hypophysis in 12 cases. The histological structure varied considerably. In some specimens, it consisted merely of a tiny strand of partly squamous differentiated cells. In other cases, single small nodules were found, with a diameter of less than 0.2 mm. The nodules consisted of undifferentiated reticular cells, mostly resembling an embryonic mesenchymal stroma (Fig. 2).

The hypophysectomies performed by Dr. Notter (1959) by means of implanting radioactive yttrium bullets in the hypophysis resulted in some cases in partial destruction of the adeno-hypophysis. In other cases, complete destruction was achieved. Such cases were considered to offer an opportunity of studying the effect of inactivation of the normal hypophysis on the cellular development in the pharyngeal hypophysis.

Of 31 patients who had died from their cancer disease more than 2 months after destruction of the hypophysis, autopsy could be performed in 25 cases. The nasopharyngeal mucosa was removed, and serial sectioning revealed a pharyngeal hypophysis in 12 of the cases. In 7 of these cases in which the post mortem examination showed complete destruction of the hypophysis, the pharyngeal hypophysis had undergone drastic changes. Thus, it was considerably enlarged and formed an elongated solid, glandular-like structure deviating from the mucosa towards the periosteum at the edge of the vomer (Fig. 3).

In the enlarged pharyngeal hypophysis in the 7 cases with destroyed sel-

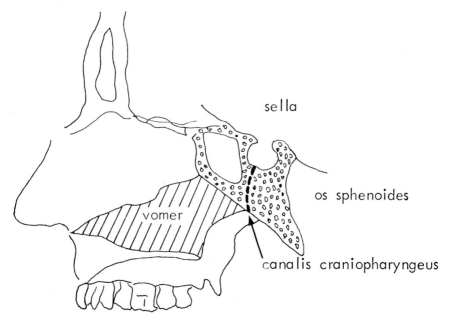

Fig. 1. Location of the canalis craniopharyngeus (Rathkes pouch).

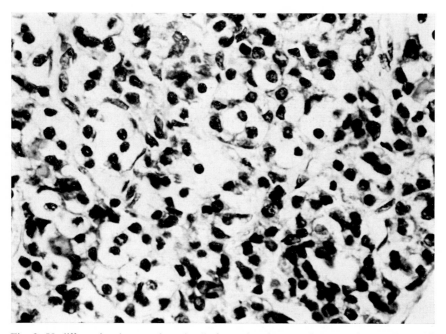

Fig. 2. Undifferentiated mesenchymal cells from the pharyngeal mucosa in a patient with normal hypophysis. Photo-micrograph × 650.

lar hypophysis, all the cellular components normally found in the anterior lobe of the hypophysis could be demonstrated, with a predominance of acidophilic chromophils (Fig. 4). A regular adeno-hypophysis had thus developed from the embryonic remnants along Rathke's pouch, mostly within the nasopharyngeal mucosa.

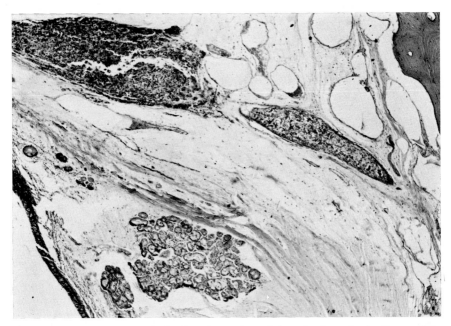

Fig. 3. Nasopharyngeal hypohysis after destruction of the sellar hypophysis. Photo-micrograph × 40.

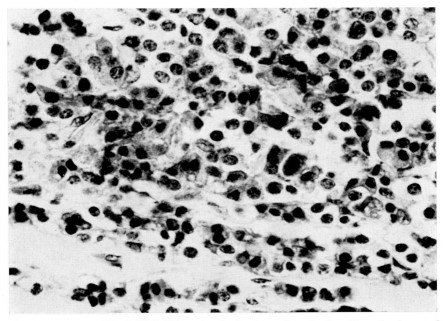

Fig. 4. The same as Fig. 3. Well differentiated adenohypophyseal cells with predominance of acidophilic chromophiles. Photo-micrograph × 650.

The biological significance of such an extrasellar hypophysis remains unknown. From a scientific point of view it may, however, be interesting to find that this cellular differentiation, and probably also cellular function, can take place distant from any direct contact with the neuro-hypophysis and the hypothalamus.

Since the area with the pharyngeal hypophysis is easily available, especially when hypophysectomy is performed by means of trans-antrosphenoidal surgery according to Hamberger, it could be questioned whether total hypophysectomy should not also involve cauterization of the pharyngeal mucosa at the site of Rathke's pouch.

General discussion

Lundberg to Backlund:

There are a few points which I think should be taken into consideration when the treatment of craniopharyngiomas is discussed.

It should be borne in mind that many craniopharyngiomas have a very irregular shape. There are sometimes isolated nodules of tumour tissue in the cyst walls, sometimes the tumour is built up as a conglomerate of several cysts and solid tumour nodules.

Furthermore, the results of surgical treatment have improved greatly during the last years. It is surprising to hear Dr. Backlund use a statement of Olivecrona from 1963 as background for the stereotaxic treatment introduced by Leksell. I think that Olivecrona's pessimistic view was at least partly based on experience from the pre-cortisone era. In any case it is by no means up to date. The fact is that nowadays craniopharyngiomas can be radically extirpated with good results. This was first convincingly shown by Matson in a report from 1964 where he presented a mixed series of 31 adults and children. The postoperative mortality was 3.2 % after primary operations. In his present material of 57 children, there are 5 postoperative deaths, all of which occurred after secondary attempts to remove tumours that had become symptomatic after a previous subtotal surgical procedure or radiation. There was no postoperative mortality after primary total extirpation in 46 cases. These results are surely due to an excellent surgical technique, but also to a meticulous endocrinological supervision during the postoperative course.

In Lund we have removed 7 tumours radically during the last 5 years without operative mortality. In one case the tumour recurred after one year and was totally removed at a second operation. Two patients are slightly incapacitated, the others are in excellent condition.

Against *this* background I think it is clear that an attempt at total removal should be made as a first step in all cases of craniopharyngioma. To start with some kind of radiation treatment is not justified.

Olivecrona to Backlund and Lundberg:

The remark, referred to by Dr. Backlund, was made a few years (6–7 years) ago, after I had reviewed the results in my series of about 120 cases. These showed a very high mortality in total extirpations. In incomplete extirpations, the immediate mortality was quite low, but the late results were disappointing, as most of them died from recurrence within a few years. I was also impressed by McKissock's article on the subject, who as well as Northfield, had a high mortality in total extirpations and therefore changed his policy, and instead of extirpation treated the craniopharyngiomas with roentgen radiation, using a rotating technique and a high-voltage machine. His results with this method of treatment were very good, with no mortality and good functional results. The doses employed were very high, up to 9000 rad, and I am a little doubtful whether these high doses really will be tolerated in the long run. Improvements in the results of total extirpations, by the use of cortisone and steroid treatment before and after the operation, have recently been reported. Nevertheless, I think that the method presented by Dr. Backlund shows excellent results, with no mortality, and will probably in the long run prove to be superior to total extirpations.

Notter to Backlund:

Was the irradiation given as a single dose or fractionated?

Backlund to Lundberg:

If one analyzes the 27 cases of craniopharyngioma which have been admitted to the Department of Neurosurgery, Karolinska Sjukhuset, since 1960— when Professor Olivecrona completed the collection of material for his series—one finds that 16 cases had a large solitary cyst, 6 were cystic or polycystic but had in addition a considerable solid component, and 5 cases were predominantly solid or had only microcysts. Thus, the majority were suitable for isotope treatment. In the polycystic group, one case had two cysts separated by a portion of solid tumour. Both these cysts were injected with isotope, on separate occasion, with a good result both clinically and radiologically.

Backlund to Notter

The patients received a single dose of radiation with an irradiation time of 10 and 25 minutes, respectively.

Padovan to Notter

I am persuaded that the stereotaxic method about which Dr. Notter has spoken gives us also a safe method of application of the isotopes into the hypophysis. Especially interesting is the application of radioactive strontium. We started with application of radioactive isotopes into the sella turcica in cases of hypophyseal tumours in 1956; first with direct application of pearls of radioactive cobalt (Co60) and later on we continued the therapy with implantation of radioactive gold and yttrium.

According to our opinion, in intrasellar tumours, the extranasal transseptal approach with application of radioactive isotope gives good results. We have tried all transnasal surgical methods, but today we personally consider as the method of choice the approach described in Archives of Otolaryngology by the group of rhinosurgeons in San Francisco (R. Netzer, E. Gordon and McCoy). This method gives, according to our opinion, the largest and the most secure approach to the hypophysis. The method consists of the following: (a) lateral rhinotomy, (b) temporary transposition of the lateral wall of the nasal cavity into the maxillary sinus, (c) the submuco-periosteal resection of the bony part of the nasal septum is performed. This is the safest way to hypophysis. When the tumour is taken out in the typical way, the radioactive isotopes (gold or yttrium) are applied into the sellar region. The covering of the sella by a piece of fascia lata and the muco-periosteum of the nasal septum prevents the endocranial complications—infection—and rhino-liquor-rhea. Our opinion is based on experience and on the material of Professor Šercer and myself. Šercer started with transnasal hypophysectomy in 1926, and all these problems have been treated from the anatomical, radiological and surgical point of view, by his collaborators, myself, Professor Krmpotić, Dr. Spaventi and Dr. Nemanić and others for the last 10 years (our material consists totally of 261 cases of hypophysectomies).

Escher to Moberger

I congratulate Dr. Moberger on his paper. The demonstration that from undifferentiated cells a differentiation and an augmentation may arise is an answer to two of my questions of this morning. (1) A compensation for a hypophysis is possible. (2) If a differentiation even from the pharyngeal cells is possible, we can also admit that a considerable regeneration of small cell remains may be possible. The unknown fact is still if these cells work again, stimulating the endocrine function.

Moberger to Escher

Thank you, Professor Escher. I agree with you that the endocrine function of the differentiated hypophyseal cell elements outside the sellar hypophysis still remains unknown. It is interesting however, that in several cases with destroyed hypophysis in our material we have also found a considerable volume of hypophyseal tissue along the pituitary stalk, as well as in the meninges beneath hypothalamus. Since it is well known that hypophyseal activity may be preserved from small amounts of adenohypophyseal tissue after incomplete destruction of the hypophysis, it is reasonable to assume that extrasellar hypophyseal tissue may exhibit endocrine function.

Chairman's summary of session IV

N. Riskaer

When trying to summarize the papers read this afternoon, I think that it is appropriate first to stress a few main points regarding Dr. Laurén's report on the sella turcica in the presence of pituitary tumours. This is because the anatomical conditions in and around the sella, especially in the sphenoid sinus, are of essential importance in relation to indication for and performance of any operation on the pituitary body, whether surgical ablation, stereotaxic implantation or ultrasonic hypophysectomy.

The normal anatomical variations will, of course, influence the direction of growth of a possible intrasellar pituitary tumour. It grows chiefly in the direction where it meets with the last resistance, a fact on which the symptomatology will depend. As for the symptomatology of pituitary tumours, Harvey Cushing, as early as 1912, set up four different categories: (1) neighbourhood symptoms, (2) general pressure manifestations, (3) secretory or glandular symptoms proper, (4) polyglandular manifestations. Deformity of the sella turcica constitutes an important factor in the group of neighbourhood symptoms which, in addition, comprise subjective discomforts and visual disturbances. It can be mentioned here that the first symptom of an intrasellar pituitary tumour is often a characteristic bitemporal, intense and persistent headache, presumably caused by tightening of the glandular membrane, before changes are visible in the sella itself. This headache, which differs completely from those incited by a general increase in intracranical tension, often decreases or even disappears when the dura of the pituitary bed has become maximally distended, and the proper enlargement of the sella starts, or the tumour stops growing. It is, however, remarkable that the sella itself may become greatly enlarged in response to a *slowly* increasing pressure, without this causing more than slight subjective troubles. Regarding the question of enlarged sella and visual disturbances, there is a reason to point out the observation first made by Cushing, i.e., that the degree of involvement of chiasm, nerves or tracts bears no direct relation to the size of the sella. In many cases of acromegaly, an enlarged sella has been found without visual disturbances. On the other hand, in patients with primary hypopituitarism and chromophobe adenoma, the visual disturbances were usually profound. The description of the pathological deformation of the sella justifies the conclusion that a correlation may exist between the pathology of a tumour and the radiographic findings in the sella, as Dr. Laurén mentioned. However, clinical observation of the patient and hormone analysis are, of course, more important aids towards establishing the existence and the type of the tumour.

Concerning the transsphenoidal treatment of pituitary tumours or destruction of the normal gland, Professor Arslan and Dr. Notter documented the possibilities of, respectively, the ultrasonic method and radiation with still more exactly calculated doses, and very accurate stereotaxic implantation of radioactive isotopes in the pituitary body. Professor Arslan has done pioneer work and achieved excellent results with ultrasonic treatment of different pituitary disorders, especially Cushing's disease. This method has, as Professor Arslan underlined, the advantages that the dura is not opened, and that the treatment can be repeated if necessary. But it seems necessary to have the assistance of a competent physicist to control and measure energy output. Moreover, experimental work on the effect of ultrasound energy on different tissues is still controversial. Dr. Notter has evidently improved his original technique for radioactive implantation treatment, so that it now seems possible to perform partial or functional complete hypophysectomy in this way without grave risks. Dr. Moberger's demonstrations of the anatomy and function of the pharyngeal hypophysis was of great clinical interest in relation to the problems of the radicality of hypophysectomy. I am sure that all doctors who try to eliminate pituitary function completely will keep his observations in mind.

The aforementioned non-surgical methods for pituitary destruction—and possibly also cryohypophysectomy as described by Dr. Grahne in the discussion—may perhaps contribute to reducing the number of surgical hypophysectomies in the future. There will doubtless still be some cases, however, which require surgical treatment, and I am here especially thinking of the otological transsphenoidal approach. In addition to cases where non-surgical treatment has proved ineffective in intrasellar tumours, certain types of visual disturbances associated with pituitary tumours may also show the best results when treated by transsphenoidal operation. Whether transfrontal or transsphenoidal removal of pituitary tumours has special advantages in cases with visual disturbances was studied by Henderson in 1939. He found that, in his series, transfrontal operation gave improved vision in most cases, and the highest frequency of freedom from recurrence over a 5-year period, 57.5 % against 32.8 % after transsphenoidal operation. Henderson nevertheless recommended transsphenoidal operation in certain cases, owing to its unquestionably greater improvement of the vision of patients with homonymous hemianopsia due to tract involvement, or with bilateral central scotoma, i.e., cases which are likely to have a prefixed chiasm. Dr. Backlund presented an interesting paper about the stereotaxic technique and implantation of radioactive isotopes as treatment in a case of craniopharyngioma. I consider this a strictly neurosurgical problem and, consequently, as an otologist have no comments.

As a conclusion of the problems dealt with in this session, I find that—from an otological aspect—the central problems to be decided on in the near future within pituitary treatment are probably the following: a more exact delimitation of the cases in which the transsphenoidal approach is preferable to the transfrontal, and clarification of the question whether stereotaxic implantation of radioactive isotopes, ultrasonic treatment, or possibly cryohypophysectomy is preferable to frank removal—always, or in special cases. A still closer collaboration with endocrinologists and neurosurgeons is required to solve the problems.

GLOMUS JUGULARE TUMOURS

Glomus jugulare tumours—introduction

By John E. Bordley

Department of Otolaryngology, The Johns Hopkins Hospital, Baltimore, Maryland, U.S.A.

On April 10, 1941, Stacy R. Guild, Ph.D. read a 225-word report before the 57th Annual Meeting of The American Association of Anatomists (1941). It was subsequently printed in the abstracts of that meeting as part of Anatomical Record 79. The title of this report was "A Hitherto Unrecognized Structure—The Glomus Jugularis in Man". He reported his observations from a study of thirty serially sectioned temporal bones. In it he described a small structure in several respects resembling the carotid body (Fig. 1). This body was usually observed in the adventitia of the dome of the jugular bulb below the bony floor of the middle ear (Fig. 2). He described the glomus as a small ovoid body consisting of blood vessels of capillary or pre-capillary caliber with numerous epithelioid cells between these vessels, and he stated that the vessels are the more prominent feature (Fig. 3). He also observed that innervation and blood supply come from the same trunks that supply the carotid body, namely the glossopharyngeal nerve and the ascending pharyngeal artery through its inferior tympanic branch. He suggested the name Glomus Jugularis.

This report was Dr. Guild's only publication on the glomus body until March 24, 1953, some 12 years later, when he wrote a definition of it for the new Gould Medical Dictionary. In his letter to Dr. Carl Francis (1953), the editor, he acknowledged one of his rare grammatical mistakes when he accepted the suggestion made by Waltner to change the name of the glomus from Glomus Jugularis to Glomus Jugulare. Dr. Guild had overlooked the fact that the Latin word in its adjective form was neuter. His definition is worthy of quotation today: "A tiny mass of tissue similar in structure to the carotid body and like it non-chromaffin paraganglion. Jugular bodies may be located anywhere along the course of the nerve of Jacobson (tympanic branch of the glossopharyngeal nerve) (Figs. 4 and 5), or of the nerve of Arnold (auricular branch of the vagus nerve). About one-half the bodies are found along the courses of these nerves in the adventitia of the dome of the superior bulb of the internal jugular vein. As many as 12 jugular bodies have been found in the sections of one human temporal bone. The average number present is slightly less than three."

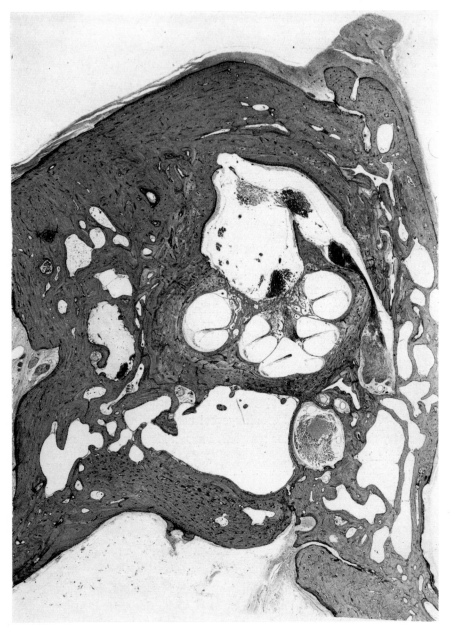

Fig. 1. Low power photomicrograph, showing a glomus body in the adventitia of the superior jugular bulb. It lies adjacent to the course of the Jacobson's and Arnold's nerves. (From Guild.)

Later in 1953, Dr. Guild presented his final work on the glomus jugulare before The American Otological Society at its annual meeting (1953). In this paper he reviewed the findings of studies on 88 serially sectioned temporal bones. He reported that 248 glomus formations had been found—135 of them closely associated with the tympanic branch of the glossopharyngeal nerve

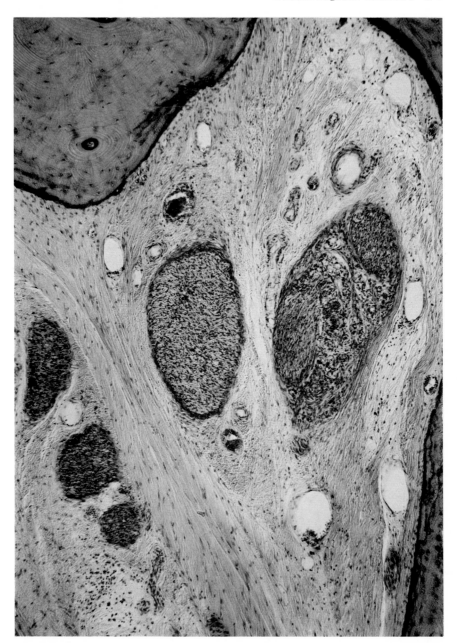

Fig. 2. Medium power photograph of glomus body in Fig. 1. It lies above Jacobson's and Arnold's nerves.

and 113 of them along the auricular branch of the vagus nerve. He pointed out the fact that most of them were seen in the adventitia of the jugular bulb. He felt that the difference in the order clinical symptoms that had been reported in glomus jugulare tumours could be accounted for by the difference in the observed location of the normal jugular bodies.

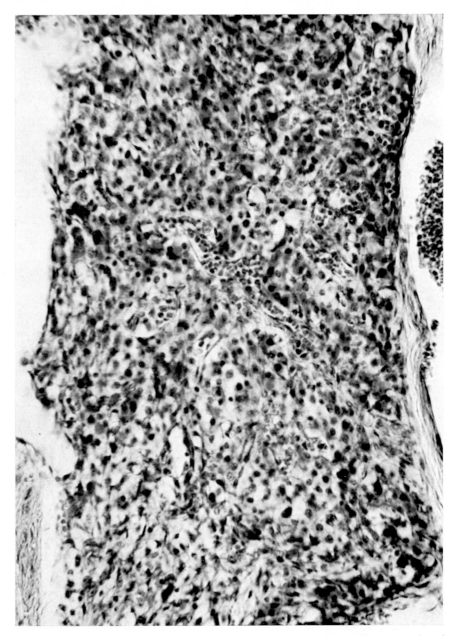

Fig. 3. High power photograph through glomus body, showing the precapillary network and epithelioid cells.

In this paper Dr. Guild discussed the reports of Valentine in 1846 and Krause in 1878. He felt that the histologic appearance of the glomus jugulare was different from those structures described by them. He drew attention to the fact that small aggregations of peripheral ganglion cells were a common occurrence along the course of the nerve of Jacobson, and these structures

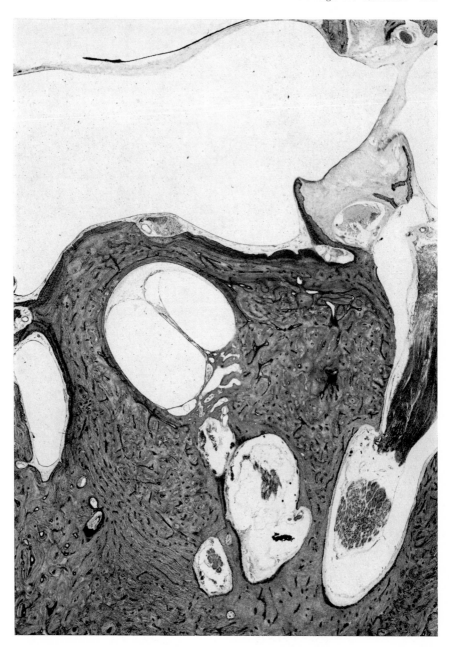

Fig. 4. Glomus body on the promontory arising in the tympanic plexus.

were what Valentine had observed. Krause's paper entitled "Die Glandula Tympanica des Menschen" concerned only the connective tissue in the osseous canal through which the nerve of Jacobson passed from the jugular fossa to the middle ear cavity.

Dr. Guild's original report in the Anatomical Record in 1941 contained

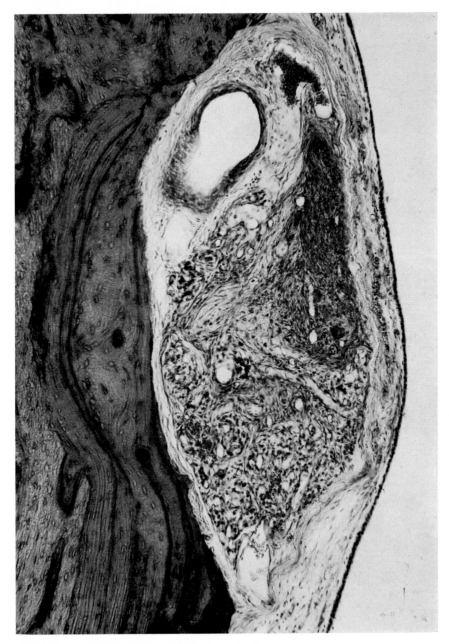

Fig. 5. Enlargement of glomus body shown in Fig. 4.

no illustrations. No reprints were obtained of this article, and it remained un-
noticed until early in 1942 when Dr. Harry Rosenwasser found a notation
concerning the report in a publication named "The Diplomate". On June 8,
1942, he wrote a note asking Dr. Guild for a complete report of the paper.
Dr. Guild replied that the 225-word report on the peculiar structure was all

that had been written and that he hoped to find some time someday to continue his study. Dr. Rosenwasser had removed a tumour from the middle ear, vascular, dark purple in color which appeared attached to the posterior canal wall. It had been reported as a carotid body-type tumour. The occurrence of a carotid body tumour in the middle ear without evidence of a carotid tumour in the neck seemed to him difficult to understand. He was looking for some other explanation for the origin of this tumour. When he reported this tumour in 1945, Dr. Rosenwasser made the following observation: "Of extreme interest and possibly providing theoretically, at least, a morphologic explanation of the presence of a carotid body tumour in the middle ear and the mastoid process is a communication of Dr. Stacy R. Guild's in which he states 'human temporal bone sections reveal structures in several respects like the carotid body for which the name glomus jugularis is proposed'. "Dr. Rosenwasser concluded, "the possibility that the tumour herein reported may have developed from the glomus jugularis first named by Guild is tentatively proposed". Upon reading this report, Dr. Guild wrote Dr. Rosenwasser a letter which the latter has used as an illustration in his recent excellent article on the glomus jugulare (Rosenwasser, 1968). In this letter Dr. Guild stated, "What I wanted to tell you was that I agree with you that the structure I reported as normal for the region may well be the basis of the tumour in your patient." The clinician and the man in the laboratory had joined hands to explain the origin of the most common middle ear neoplasm.

Dr. Guild's correspondence following Dr. Rosenwasser's publication includes many letters from all over the world by otologists and pathologists describing tumours of the middle ear and asking his advice concerning publication. Unfortunately, much of this correspondence has not yet been made available. However, the letters catalogued to date are a veritable roll call of the early authors; such names as Le Compte, Strauss, Winship, Waltner and Riemenschneider are but a few of those authors with whom he corresponded on this subject. He was always interested and enthusiastic, but his weakness for procrastination is evidenced in these records. A note from Professor Terracol, who dedicated his fine monograph (1956) to Dr. Guild, Dr. Rosenwasser and Dr. Masson, illustrates Dr. Guild's lack of concern over the passage of time. He received the note in mid-October of 1956. In it Professor Terracol inquired of him if he had ever received copies of his work on the glomus jugulare which had been forwarded from France. In mid-November 1956, Dr. Guild replied that indeed he had received two copies of the monograph sometime during the early summer; and he apologized for the fact that somehow they had been overlooked, and he had even forgotten to send the second copy to Dr. Rosenwasser as Professor Terracol had directed. He freely accepted the blame for the five month's delay.

The 225-word report read in 1941 is remarkable in a number of ways. It typifies the brevity of Dr. Guild's communications and comments. In it he reported his greatest contribution to otology; and in it he committed one of his few published grammatical mistakes. With this brief statement a new concept concerning the origin of a middle ear tumour was born. It is surely fitting that his name and his splendid histological observations be recalled as we here today undertake to develop a broader understanding of glomus jugulare tumours.

References

Guild, S., *Anat. Rec., 79,* suppl. 2 (1941).

Guild, S., *Correspondence to Carl Francis, M.D.* (March 1953).

Guild, S., *Ann. Otol., 62,* 1045 (1953).

Krause, W., *Zbl. Med. Wiss.* (1945).

Rosenwasser, H., *Arch. Otolaryng.* (Chicago), *41,* 64 (1945).

Rosenwasser, H., *Arch. Otolaryng.* (Chicago), *88,* 3 (1968).

Terracol, J., *Le Glomus Jugulaire.* Monographie Oto-Rhino-Laryingologie Int. Masson Cie, Paris (1956).

Valentine, G., *Arch. Anat. Physiol. Wiss. Med.,* 287 (1846).

Catecholamines in glomus tumours

By Bertil Hamberger

Department of Histology, Karolinska Institutet, Stockholm, Sweden

Biogenic monoamines seldom occur in tumour tissue. The best known examples are the noradrenaline and adrenaline-containing phaechromocytomas and 5-hydroxytryptamine-containing carcinoid tumours. It has also been reported that tumours arising from the carotid body, glomus jugulare and related structures contain catecholamines (Berdal *et al.,* 1962, Glenner *et al.,* 1962, Pryse-Davies *et al.,* 1964). These organs are generally included in a group of structures named non-chromaffin paranganglia, where the term non-chromaffin is meant to denote that they do not contain any appreciable amounts of catecholamines or indole amines. The chromaffin reaction is, however, a fairly unspecific and unsensitive one, which reacts on phenolic amines (Pearse, 1961). In 1962, a new histochemical method was developed by Falck and Hillarp, which permits an extremely sensitive and exact cellular localization of certain catecholamines and indole amines (Falck *et al.,* 1962; Corrodi and Jonsson, 1967). The method is based on the findings that catecholamines, e.g. noradrenaline, react with formaldehyde gas to give products with strong green fluorescence (fluorescence peak at 480 mμ), while serotonin or 5-hydroxytryptamine with formaldehyde gives a product with strong yellow fluorescence (fluorescence peak at 520 mμ).

With this method, we studied the carotid body from humans, operated on because of bronchial asthma (Hamberger, Ritzén and Wersäll, 1966). As is well known, the cells, generally recognized as chemosensory cells, are arranged in balls or cords. In the fluorescence microscope, the cells exhibited a strong formaldehyde-induced fluorescence, which was localized to the cytoplasm, whereas the nucleus was non-fluorescent. Part of the cells had a green fluorescence, while others had a yellow fluorescence (Fig. 1). Microspectrofluorimetry and other specificity tests were performed, and it was concluded that the green-fluorescent cells contained noradrenaline, and the yellow-fluorescent cells 5-hydroxytryptamine. The presence of noradrenaline in the carotid body has earlier been reported (Pryse-Davies *et al.,* 1964), but the finding of another potent monoamine is new. It is likely that these biogenic monoamines have a local effect in the organ, and can be released and influ-

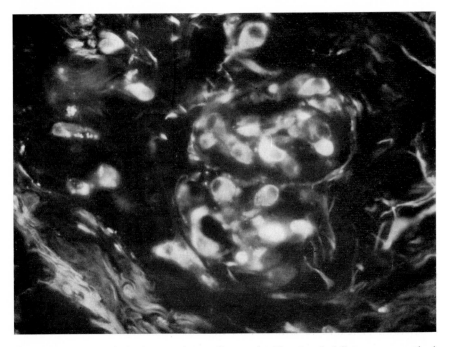

Fig. 1. Human carotid body treated according to the histochemical fluorescence method. Several strongly fluorescent cells are seen, surrounded by connective tissue with non-specific fluorescence. Some cells have a green fluorescence specific to catecholamines, while others have a yellow fluorescence specific to 5-hydroxytryptamine ×450.

ence sensory nerves which are known to exist around the chemosensory cells (Hamberger, Ritzén and Wersäll, 1966; Grimley and Glenner, 1968).

Some tumours arising from the glomus jugulare (Hamberger et al., 1967) and the carotid body were also studied with the histochemical method. These tumours have a microscopical appearance which greatly resembles the normal architecture of the organs, and are composed of cell balls surrounded by connective tissue (Fig. 2, Le Compte, 1951). In the microscope, it is impossible to distinguish glomus jugulare and carotid body tumours, and the malignancy cannot be determined (Moberg, 1961). In some of these tumours, the tumour cells had a strong green fluorescence specific to catecholamines. The fluorophore was localized to the cytoplasm, while the nucleus was non-fluorescent (Fig. 3). The fluorescence was concluded to be due to the presence of noradrenaline. From electron microscopy, it is also known that the carotid body, as well as glomus tumours, contain special storage granules which are typical of catecholamines (see Grimley and Glenner, 1968). No tumours with yellow fluorescence specific to 5-hydroxytryptamine were found. It may thus safely be concluded that there exist both carotid body and glomus jugulare tumours which contain large amounts of catecholamines. These tumours may

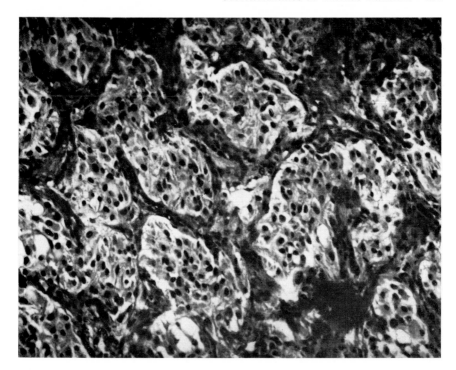

Fig. 2. Glomus jugulare tumour, routine staining. Several strands of tumour cells are seen, surrounded by connective tissue × 330.

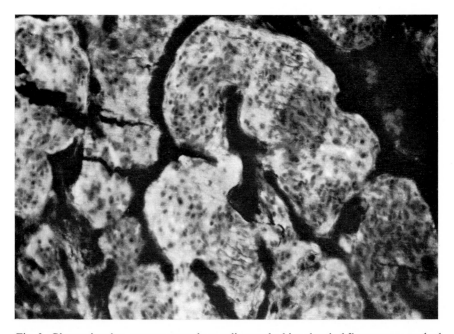

Fig. 3. Glomus jugulare tumour treated according to the histochemical fluorescence method Strong fluorescence, specific to catecholamines, is found in the tumour cells. The surrounding. connective tissue has no fluorescence, and thus appears dark × 210.

produce severe symptoms from the cardiovascular system, and high levels of metabolites in the urine (Berdal *et al.*, 1962; Hamberger *et al.*, 1967) which shows that potent monoamines can be released in large amounts from these tumours under physiological conditions.

References

Berdal, P., Braaten, M., Cappelen, Chr., Jr., Mylius, E. A. & Walaas, O., *Acta Med. Scand., 172,* 249 (1962).

Le Compte, P. M., *Atlas of tumor pathology,* Washington D.C. (1951).

Corrodi, H. & Jonsson, G., *J. Histochem. Cytochem., 15,* 65 (1967).

Falck, B., Hillarp, N.-Å., Thieme, G. & Torp, A., *J. Histochem. Cytochem., 10,* 348 (1962).

Grimley, P. M. & Glenner, G. G., *Circulation, 37,* 648 (1968).

Glenner, G. G., Craut, J. R. & Roberts, W. C., *Arch. Path.* (Chicago), *73,* 230 (1962).

Hamberger, C.-A., Hamberger, C. B., Wersäll, J. & Wågermark, J., *Acta Path. Microbiol. Scand., 69,* 489 (1967).

Hamberger, B., Ritzén, M. & Wersäll, J., *J. Pharmacol. Exp. Ther., 15,* 197 (1966).

Moberg, A., *Acta Otolaryng.* (Stockholm), *53,* 590 (1961).

Pearse, A. G. E., *Histochemistry,* Churchill, London (1961).

Pryse-Davies, J., Dawson, I. M. P. & Westbury, G., *Cancer, 17,* 185 (1964).

Roentgen diagnosis of glomus jugulare tumours

By Tore Laurén

Department of X-ray Diagnosis, Kronprinsessan Lovisa's Children's Hospital, Stockholm, Sweden

At Karolinska Sjukhuset, 28 cases of histologically verified glomus jugulare tumours have been seen during the period 1960–1968. The name "glomus jugulare tumour" has been used in the traditional way, and some cases are therefore included with obvious tumour origin from the glomus tympanicum. In most cases, an elaborate radiologic investigation was performed, including skull examination with special attention to the jugular foramen, angiography of the common or external carotid arteries, and retrograde phlebography of the internal jugular vein. In some cases, vertebral angiography was also performed. Pneumoencephalography with filling of the basal cisterns was used only in exceptional cases. Some examinations were carried out at other hospitals, and the films were generously put at our disposal.

Fig. 1 demonstrates the satisfactory roentgen examinations performed in 20 cases during the period 1960–1967.

Positive findings were present at examination of the jugular foramen in 10 of 19 cases. Of the pathologic jugular foramina, all had ill-defined or slightly sclerotic margins (Fig. 2), and 6 were considerably expanded, with the expanding centre corresponding to the vascular portion of the foramen, and the intrajugular process of the temporal bone was destroyed. Two of the cases with apparently normal foramina had a very large tumour, and in one of them (Fig. 5) the size of the foramen was within normal limits. The posterior contour was, however, slightly ill-defined.

At angiography of the common or external carotid arteries, positive findings were noted in 12 of 13 cases. The tumours were visualized as highly vascular areas with homogenous staining, suggesting a capillary network rather than irregular tumour vessels (Fig. 5). The tumours were supplied exclusively by the external carotid artery, and in some cases the inferior tympanic branch of the ascending pharyngeal artery could be identified. Arteriovenous shunting was always present. The angiographies must be performed with special attention to the temporal bone because in routine carotid angiography—suitable for a study of the intracranial vessels—the temporal region will be underexposed. In only one case was common carotid angiography

Case	Jug. for.	Car. ang.	Vert. ang.	Int. jug. phlebogr.
1	+			+
2	−	+	+	+
3	+	+		+
4	+			+
5	−	+		+
6	+	+	+	+
7				+
8	−			+
9	−	+		
10	−		−	
11	+			+
12	+	+	+	+
13	+	+	−	+
14	−	+	−	+
15	+	+	−	+
16	+	+		+
17	+	+		
18	−			−
19	−	+	−	−
20	−			+
	10/19	12/13	3/7	16/18

Fig. 1. Positive and negative findings in 20 cases of glomus jugulare tumour (see text).

negative, and this is explained by previous ligation of the external carotid artery.

Vertebral angiography was performed in 7 cases, and 3 were positive, exhibiting an additional arterial supply from the anterior meningeal branch. In no case did intracranial branches from the vertebral artery supply the tumour, as has been described in a few cases in the literature.

Carotid and vertebral angiography was not performed in 7 and 13 cases, respectively, since the diagnosis was already established, or because the patients were in too poor condition to benefit practically from a detailed topographic diagnosis.

Internal jugular phlebography was positive in 16 of 18 cases, and was not performed in 2. The positive findings were of three kinds: (1) intravascular filling defect with convex distal contour and expansion of the vein (Figs. 2 and 6). This finding is regarded as highly characteristic. (2) non-expansive filling defect, resembling a thrombus. (3) external compression of the vein. The last two types of change have also been seen in cases af sinus thrombosis and other tumours in this region.

Judging from our present experience, plain examination of the jugular foramen is positive in about 50 % of the cases. It indicates the size of the tumour at the level of the foramen, but gives little indication as to its size above or below this level. Pathologic foramina have so far been seen only in advanced tumours.

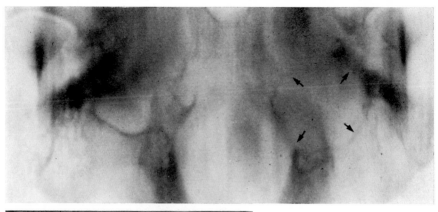

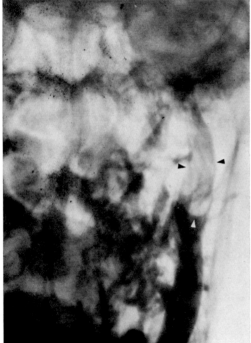

Fig. 2. Case 6. Tomography of the jugular foramina in submentotemporal projection (upper film), demonstrating almost circular expansion on the left side. The margins are slightly sclerotic.
Internal jugular phlebography in a.p. projection (lower film), demonstrating slightly expansive filling defect in the vein.

In most cases, angiography of the common carotid artery gives information about the nature of the tumour, as well as its extent, apart from the small portion supplied by the vertebral artery. When marked arteriovenous shunting to the jugular vein is present, the intravascular growth can be exactly determined.

Angiography of the vertebral artery may demonstrate additional extent of the tumour.

Phlebography of the internal jugular vein gives the best information as to intravascular growth, which seems to be present far more often than has been realized before.

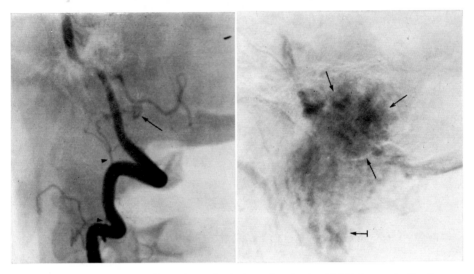

Fig. 3. Case 6. Common carotid angiography in lateral projection (right), demonstrating the tumour as a large vascular area, occupying the temporal bone (→). The part which extends below the base of the skull (←+) corresponds to the intravenous expansion seen in Fig. 2. Vertebral angiography in the same projection (left) with the anterior meningeal branch (▶) supplying a small part of the tumour (←).

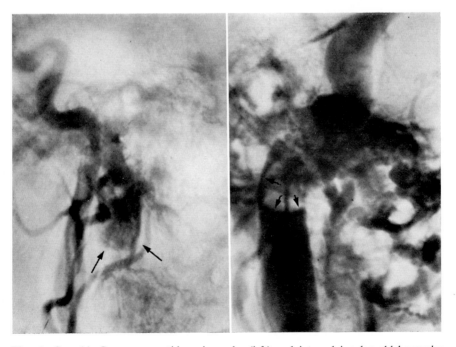

Fig. 4. Case 14. Common carotid angiography (left) and internal jugular phlebography (right). A tumour with a diameter of about 1 cm is seen stained with contrast medium and as a filling defect.

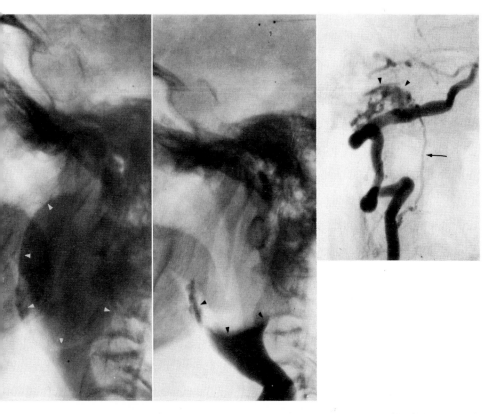

Fig. 5. Case 12. Common carotid angiography, late arterial phase (left). A large, evenly stained tumour is seen in the internal jugular vein, which is enormously expanded. Marked shunting to the lower portion of the vein.
Internal jugular phlebography (middle) demonstrates the lower pole of the tumour.
Vertebral angiography (right) demonstrates an additional arterial supply to the tumour (▼) from the anterior meningeal branch (←).

The following sequence of roentgen examination can be recommended:

1. Routine examination of the skull with special attention to the jugular foramen.

2. Common carotid angiography, if necessary supplemented by selective examination of the external carotid artery. The examination must be performed with special attention to the temporal region, and the subtraction technique is essential.

3. If the extent of the tumour is not obvious from those two examinations, internal jugular phlebography should be made.

4. Vertebral angiography should be performed when the complete extent

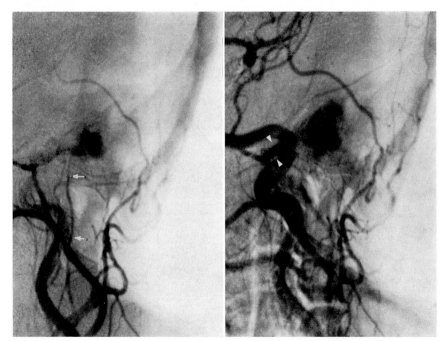

Fig. 6. Case 19. Common carotid angiography in oblique projection. The size and location of the tumour correspond exactly to the middle ear, and a tail of the tumour extends into the Eustachian tube (▼). The main supply is derived from the ascending pharyngeal artery (←). This tumour obviously originates from the glomus tympanicum.

of the tumour must be determined, for instance, when radical surgery is planned, or when ligation of the external carotid artery is considered, for relief of pain and tinnitus.

Complete angiographic mapping appears to make pneumoencephalography superfluous in assessing the intracranial extension of the tumour.

References

Alford, B. R. & Guilford, F. R., *Laryngoscope, 72,* 765 (1962).
Bateson, E. M. & Bull, T., *Brit. J. Radiol., 40,* 120 (1967).
Capps, F. C., *J. Fac. Radiol.* (London), *8,* 312 (1957).
Di Chiro, G., Fischer, R. L. & Nelson, K. B., *J. Neurosurg., 21,* 447 (1964).
Gastpar, H., *Acta Otolaryng.* (Stockholm), suppl. 167 (1961).
Gejrot, T. & Laurén, T., *Acta Otolaryng.* (Stockholm), *57,* 556 (1964).
Gejrot, T. & Laurén, T., *Acta Otolaryng.* (Stockholm), *58,* 191 (1964).
Gejrot, T. & Laurén, T., *Pract. Otorhinolaryng.* (Basel), *26,* 71 (1964).
Gejrot, T. & Lindbom, Å., *Acta Otolaryng.* (Stockholm), suppl. 158, 180 (1960).
Greitz, T. & Laurén, T., *Acta Radiol.* [Diagn.] (Stockholm), *7,* 219 (1968).
Hawkins, T. D., *Clin. Radiol., 12,* 199 (1961).
Hooper, R. S., *J. Fac. Radiol.* (London), *7,* 77 (1955).
Porchet, P., Porot, J. & Rossand, L., *J. Radiol. Electr., 34,* 18 (1953).
Rice, R. P. & Holman, C. B., *Amer. J. Roentgen., 89,* 1201 (1963).
Rucker, T. N., *Radiology, 81,* 807 (1963).

Jugular foramen syndromes

By Tomas Gejrot

Department of Otolaryngology, Lasarettet, Kristianstad, Sweden

The jugular foramen, formed by the jugular notch on the occipital bone and the adjacent temporal bone, consists of two parts. The posterior lateral component transmits the initial part of the internal jugular vein. The medial anterior part, which is known as the pars nervosa, transmits the IXth, Xth and XIth cerebral nerves. The glossopharyngeal nerve lies anterior and medial to the other two nerves, from which it is separated by a fibrous septum.

The glossopharyngeal nerve gives off the tympanic nerve, which distributes sensory fibres to the mucous membrane lining the tympanic cavity and auditory tube, and the parasympathetic secretomotor fibres to the parotid gland.

Efferent fibres originating in the nucleus ambiguus pass in each of the three nerves. Those running in the glossopharyngeal nerve end in the stylopharyngeus muscle, those in the vagus are joined outside the skull by similar fibres from the cranial division of the accessory nerve, and terminate in the intrinsic muscles of the pharynx and larynx.

Afferent fibres from the larynx, pharynx and posterior third of the tongue run in the glossopharyngeal nerve to the tractus solitarius. Sensory fibres from the tympanic cavity and auditory tube pass, via the tympanic nerve, to the glossopharyngeal nerve. Sensory fibres from the pharynx, larynx, trachea and thoracic and abdominal viscera run in the vagus nerve, and terminate in the tractus solitarius and its nucleus.

The spinal portion of the accessory nerve joins the cranial fibres of the nerve (functionally part of the vagus) before they course through the jugular foramen. The cranial root joins the vagus nerve below the superior ganglion. The spinal root descends laterally and backwards, crossing the internal jugular vein, piercing the deep surface of the sternocleidomastoid muscle and continuing to the trapezius. The hypoglossal nerve is often damaged with the aforementioned cranial nerves. It is transmitted by the hypoglossal canal, and its initial stretch is situated medially and posterior to the vagus nerve.

The symptoms resulting from damage to the glossopharyngeal nerve include impairment of the sensitivity of the posterior third of the tongue, the tonsils and the pharynx, and of the sense of taste in the affected part of the tongue.

The salivary secretion is also affected. The condition is diagnosed by tests of taste and pharyngeal reflex.

Isolated damage to the vagus nerve in the posterior cranial fossa is rare, the aforementioned nerves usually also being involved. The cause generally lies in a tumour, in most cases a glomus tumour (Brain, 1960). The signs consist of unilateral paralysis of the palate and pharynx, which, though not necessarily giving rise to subjective symptoms, is manifested in the intonation and in tests of the pharyngeal reflex. The chief sign is paralysis of the recurrent laryngeal nerve. Autonomous symptoms in cases of unilateral damage to the vagus nerve are usually of a minor nature.

Involvement of the accessory nerve results in paralysis of the sternocleidomastoid and trapezius muscles. The outline of the former muscle on the neck is abnormal, the shoulder drops and the border of the trapezius muscle is not so easily recognizable by palpation as usual. The power of the shoulder and arm is reduced.

Because of the relation of these four nerves, not only at the base of the skull but also intracranially, a lesion affecting one of the nerves is likely to involve one or more of the others. As a result, several syndromes due to various combinations of nerve involvement have been described.

Fig. 1 is a schematic picture illustrating the syndromes. Of these, many textbooks list Jackson's and Schmidt's syndromes as being purely nuclear. Vernet's syndrome, the true jugular syndrome, denotes the group of symptoms arising from paralysis of the IXth, Xth and XIth nerves.

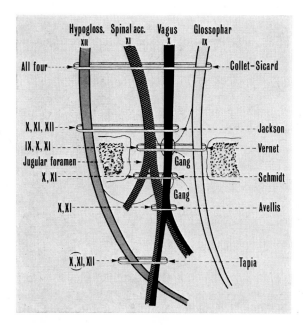

Fig. 1. Schematic representation of the jugular syndromes.

The pathologic conditions known to produce the jugular foramen syndrome may be fractures of the skull inflammations, aneurysms and other vascular lesions. A case of sinus thrombosis and fully developed jugular syndrome has been reported, in which the neurologic symptoms had regressed completely 4 months after operation (Šuster, 1960). In another case, the jugular foramen syndrome was caused by a bullet wound; paralysis of the IXth, Xth and XIth cranial nerves regressed after removal of the foreign body (Bauer, 1962). Carcinoma of the middle ear, acoustic neuroma, neurofibromas, chordomas, metastases and lymphadenitis are reported to cause the syndromes.

The tumours causing a jugular foramen syndrome may be intracranial, extracranial, or originating from the fossa jugulare itself, then especially the superior bulb of the internal jugular vein.

Svien *et al.* (1963) described 29 cases from the Mayo Clinic with several kinds of jugular syndromes. Fifteen of these patients had a neoplasm, mostly a meningioma or neurofibroma. Five of them were intracranial, 7 extracranial and 3 intracranial with extracranial extension. Of the other 14 patients, an aetiological factor could be discovered in 9 of them (tuberculosis, diabetes mellitus, syphilis, meningitis, aneurysm, hypertension and cerebrovascular disease). In all cases with a jugular syndrome, the XIIth cranial nerve was involved. The main initial symptom was hoarseness or difficulty in swallowing.

The tumour that is most likely to be present in the region of the jugular foramen is a glomus tumour. It may originate from the middle ear and grow out towards the sigmoid sinus, or it may arise from the jugular bulb or the vagal ganglion just beneath the foramen.

Neurologic manifestations of tumours of the glomus jugulare have been reported by several authors. Siekert (1956) reported 14 neurologic abnormalities among 33 described cases. Eight of them had involvement of the IXth, Xth, XIth and XIIth cranial nerves. No true Vernet's syndrome, was seen in any case. The earliest symptom after tinnitus, hearing impairment and aural discharge was involvement of the facial and vagus nerves.

Alford and Guilford (1962) found, among 277 suitable cases of glomus jugulare tumours in the literature, involvement of the IXth, Xth, XIth and XIIth cranial nerves in 20%.

Since 1960, we have examined and treated 28 cases of glomus jugulare tumours at Karolinska Sjukhuset. Of these, 10 had a jugular syndrome and 7 partial paralysis of the VIIth–XIIth cranial nerves. The most common initial neurologic symptom was hoarseness and difficulty in swallowing.

To the former diagnostic methods we have added radiography of the jugular foramen in special positions, cerebral angiography of the external carotid and vertebral arteries and, if necessary, pneumoencephalography. Among the

		For. Jug.		Retr. Jug.	
		Path.	Normal	Path.	Normal
Vernet's S.	(1)	1		1	
Collet-Sicard's S.	(9)	8	1	9	
Partial paral.	(7)	1	6	4	3

Fig. 2. Results of radiographic examinations of the jugular foramen and the superior jugular bulb in cases of glomus tumours with jugular syndromes or partial paralysis of the last four cranial nerves.

jugular syndrome cases, we found pathologic changes in the jugular foramen in all but one case. At retrograde jugularography, intravascular expansive growth or obliteration of the internal jugular vein or sigmoid sinus was seen in every case. A visible change, either in the jugular bulb or the jugular foramen, was observed in every case with partial involvement of the last four nerves. These findings indicate the necessity of examination of the jugular foramen or jugular bulb in cases with paralysis of one or more of the last four cranial nerves.

In view of the radiological findings, especially the angiographic ones, operative treatment must be more radical than the current ones, for complete removal of the tumour and its intravascular extensions. Fig. 3 recalls the methods devised by Voss and Grunert in sinus thrombosis. The mastoid process is evacuated, and the VIIth and IXth–XIIth cranial nerves are exposed. The external carotid artery and ascending pharyngeal artery are ligated, in order to diminish bleeding. After packing the proximal part of the sigmoid sinus, its lateral wall is exposed down to the jugular bulb and the site of the tumour. After packing towards the inferior petrosal sinus and ligating the internal jugular vein, the intravascular tumour is removed together with the lateral venous wall. Remaining tumour tissue in the middle ear and hypotympanum is excised. The wound is left open until the packing has been removed.

Totally 14 cases were operated upon because of the phlebographic findings. In glomus jugulare cases with a normal retrograde jugularogram, radical mastoidectomy was performed. Radiation treatment was given after discussion with the radiologists, with regard to the localization and growth of the tumour.

One postoperative bleeding was the only complication. Postoperative improvement of paralysis was seen in three cases.

Because of the slow growth of a glomus jugulare tumour, it is difficult to make any statement about the prognosis. A 10-year freedom from symp-

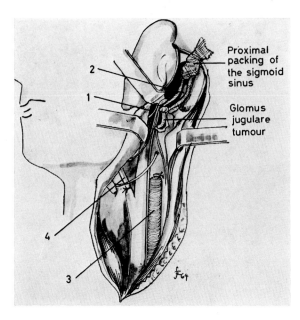

Proximal
packing of
the sigmoid
sinus

Glomus
jugulare
tumour

2

1

4

3

Fig. 3. Schematic drawing of the surgical procedure. The mastoid process is evacuated down to the mastoid tip. Nerves and vessels around the jugular foramen are exposed. The external carotid artery is ligated. The sigmoid sinus is exposed and packed, the lateral wall opened down to the site of the tumour. 1. Facial nerve. 2. Sigmoid sinus. 3. Internal jugular vein. 4. External carotid artery.

toms does not necessarily imply full healing. The object of a radical intervention is to stop further expansion, and rule out the risk of the tumour becoming malignant, in addition to relieving the patient of a troublesome discharge, due to inflammation of the tumour, as well as tinnitus and dullness. Complete regression of existing paralysis with a duration of 1–3 months seldom occurs.

References

Alford, B. R. & Guilford, F. R., *Laryngoscope, 72,* 765 (1962).
Bauer, F., *J. Laryng., 76,* 367 (1962).
Brain, R., *Clinical Neurology,* Oxford University Press (1960).
Gejrot, T., *Acta Otolaryng.* (Stockholm), *57,* 450 (1964).
Gejrot, T. & Laurén, T., *Acta Otolaryng.* (Stockholm), *58,* 191 (1964).
Gejrot, T. & Hamberger, C.-A., *Laryngoscope, 74,* 1029 (1964).
Gejrot, T., *Acta Otolaryng.* (Stockholm), *60,* 150 (1965).
Siekert, R. G., *Arch. Neurol. Psychiat.* (Chicago), *76,* 1 (1956).
Šuster, M., *Cesk. Otolaryng., 9,* 50 (1960).
Svien, H. J., Baker, H. L. & Rivers, M. H., *Neurology* (Minneap.), *13,* 797 (1963).

Needle biopsy in skull base tumours

By Sixten Franzén

Department of Radiopathology, Karolinska Sjukhuset, Stockholm, Sweden

Before embarking on treatment of any tumour, it is of importance to have a microscopic diagnosis. We have done thin-needle aspiration of tumours in an increasing number of cases for the past 15 years. Last year, we did 8000 punctures of a variety of tumours. For example, the majority of mammary tumours were diagnosed cytologically before any intervention. In most cases, the same doctor performed the aspiration, made the smears and read the microscopic cell picture. The method is a cytologic one, analogous to bone marrow aspiration in haematology.

Concerning skull base tumours, tissue for microscopic diagnosis is not easily obtained surgically. However, the skull base can be reached with needles via several portals; for example, through the mouth and soft palate, through the nose, through the cheek inferior to the maxilla, or retromandibularly. I would like to demonstrate the potentialities of thin-needle biopsy in the skull base, and I have selected three cases.

The first was a man aged 60, presenting with left-sided headache. Physical examination was negative. X-rays revealed a destructive process involving the left occiput, including the rim of the foramen magnum. Aspiration was performed through the soft palate in the direction of the lesion, using a one-handed syringe with a long thin needle attached (Esposti *et al.*, 1968). Material was easily aspirated, smeared on slides, air-dried and stained with May-Grünwald-Giemsa. The cell picture was typical of plasma cell sarcoma (Fig. 1). Three years later, new lesions of multiple myeloma appeared.

The second case was a 36-year-old woman with deep-seated, non-specific head-pain present for several years. X-rays demonstrated a lytic lesion in the region of the left occiput and clivus (Fig. 2). A thin needle was passed through a guide needle, placed behind the ramus of the mandible on the left under fluoroscopic control. Mucoid material was easily obtained. The cell picture was typical of chordoma (Fig. 3).

The third case was a woman with a suspected glomus jugulare tumour. On a venous angiogram, a filling defect was seen. Aspiration performed be-

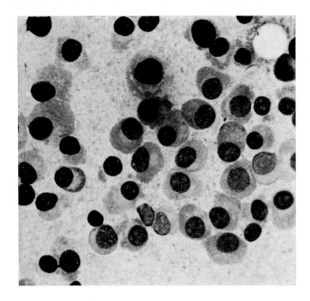

Fig. 1. Typical plasma cells with slight polymorphism. Highly differentiated plasmacytic sarcoma.

hind the ramus of the mandible during fluoroscopy yielded bloody material. The cell picture was typical of a glomus tumour (Fig. 4). These tumours are rare, but experience has previously been obtained from the aspiration smears of 10 carotid body tumours, which cytologically are the same (Franzén).

Summary

A technique for thin-needle aspiration of deep-seated masses of the skull base is presented. Material was easily obtained, allowing precise diagnosis of three diverse tumours.

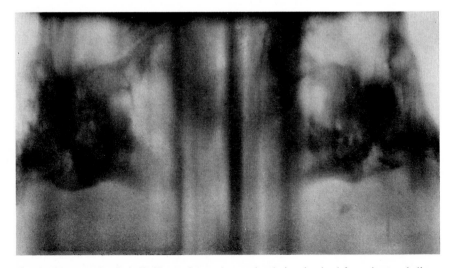

Fig. 2. Tomograph of skull, illustrating a destructive lesion in the left occiput and clivus.

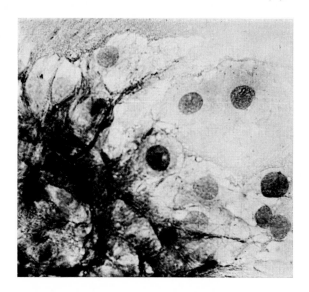

Fig. 3. Chordoma cells characterized by small, uniform nuclei and abundant bubbly cytoplasm, embedded in mucoid substance.

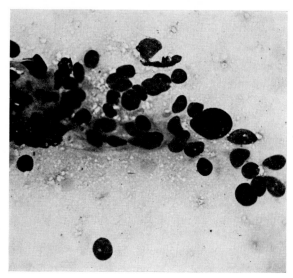

Fig. 4. Cells of glomus tumour, characterized by tight clusters and polymorphous, free nuclei. The cytoplasm is greyish violet.

References

Esposti, P., Franzén, S. & Zajicek, J., In *Diagnostic Cytology* by Leopold G. Koss, 2nd ed., Lippincott Co., Philadelphia (1968).

Franzén, S., to be published.

General discussion

Portmann to Bordley

I want to thank Dr. Bordley for this very interesting introduction. Stacy Guild is definitely the first who opened this field. Although it is true so say that Valentine in the XIXth century described a similar structure, we recognize now that it was not exactly the glomus jugulare. I again thank Dr. Bordley for this fine presentation.

Berdal to B. Hamberger

Did you find an increased urinary excretion of catecholamines in the patients you have examined?

House to B. Hamberger

Any correlation of preoperative and operative blood pressure and amount of noradrenaline in tumour by histochemistry?

Wersäll to Berdal and House

In a case of a malignant carotid body tumour, we have reported a markedly increased urinary excretion of catecholamines.

We have had no significant rise in blood pressure in cases of glomus jugulare tumours where this has decreased after operation. We have, however, observed this in a couple of carotid body tumours. It might be wise to record the arterial blood pressure during the operation, considering the large amount of catecholamines present in the tumour.

Padovan to Laurén

Dr. Laurén, I would like to ask you: Did you have difficulties in differential diagnosis with the angiographic radiography in this region? We made (Professor Krmpotić and I. Padovan) investigations of the sinus transversus and sigmoides. We have established that the width of the sulcus transversus is, on the average, smaller than that of the sulcus sigmoides, the right sulcus being always larger than the left one. The sulcus sigmoides shows large variations in its width as well as in its depth. Its width varies from 2 to 16 mm and its depth from 0.5 to 18 mm.

Hitselberger to Laurén

Comment on the difference between the cadaveric appearance of the lateral and sigmoid sinuses and the appearance one obtains on a venogram: Except in those part with obstruction due to tumour, such as in glomus tumours, we have always been able to demonstrate bilateral filling of the sinuses with jugular venography.

Aschan to Laurén

You talked about the size of the foramen jugulare as a diagnostic tool. But since there is a large normal "asymmetry", where do you put your "normal" limits?

Naumann to Laurén

How often could you observe in your material *larger* communications between the carotid artery system and the jugular vein system acting as an important shunt? I am asking because just recently we could observe a case with an astonishingly large communication between the two vascular systems.

Laurén to Padovan and Hitselberger

The numerous anatomical variations of the transverse-sigmoid sinuses, the torcular and the emissary veins may cause diagnostic problems, but I think that the usual pitfalls connected with phlebography are of greater importance. When the patient is in the supine position, blood from a wide inferior petrosal sinus may give filling defects in the anterior part of the bulb, which can easily be misinterpreted as a tumour. Similar poor mixing of contrast medium and blood from dural sinuses, emptying in the transverse sinus, may simulate thrombosis. As a rule, I think that it is more convenient to study the transverse and sigmoid sinus in the venous phase of carotid angiography with the subtraction technique, and reserve jugular phlebography for the bulb region.

Unlike Dr. Hitselberger, I have failed to fill the contralateral transverse sinus on several occasions in spite of rather high injection pressure and compression distally during the injection. This has happened in cases which undoubtedly had free passage on both sides. In one case this was due to excessive filling of the deep cervical plexus through an unusually wide condylar emissary vein. Besides, there are cases with narrow or even absent communications between the two sides in the torcular. If, however, the contralateral transverse-sigmoid sinus fills, but the contrast medium fails to pass further into the jugular vein, I think that it strongly indicates a tumour.

Laurén to Aschan

I cannot give any normal values, but I have seen a normal case published with the diameter of the jugular foramen exceeding 2 cm. They can also be asymmetrical as to the shape, so very little help can be obtained comparing the two sides. The appearance of the bony margins seems to be of greater diagnostic importance. In doubtful cases, phlebography always seems justified, to see if the vein fits well into the foramen.

Laurén to Naumann

All carotid angiographies in our glomus tumour cases showed arteriovenous shunting, but large communications were seen only in large tumours. At the Neuroradiological Department, I saw a few cases with arteriovenous malformations who presented rather striking communications. I do not know if they were of cardiovascular importance.

Fisch to Gejrot

Siebenmann described a syndrome of the foramen jugulare occurring after a cranial trauma, often even without evidence of a fracture. In the literature, about 14 cases of this disabling syndrome are described. Did you observe similar cases in your material? We had the opportunity to see 2 of them and to operate on one of these cases, decompressing the foramen jugulare, with an excellent functional result.

Gejrot to Fisch

A jugular syndrome following skull damage without signs of fracture may be a posttraumatic vascular lesion, e.g. an aneurysm.

Palva to Franzén

I should like to ask Dr. Franzén how much material he obtains with the thin needle punctures, whether or not it is sufficient for staining of several slides. I noticed that the stain used was that of Giemsa, and should like to ask whether he also uses Papanicolau staining and possibly some other stains in order to obtain different views of cellular details.

Naumann to Franzén

How do you estimate the chance or the danger of getting metastases along the route by which your needle came?

Ketcham to Franzén

Needle biopsy at the time of first seeing the patient has become a relatively routine procedure on our service at Bethesda. This includes both bone and soft tissue tumours. The needle tract is directed through an area which we expect to remove with definitive surgery, although surprisingly enough seeding of tumour along the needle tract is a rare phenomenon. The limited number of pathology reports which state "insufficient for diagnosis" have encouraged us to continue using a No. 14 to 18 gauge needle so that we have tissue for blocking and microscopic examination as well as a smear for cytological study. Finally, there is much debate even between pathologists about the validity of cytology alone, and therefore in the United States few surgeons would feel nor should feel competent to make the diagnosis, whether it be from tissue block or cytology. It would be manditory to have an official pathology examination by a qualified pathologist.

Hallén to Franzén

Do you do transmeatal aspiration biopsies from the middle ear?

Portmann to Franzén

Do you have some risks of haemorrhage if you do a needle biopsy for a very haemorrhagic disease like a glomus jugulare tumour?

Franzén to Palva

Sufficient material is obtained for several smears, and repeated punctures may be done. Giemsa stain is generally preferred. Papanicolaou staining may also be done to demonstrate nuclear details.

Franzén to Naumann

This question is frequently asked. We have seen tumour implantation once in over 50,000 punctures. It was a case of generalized melanoma.

Franzén to Ketcham

I wish to thank Dr. Ketcham for his interesting comments. Our experience based on extensive follow-up has demonstrated beyond doubt the usefulness and validity of aspiration cytology.

Franzén to Hallén

We have not done any transmeatal aspirations.

Franzén to Portmann

All glomus tumours bleed easily. One death occurred two days after aspiration. Autopsy revealed nearly total occlusion of the carotid by tumour with superimposed clot. Whether the puncture was a cause was not clearly determined.

Diagnosis and treatment of glomus jugulare tumours—Movie

By Tomas Gejrot, Carl-Axel Hamberger, Tore Laurén and Jan Wersäll

Department of Otolaryngology, Karolinska Sjukhuset, Stockholm, Sweden

Operative treatment of glomus jugulare tumours—Movie

By William House

Otologic Medical Group, Los Angeles, California, USA

General discussion

Grahne to Gejrot

In your retrograde phlebography do you always make the puncture of the jugular vein percutaneously, or do you sometimes have to explore a part of the vein? How about preservation of the facial nerve? Do you cut it sometimes by operating upon the very large tumours? How about the recovery of the function of the facial and the other cranial nerves postoperatively? Do you sometimes see recovery of the nerve function?

Engström to Gejrot

From my point of view, one of the most important areas of interest in the surgical handling of the glomus tumour is the area of tumour origin, and that is the region where the maximum of radicality should be used. Can you from your venography be certain where that origin is? Another question: Can you be quite certain that a glomus tumour is not sometimes encapsulated in one region and more diffusely growing in another?

Meurman to Gejrot and House

I would like to ask the speakers how many recurrences they have seen among their patients.

Arslan to Gejrot and House

Would it not be better to maintain for the tumours of the jugular glomus the old and the more precise term "non-chromaffin paraganglioma"?

Aschan to Gejrot and House

The movies dealt with surgery. Irradiation was mentioned by House. Would he and Gejrot comment further on irradiation therapy in these cases *versus* surgery.

Bordley to Gejrot

What has been the experience in this group of the longterm of X-ray therapy for glomus tumours upon the hearing and upon the brain tissue, especially in the posterior fossa? We have had two patients treated by radiation who have shown signs many years later suggesting brain damage. There have also been reports that X-ray therapy may result in some sensory neural hearing loss.

Escher to Gejrot and House

According to Professor Zuppinger in Berne, conventional X-ray irradiation has no effect. On the other hand, the Betatrone irradiation gives good results in cases which grow quickly; these may be arrested, but not cured.

Jongkees to Gejrot and House

To the comments made upon the effect of X-ray treatment of glomus jugulare tumours, I should like to add one about our results. In general, we operate upon those tumours that can be removed radically (probably mostly the glomus tympanicum type). In other cases we prefer irradiation, and have some good results, even over a period of approx. 15 years. I must state, however, that the tumour does not disappear but seems to come to a standstill.

Engström to Gejrot and House

In several cases of glomus tumours treated with operation and irradiation, good results have been observed, but in two cases, necrosis of the bony and membraneous labyrinth has been seen. In one case the promontory and the bone around the semicircular canals slowly sequestrated, and could be lifted out without vestibular reaction or liquorrhoea. A similar case was shown to me by my colleague Lidén working in the Gothenburg clinic.

Ketcham to House

It is my understanding that this group of tumours are slow growing, benign and with little tendency to developing local recurrence. I would suggest that this must be true because it seems that you are removing tumour in a "piece meal" manner and by curettement. Most other tumours, as we ordinarily think of them and observe their behaviour, certainly are seldom controlled without *en bloc* resection. This radical surgical approach to the tumour has been only recently popularized, and I would guess that the 5–10-year and maybe even 15-year local recurrence rate will be alarmingly high.

Denecke to Gejrot and House

Das Hauptproblem bei der vollständigen Entfernung ausgedehnter Glomustumoren ist die Beherrschung der ausserordentlich starken Blutung. Bei diesen Tumoren ist es nicht nur zu einem Eindringen längs der V. jugularis int. caudalwärts und längs des Sinus sigmoideus cranialwärts gekommen, sondern auch zu einem Vorschieben längs der transbasalen Venen nach medial.

1. das Rete jugulare, das vom Bulbus aus zum Knie der Carotis int. im lateralen horizontalen Felsenbeinkanal zieht,

2. den Sinus petrosus inf. accessorius, der vom Rete jugulare zu den medial gelegenen cavernösen Räumen an der Carotis int. im Felsenbein führt,

3. den Sinus petrosus inf., der zum Sinus cavernosus zieht und

4. den Venenplexus an der A. carotis int. selbst, der von der Einmündung des Rete jugulare an der Carotis int. — entlang dieser — bis zum Sinus cavernosus verläuft.

Diese Venenwege müssen beim operativen Vorgehen in Rechnung gestellt werden. Ein Verfahren, das sich zur Blutstillung hervorragend bewährt hat, ist die Verwendung eines grossen gestielten Muskellappens aus dem M. sternocleidomastoideus. Hat nämlich der Tumor die cavernöse Verbindungsstrecke an der A. carotis int. erreicht, so ist es zu seiner radikalen Entfernung nach Abtragung des knöchernen Carotiskanals erforderlich, die totale Petrosektomie durchzuführen. Um in der Tiefe unter guter Sicht arbeiten zu können, werden dabei die Dura der hinteren Schädelgrube, das Gebiet des ehemaligen Foramen jugulare und das Knie der A. carotis int. zur Blutstillung mit dem Muskellappen abgedeckt. Ein Duraschützer hält den Lappen in seiner Position. Durch das Tumorwachstum und infolge der Knochenabtragungen bei der Herstellung des Zugangsweges finden sich alle Knochenverbindungen mit der restlichen Pyramidenspitze gelöst. Der bewegliche Knochenanteil darf nun auf keinen Fall mit Gewalt entfernt werden, da sonst der Ast der Carotis int. im Sinus cavernosus abreissen und es zu einer arterio-venösen Fistel kommen kann. Ausserdem kann bei unvorsichtigen Manipulationen der N. abducens abgerissen werden. Die Zerkleinerung der verbliebenen Pyramidenspitze muss deshalb vorsichtig mit Bohrern und Spezialzangen und unter Lagefixation der sich bei der Bearbeitung bewegenden Knochenpartie vorgenommen werden. Beim Auslösen der letzten dünnen Knochenschale reissen zwar die laterale Cavernoswand und die Wände des Sinus petrosus sup. und inf. infolge der anatomischen Verhältnisse ein, doch hat man nun den vorgebildeten Muskellappen zur Abdeckung des sich ergiessenden Blutstroms zur Verfügung. Nachdem durch diese Lappen auch der Liquorfluss zum Stehen gekommen ist, kann die Arbeit an der Carotis int. fortgesetzt werden, die vorsichtig aus dem Tumor herausgelöst wird. Die Blutung aus der Flügelgaumengrube stört dabei manchmal und ist durch Tamponade zu stillen. Im medialen

Anteil des horizontalen Abschnittes der A. carotis int. (Curvatura fibrocartilaginea) kommt noch ein kleines arterielles Gefäss, die A. Canalis pterygoidei, zum Bluten. Auch dieses steht auf Tamponade. Nun kann die Dura, die hier schon die A. carotis int. umscheidet, stumpf abgelöst und mit dem daraufsitzenden Tumor entfernt werden. Erst wenn die A. carotis int. völlig gesäubert ist, wird der restliche Tumor mit der befallenen Dura im Bereich der hinteren Schädelgrube entfernt. — Nachdem auch die das Foramen jugulare passierenden Nerven entsprechend im Gesunden reseziert sind, wird der Tampon aus der Flügelgaumengrube herausgezogen. — Nun wird die Hautwunde, am Warzenfortsatz beginnend, vernäht. Es wird dabei sorgfältig darauf geachtet, dass sämtliche Duradefekte, auch die an den Hirnblutleitern, durch die Muskelplastik gedeckt sind. Auch der freiliegende Abschnitt der A. carotis int. wird durch den Muskellappen zuverlässig geschützt. Diese Gefässprotektion ist bei bestrahlten Fällen von besonderer Bedeutung. Sollte die Muskeldeckung ausnahmsweise nicht ausreichen, so kann man die Defekte in den Sinuswänden auch durch gestielte Hautlappen decken, wie wir das seit einigen Jahren bei Verletzungen des Sinus sigmoideus vorgenommen haben. — Zur Deckung der Duradefekte in der hinteren Schädelgrube kann man sich zusätzlich auch der Fascia lata-Plastik bedienen. Es muss dabei aber darauf geachtet werden, dass die Fascia lata nicht zu weit nach vorn vernäht wird, und die restliche Tubenöffnung freibleibt. Der Patient presst sonst postoperativ infektiöses Material aus dem Nasopharynx längs der Tube in die hintere Schädelgrube.

Ist es durch Atrophie der Pharynxmuskulatur der einen Seite und durch Insuffizienz des Glottisschlusses zur erschwerten Nahrungsaufnahme gekommen, dann sollten unverzüglich die von mir angegebenen rekonstruktiven Eingriffe an Pharynx und Larynx zur Wiederherstellung des Schluckaktes und der Stimme durchgeführt werden (Arch. Ohr. Nas. Kehlkopfheilk. 178, 538, 1961). Danach kann das Dekanülement erfolgen. Die Exstirpation ausgedehnter Glomus-Tumoren ist also nur mittels eines kombinierten oto-neuro-halschirurgischen Eingriffs möglich.

Gejrot to Grahne

We always puncture the internal jugular vein percutaneously. This causes no trouble when we do it distally in the inferior jugular bulb. We have never been forced to cut the facial nerve. Recovery of function has been seen in two cases. In both the history was very short, only one month.

Gejrot to Engström

One of our first patients had an encapsulated glomus tympanicum tumour, which was extirpated by tympanotomy. Postoperative jugularography showed a tumour in the jugular bulb. Another operation showed a diffusely growing tumour in the hypotympanum, growing into the jugular bulb.

Gejrot to Arslan

We agree that there are too many names for these tumours. As they arise from Guild's glomus formations, we like to call them glomus tumours. Irradiation therapy we discuss in every case with the radiologists. I think that Dr. Notter will comment on the irradiation therapy.

Notter to Gejrot and House

To the question of radiosensitivity of glomus jugulare tumours: According to the two components of the tumour, fibrous and angiomatous tissue, the radiosensitivity may vary. The tumour is, however, relatively radiosensitive and reacts to radiation doses of 3000–4500 rads/during 3–4 weeks. If operation is radical, postoperative irradiation is not indicated. If it is to be given in not radically or inoperable cases, higher doses may be given, but then with respect to the radiosensitivity of the surrounding nerve and brain tissue.

Jongkees to Notter

I am sorry that I am not an expert at all, and that I can only try to explain what I believe to be the true facts. About 5000 rads are given in 42 sessions (about 5 per week), high-voltage, rotation or multiple-field techniques.

House

There are some tumours that are susceptible to irradiation and they do seem to shrink following irradiation. However, I am not aware that irradiation actually cures the tumour. I believe that the decrease in size of the tumour is due to sclerosis of the blood vessels. The amount of vascularity of the tumour and the degree of shrinkage in response to X-ray treatment should be correlated. If we find that those tumours which are quite vascular do, indeed, decrease considerably in size, then it would seem valuable to irradiate these and follow irradiation with surgery. It seems to me that, clinically, those tumours which are primarily cellular do not respond readily to irradiation. On the other hand, they are much easier to operate on because of their relative lack of vascularity.

In response to Dr. Engström's question, it is possible to remove the jugular bulb. We feel that if surgical removal is possible, this is preferable to freezing of the tumour, since freezing often involves the IXth, Xth, XIth and XIIth nerves and gives a defect of considerable magnitude. Our present technique is to locate the accessory nerve in the neck and follow this up across the jugular vein. At about the point where it crosses the vein, we ligate the vein and then follow along the plane between the XIth nerve and the jugular vein. This separates the wall of the vein away from the IXth, Xth and XIth nerves and then allows us to dissect tumour and the bulb away from the nerves with a minimum amount of injury. The bone around the jugular bulb can then be removed with curette and diamond stone methods.

Chairman's summary of session V

M. Portmann

Now, it is my duty to summarize this very fascinating morning. I want first of all to thank the speakers who took part in this discussion. The organizers were very clever to divide this morning into three parts:

1. *History, histology and histophysiology.* Two articles (Bordley and Hamberger, Jr.) were remarkably written on this subject.

2. *Clinical symptoms and several examinations.* The needle biopsy presented by Dr. Franzén: I think that this technique is very interesting, but difficult to popularize. Handled by Dr. Franzén, I heard that it was excellent, but I do not think that other pathologists would be so successful.

The second examination which was pointed out is direct jugular phlebography. I am sure that it is a very important improvement to know the intravenous extension of the tumour, and the method should definitely be adopted everywhere, to help the surgeon to recognize the position of the tumour. We must thank Professor C.-A. Hamberger and his group for this study.

3. *Treatment.* We spoke specially about the surgical treatment, which must be chosen in all cases where it is possible. Of course, we can sometimes stabilize the process with Cobalt treatment, when operation is not suitable.

I agree completely with Dr. House when he said that there were two sorts of tumours: tympanic glomus and glomus jugulare tumours. Theoretically, both are purely otological diseases, but when the tumour has extended too far into the intracranial space, we are obliged to recognize that it is a combined problem, and that the neurosurgeon must help us to solve the surgical intracranial difficulties.

The main message of this morning is the following. Even for a special otological disease, like glomus jugulare tumours, we must form an oto-neuro-surgical team, not only for diagnosis but also for the operation itself.

To emphasize this point, I want to recall a case in my series where the combined work was definitely necessary to do the best for the patient. The patient was a young worker who came with paralysis of the VII, VIII, IX, X, XI and XII nerves, a glomus tumour in the canal, a subtotal destruction in the pyramid on X-ray film and very important and numerous vascular pedicles from vertebral and carotid arteries and from the venous intracranial sinus. This tumour had a large extension in the posterior fossa. We decided with the neurosurgeon of our oto-neurosurgical group to do a two-stage operation: one to clip vascular pedicles from the intracranial sources, to recognize the importance of the extension in the posterior fossa, and a second one very quickly made to ligate some cervical arteries (the subclavicular artery, the external carotid artery), to pack the lateral sinus, and perform a subtotal petrectomy and, moreover, to follow the tumour further than the jugular foramina, until we reach the region of the XIIth nerve. This operation, performed 2 years ago, was very successful. Probably, the neurosurgeon or myself could not have done it alone, but working together made it safe and efficient. Only the combination of two sorts of surgeons is suitable for this kind of operation.

Finally, I think that the most important message of this meeting is to prove that we are compelled to work together for special cases. But if it is easy to discuss together, to examine the patient together, yet to operate in the same team is sometimes very difficult. We must have a good human and sympathetic relation between both surgeons.

It is in such a way that we can give the best of our knowledge and ability to our patients.

MISCELLANEOUS SKULL BASE TUMOURS

Clinical aspects of parapharyngeal tumours

By Erik Fluur

Department of Otolaryngology, Karolinska Sjukhuset, Stockholm, Sweden

The parapharyngeal space is a region below the base of the skull which the surgeon approaches with the greatest respect. This is partly because of its inaccessibility, and partly because it is crossed by the large vessels to and from the brain, with a rich network of branches.

To understand the clinical features and therapy of these tumours, it is necessary to be acquainted with the anatomy of the region where they are found. The space between the spinal column and the visceral cranium is denoted as the craniovertebral space. In this region, the styloid process is perhaps the most important keystone for the surgeon. This is because it is the site of origin of the stylopharyngeal septum, which is a musculofibrous sail, running between the styloid process and the lateral pharyngeal wall. This septum divides the craniovertebral space into two parts; one anterior, which is known as the parapharyngeal space, and one posterior, denoted as the retropharyngeal space. In its lateral border, the septum is strengthened by the styloglossal and stylopharyngeal muscles and the stylomandibular ligament. The stylopharyngeal septum serves as a supporting plate for those nerves and vessels running towards the pharynx. The vessels running in this direction are usually given off from the external carotid artery. Only in rare cases does the ascending pharyngeal artery arise from the internal carotid artery, after which it follows the septum in the medial direction.

Hidden behind the fairly thick stylopharyngeal septum and medial to the styloid process, the internal carotid artery ascends towards the skull (Fig. 1). Here is also the opening of the jugular foramen, with the internal jugular vein. Initially, it has no contact with the septum, but further caudally it touches on the muscles given off from the styloid process. The anterior part of the jugular foramen is crossed by three nerves coming from the skull, namely, the glossopharyngeal, vagus and accessory nerves. The hypoglossal nerve also enters from behind the vein. At their exit from the skull, all four nerves lie behind the internal carotid artery, whereas laterally they run in different directions. Thus, the glossopharyngeal nerve passes downwards, lateral to the internal carotid artery, to the inferior border of the stylopharyngeal muscle,

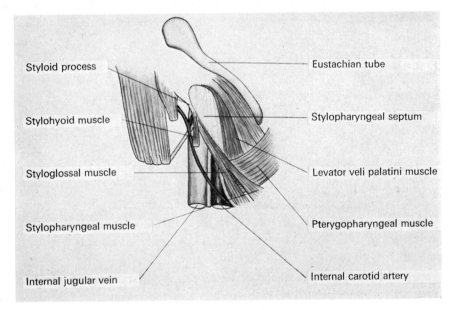

Fig. 1

after which it accompanies the stylopharyngeal septum to the tongue and throat.

The only one of the nerves which follows the sheath of the vessels is the vagus nerve, which lies between the artery and the vein. Via the stylopharyngeal septum, it sends small branches to the throat. High up in the retropharyngeal space, it also gives off the superior laryngeal nerve which runs, behind the internal carotid artery, forwards and downwards to the larynx.

The accessory nerve runs laterally from the jugular foramen, in front of the internal jugular vein, and emerges—below the styloid process—between the digastric and sternocleidomastoid muscles, after which it passes downwards towards the trapezius muscle.

Close to its exit from the hypoglossal canal, the hypoglossal nerve crosses the posterior part of the internal carotid artery, and passes forwards in the direction of the tongue, in a superficial arch lying on the arterial branches.

The sympathetic chain extends from the base of the skull in the caudal direction, situated in front of the prevertebral fascia, but all the time behind the internal carotid artery.

Since this relatively narrow space is occupied by several different tissue elements, it is not surprising that the tumours involving it may be of varying origin. The parapharyngeal space is bordered both medially and laterally by tissue which contains salivary glands, and these may give rise to both benign and malignant tumours which penetrate into it. The literature contains

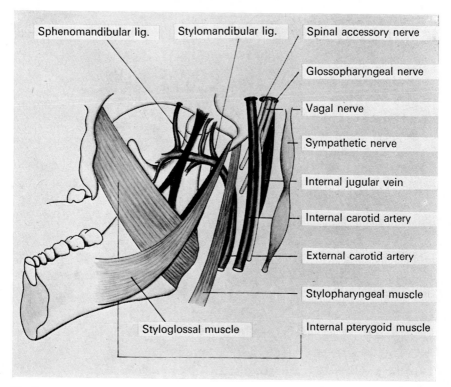

Fig. 2

fairly lively discussions of whether these tumours have issued primarily from the pharynx or from the parotid gland (Patey and Thackray, 1957, Patey and Ranger, 1957). However, there has been an increasing tendency to believe that the tumours generally arise from the parotid gland. From the parotid gland is given off a parapharyngeal process, which extends around the posterior margin of the mandible, and then for a varying distance in the medial direction. The parotid gland is delimited laterally by a firm fibrous capsule, but the deeper medial portion, the parapharyngeal process, is covered only by a thin connective tissue fascia. Consequently, according to the law of least resistance, a tumour of the deep parotid lobe will grow deeply into the parapharyngeal region. On its way inwards, the tumour must pass through the stylomandibular tunnel (Patey and Thackray, 1957). This is bordered upwards by the base of the skull, anteriorly by the ascending ramus of the mandible and the internal pterygoid muscle, and posteriorly by the styloid process and the stylomandibular ligament (Fig. 2). The tumour will therefore grow behind the internal pterygoid muscle, but in front of the stylopharyngeal septum.

When the tumour has extended into the parapharyngeal space, it is confined by the relatively indistensible walls, so that its subsequent growth can take place only at the cost of the medial wall, which consists of the constrictor pharyngis superior muscle. This gradually produces an indentation in the lateral pharyngeal wall, with associated medial displacement of the tonsils and anterior palatal arch.

Mixed tumours may occur not only in the three large salivary glands, but also in smaller salivary glands. Rarely, a tumour arising in the mucosa of the lateral pharyngeal wall may invade the parapharyngeal space and there become so large that it can be palpated below the mandible. In such a case, it is naturally difficult to decide whether the tumour has derived primarily from the parotid lobe or from the pharynx. A parapharyngeal parotid tumour lies outside the constrictor musculature, which implies that the pharyngeal mucosa is freely mobile towards the tumour. A primarily pharyngeal mixed tumour has, on the contrary, arisen in the mucosa and is located medial to the constrictor pharyngis muscle. The mucosa and muscles are therefore considerably more adherent to the tumour than in the former case. As the latter tumour grows, it pushes the musculature in front of it in the lateral direction, and stretches it until it divides and allows the tumour to invade the parapharyngeal space. Despite this, the tumour will lie medial to the pharyngeal fascia, which thus encloses it in a kind of pseudocapsule.

The neurogenic tumours, which are as uncommon as the salivary gland tumours, may also invade this region. A common localization of the neurogenic tumours is precisely the retropharyngeal space, i. e., behind the stylopharyngeal septum. The extension of the tumour is, naturally, determined by its site of origin. Thus, a tumour originating in the sympathetic chain is primarily situated behind the internal carotid artery, but later usually tries to expand on the medial side of the vessel, and then gradually continues to grow behind the stylopharyngeal septum, towards the throat (Fig. 3). Here, it presses the posterior part of pharyngeal wall behind the tonsillar region and above it.

Sometimes, however, the tumour may also expand on the lateral side of the internal carotid artery, especially if the tumour arises in any one of the last four cerebral nerves. It extends laterally between the artery and the vein, and when it reaches the styloid process it is diverted in the posterior direction towards the mastoid process and the spinal column (Fig. 4). In this case, the tumour is located below and behind the insertion of the sternocleidomastoid muscle.

The symptomatology of a tumour in the parapharyngeal space naturally depends on the type of tumour growing there. The mechanical distension may produce a feeling of pressure and swelling in the throat, and sometimes irritation or even pain. Other symptoms are dysphagia and deafness. In neurogenic tumours, we also have neurological symptoms from the different nerves involved in the process.

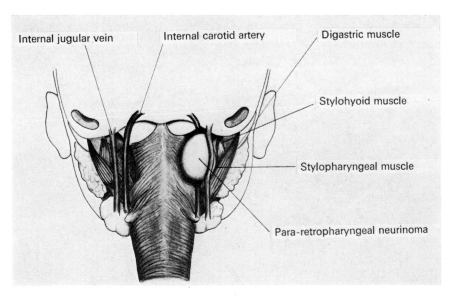

Fig. 3

Even if salivary gland tumours and neurogenic tumours are the most usual types of neoplasm occurring in the parapharyngeal space, other types are also seen. Reports are found of fibrolipoma (Howarth, 1930), lymphoma (New and Childrey, 1931), lymphatic leucomia (Patey and Thackray, 1957), aneurysm, carotid body tumour (Morfit, 1955), chordoma (André and Lacourreye, 1962), congenital cysts (Ombrédanne and Goddé, 1962) and cholesteatoma (Goddé, 1962).

Once a tumour extending into the parapharyngeal space has been detected, it is important to try to ascertain its site of origin. Bimanual palpation may be helpful, and should be performed in every case of parapharyngeal tumour. Carotid angiography and retrograde jugular angiography are valuable tools for establishing the location of the tumour. In addition, a roentgenologic examination of the skull should be made, to determine whether the bones at its base have been invaded. This is especially the case in malignant tumours. The histological diagnosis is established by puncture or biopsy.

Tumours appearing in a region that is so inaccessible as the parapharyngeal space have often been regarded as inoperable, and irradiation therapy has therefore been recommended instead of operation. However, since these tumours are seldom radiation-sensitive, surgical excision has become the most effective form of treatment. Because a tumour occurring in the parapharyngeal space generally bulges into the lateral wall of the pharynx, many surgeons have preferred a pharyngeal approach. This technique is practicable only in a case where a very small salivary gland tumour arises in the phar-

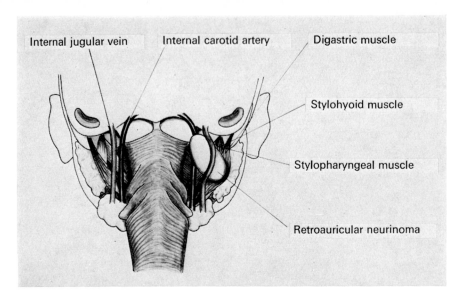

Internal jugular vein   Internal carotid artery   Digastric muscle

Stylohyoid muscle

Stylopharyngeal muscle

Retroauricular neurinoma

Fig. 4

yngeal mucosa, i.e., when the mucosa is not freely mobile towards the tumour.

Nowadays, most surgeons favour the external approach, in view of the smaller risk of haemorrhage and infection.

In the presence of a parapharyngeal parotid tumour, the facial nerve is sought in the angle between the external auditory canal, the mastoid process, and the digastric muscle. The retromandibular process of the lower lobe is freed from the rest of the gland, and followed round the angle of the mandible toward the stylomandibular tunnel. The anterior border of the digastric muscle is followed downwards, and the interglandular septum, a double layer of fascia which separates the parotid gland from the submandibular gland, is divided laterally, to provide a good view of the parapharyngeal space. To facilitate removal of the tumour, the space behind the mandible should be enlarged by fracturing the styloid process backwards towards the spinal column. It should be borne in mind that this type of tumour lies anterior to the stylohyoid, styloglossus and stylopharyngeus muscles, so that this fracture will cause all of them to relax. These muscles lie protectively in front of the internal carotid artery, except in the region directly medial to the styloid process, where the tumour may lie immediately beside the vessel. The posterior margin of the tumour is fairly easily freed by following with the finger along the aforementioned muscles and septum. The anterior and lower margins are freed by digital extracapsular dissection along the posterior surface of the internal pterygoid muscle. After severing the superior temporal artery, the tumour is mobilized during cautious, concurrent downward traction.

In excision of neurogenic tumours, the procedure differs in several respects from the aforegoing description. Because such a tumour lies behind the stylopharyngeal septum, one must, for visual inspection of its site of origin, proceed in a somewhat different way.

In order to excise the tumour under visual control, it is necessary to penetrate behind the septum. This is most easily done by ligating and dividing the external carotid artery. The proximal stump is then lifted up towards the mandible, which implies that all its branches, as well as the stylopharyngeal septum, will be lifted up towards the internal pterygoid muscle. When the internal carotid artery has been retracted backwards, a large space presents in front of the vertebral column. Here, the sympathetic chain can then easily be exposed and traced upwards in the direction of the tumour, under visual control. To avoid a fall in blood pressure on traction of the vagus nerve, the conduction of the nerve should be blocked by local anaesthesia. It is then easy to excise the tumour, irrespective of whether it extends in the medial or the lateral direction. With this approach, the nerve can be sutured after excision, should this prove necessary.

In the presence of a malignant tumour of the parapharyngeal space, it is often impossible to perform a completely radical operation. In view of the limited space, the tumour rapidly penetrates the fascia and muscles and then infiltrates the large vessels of the neck. When the tumour is suspected to be malignant, it is recommended always to place a loop around the common carotid prophylactically, to avoid profuse haemorrhage if the internal carotid has been injured during dissection. Postoperative irradiation therapy should be considered.

References

André, P. & Lacourreye, *Ann. Otolaryng.* (Paris), *79,* 312 (1962).
Goddé, M. D., *Ann. Otolaryng.* (Paris), *79,* 619 (1962).
Howarth, W., *J. Laryng.,* *45,* 673 (1930).
New, G. B. & Childrey, J. H., *Arch. Otolaryng.* (Chicago), *14,* 596 (1931).
Ombrédanne, M. & Goddé, C., *Ann. Otolaryng.* (Paris), *79,* 613 (1962).
Patey, D. H. & Ranger, I., *Brit. J. Surg.,* *45,* 250 (1957).
Patey, D. H. & Thackray, A. C., *Brit. J. Surg.,* *44,* 352 (1957).

Histological aspects of parapharyngeal tumours

By Carl-Magnus Eneroth

Department of Otolaryngology, Karolinska Sjukhuset, Stockholm, Sweden

Parapharyngeal tumours arise from tissue structures in the parapharyngeal space itself, or from surrounding organs.

Different types of head and neck tumours, as well as pharyngeal tumours, can involve the parapharyngeal space.

Here, however, I shall discuss only the clinically parapharyngeal tumours —that is, those bulging into the pharynx from the parapharyngeal space. Parapharyngeal tumours in this limited sense are extremely rare.

In an analysis of operated tumours of the head, neck and pharynx from the Department of Otolaryngology of Karolinska Sjukhuset during the period 1950–1968, 32 proved to have been clinically parapharyngeal. The majority of them—namely, 27—had been operated on after 1960.

A characteristic feature of the tumours of the parapharyngeal space is a pronounced variation in the histological picture. This is illustrated by the fact that the 32 tumours are distributed among 12 different types. Mixed tumours (12 cases) and carotid body tumours (5 cases) are the most common, and together comprise more than half of all the parapharyngeal tumours. The remaining 15 tumours are distributed among 10 different types, most of which are exceedingly rare, and therefore may cause diagnostic difficulties.

To permit a more accurate evaluation of the material from the histological and clinical point of view, a histological re-examination and reclassification were made. Following this reclassification, the parapharyngeal tumours in the 32 patients comprising the material were distributed as shown in Table 1.

For the sake of clarity, the various salivary-gland tumours and neurogenic tumours are assembled in two collective groups, which differ pathogenetically and histologically from other types, accounted for separately. Pathogenetically, tumours of the ganglion nodosi vagi should actually be denoted as neurogenic. They will, however, be discussed together with carotid body tumours, since these two types of tumour have similar histological features.

It is seen that the group of salivary-gland tumours is the largest, more than one in three of all parapharyngeal tumours being of this type. These

Table 1. *Parapharyngeal tumours. Distribution after reclassification.*

Salivary-gland tumours	13
Neurogenic tumours	8
Carotid body tumours	5
Ganglion nodosi vagi tumours	2
Synovial sarcoma	1
Lipoma	2
Lymph node metastases	1
Total	32

tumours can arise primarily either from the pharynx, or from the parotid or submandibular gland.

At operation of the 13 patients with a salivary-gland tumour, a connexion with the deep parotid lobe could be established in 9, and with the submandibular gland in one. In the remaining 3 cases, the parapharyngeal tumour seemed to be well delimited from both the parotid and the submandibular gland. Consequently, it probably arose primarily in the pharyngeal mucosa.

The great majority of parotid tumours ($> 80\%$) are localized in the superficial lobe. Of the tumours in the deep lobe, only a few attain such a size that they fill the parapharyngeal space, causing the pharyngeal wall to bulge in medially.

With a view to studying the incidence of parapharyngeally growing parotid tumours, 1108 cases of such operated tumours were analyzed. Nine of them—thus, $< 1\%$—proved to be clinically parapharyngeal. The incidence of submandibular tumours with parapharyngeal growth was just as low—1 of 129 cases.

Table 2 shows the incidence of the various types of salivary-gland tumours after reclassification.

Eleven of the 12 mixed tumours were benign. Acinic cell carcinoma is a low-malignant type of tumour. A remarkable fact is the high incidence of mixed tumours, and the absence of all other types, apart from the one case of acinic cell carcinoma. This can be explained by the types of tumour represented here being slow-growing, and usually asymptomatic on growth into the parapharyngeal space, until they have reached such a size that they

Table 2. *Parapharyngeal salivary-gland tumours. Distribution after reclassification.*

Diagnosis	No.
Mixed tumours	12
Acinic cell carcinoma	1
Total	13

Table 3. *Parapharyngeal neurogenic tumours. Diagnosis after reclassification.*

Diagnosis		No.
Neurofibroma		3
Neurofibrosarcoma		1
Neurilemmoma		2
Chordoma		1
Ganglioneuroma		1
	Total	8

bulge into the pharynx. The high-malignant types of tumour come under treatment before they have reached such a size. This is because of their greater variety of symptoms, in the form of, for example, nerve infiltration and metastasis.

Parallel with the salivary-gland tumours becoming increasingly well defined histologically, preoperative cytologically diagnosis has become more reliable. In every case in which a preoperative cytological examination of puncture biopsy material was made (9 of 13 cases), the diagnosis was correct.

The incidence of the various types of parapharyngeal neurogenic tumours can be inferred from Table 3.

Neurofibroma, neurofibrosarcoma, neurilemmoma and chordoma are histologically well-defined types of tumour. Preoperative diagnosis by cytological examination presented no difficulties. Ganglioneuroma is a tumour of the sympathetic nervous system, characterized by the presence of ganglion cells and neurofibrils.

The whole material contains 12 carotid body tumours. Five of them had such extensive growth into the parapharyngeal space that they bulged into the pharynx. A carotid body tumour arises at the bifurcation of the carotid artery, and is composed of nests of fairly large und uniform epithelioid cells in a vascular fibrous stroma. Both cytologically and histologically, this type of tumour presented certain diagnostic difficulties. Cytologically, the correct diagnosis was made in 6 of the 10 cases in which puncture biopsy was performed. The others were denoted cytologically as neurofibroma, neurofibrosarcoma or thyroid carcinoma. However, in view of the localization of this type of tumour, the preoperative diagnosis is easy to establish, particularly by carotid angiography.

Tumours structurally similar to carotid body tumours may arise in other organs in the neck, such as the ganglion nodosum of the vagus, and glomus jugulare. Only a few cases of tumour of the ganglion nodosi vagi have previously been described in the world literature. Two such were diagnosed in the present series. Histologically, both tumours showed a great resemblance to a carotid body tumour. However, in both cases brown, non-chromaffin pigment was demonstrable, which has been described as characteristic of this type of tumour.

None of the 28 glomus tumours in the material was clinically parapharyngeal.

A synovial sarcoma is of mesothelial origin. It has a fibrosarcoma-like stroma, and an epithelial-like component. The neck is an extremely rare localization of this type of tumour; in fact, only 5 cases of cervical synovial sarcoma have been reported in the literature. Another case of interest is that of parapharyngeal lymph-node metastasis (poorly differentiated carcinoma without known primary tumour).

Finally, if we consider the whole series of pharapharyngeal tumours, it is found that the overwhelming number were benign, namely, 26 of 32 tumours.

In most cases, a correct preoperative diagnosis can be made by means of puncture biopsy. A remarkable feature is, nevertheless, the occurrence of occasional cases of exceedingly rare types of tumour. These presented diagnostic difficulties, both cytologically and histologically.

Carotid body tumours

By Peter Berdal

Department of Otolaryngology, Rikshospitalet, Oslo, Norway

Based on histological and histochemical findings and on functional properties, the following grouping of carotid body tumours can be suggested:

1. Tumours with numerous cells containing argentaffin granules (Fig. 1). Catecholamines are produced in considerable amounts.

2. Tumours with argentaffin granules in small number (Fig. 2). Hormone production is questionable.

3. Tumours with a vascular pattern without argentaffin cells and with no hormone production of clinical importance (Fig. 3). This is the most usual type.

Having listened to the excellent lecture of Dr. B. Hamberger today, I think that the new histochemical method will permit a broader basis for classification, and that the grouping will perhaps be another one.

At Rikshospitalet, 8 cases of carotid body tumours have been hospitalized during 1960–1968 (see Table 1). One patient had a coincident tumour of the glomus jugulare-tympanicum. One patient had a recurrence following removal of a carotid body tumour 10 years previously. Two of the cases were definitely malignant, with lymph node metastases and distant metastases. In one case, a pronounced production of noradrenaline was demonstrated. Excision of the tumour was performed in 7 cases. In two of them the carotid bifurcation was resected. The postoperative course was uneventful in all patients except case 1, in whom vagus paralysis occurred. Of the operated patients, four of those with a benign tumour are alive and in good health. In case 2, radiological treatment was followed by a considerable reduction of the tumour, and its growth seems to have stopped.

Approximately 700 cases of carotid body tumours have been reported in the literature, occurring with the same frequency in males and females. Familial occurrence, bilateral carotid body tumours, separate or coincident with familial occurrence, have been reported by many authors. Unilateral and bilateral carotid body tumours coincident with a glomus jugulare tumour are also reported (e.g. Lubbers, 1937, Kipkie, 1947). Other interesting combinations include a case of Zacks (1958) in which the patient had one carotid

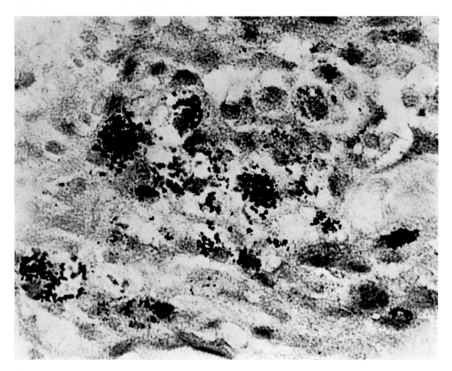

Fig. 1. Numerous argentaffin cells in tumour with hormone production. Hexamine-silver.
× 160.

body tumour, one glomus jugulare tumour and two retroperitoneal chemo-dectomas.

The tumour appears in typical cases as a slowly growing lump in the neck, close to the carotid bifurcation. There may be involvement of the cervical sympathetic chain, the vagus nerve and the hypoglossal nerve. Dysphagia may occur, due to medial growth with displacement of the pharyngeal wall and the tonsil. The tumour may be pulsating, and in some cases a stethoscopically audible bruit is produced.

Differential diagnosis includes branchial cyst, neurinoma, ganglioneuroma, infiltrating haemangioma, parotid tumour, lymphoma, and metastatic tumour.

Aspiration biopsy may provide the correct diagnosis, but the result is not always conclusive. An aspiration biopsy yielding blood only is strongly suggestive of a carotid body tumour. A biopsy by direct exposure of the tumour under general anaesthesia may then be required.

A most valuable aid to diagnosis is carotid angiography, which was employed by Engström and Hamberger (1957) and later by many authors. This may disclose a displacement of the external and internal carotid arteries, and the tumour itself may be outlined by a rich vascular network. In some cases,

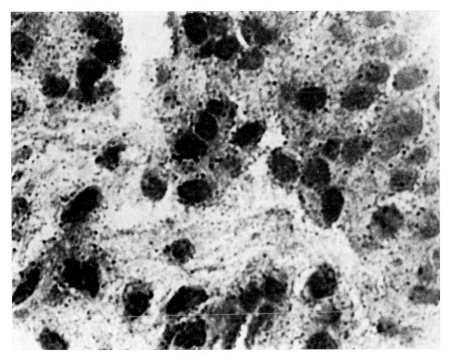

Fig. 2. Widespread single argentaffin cells (centre) in tumour with questionable hormone production. Hexamine-silver. × 480.

a blood supply from the vertebral and thyrocervical arteries has been demonstrated (von Leden, 1965).

Since a production of noradrenaline is demonstrated in some cases, repeated blood pressure measurements and a search for increased urinary excretion of catecholamines are necessary. In cases with a pronounced noradrenaline production, surgical removal of the tumour may lead to a severe or even fatal drop in the blood pressure (Glenner *et al.*, 1962).

The incidence of malignancy varies considerably among the different observers. Some report a very low malignancy rate, others up to 50%. The criteria of malignancy may be difficult to evaluate. Romanski (1954) described a tumour with a fairly benign histological picture and distant metastases to vertebral bodies, the lungs and the mediastinum. Evidence of malignancy are metastases to lymph nodes and distant dissemination. Twenty-eight definitely malignant cases observed by different authors were summarized by Reese and associates (1963). Later 7 additional cases have been reported, including 2 of our own. Based on clinical and histological criteria, I think that the incidence of malignancy may be estimated at about 20%. It would appear that the slow growth of some of these tumours during several years may endanger the patient by local extension and the possibility of metastases.

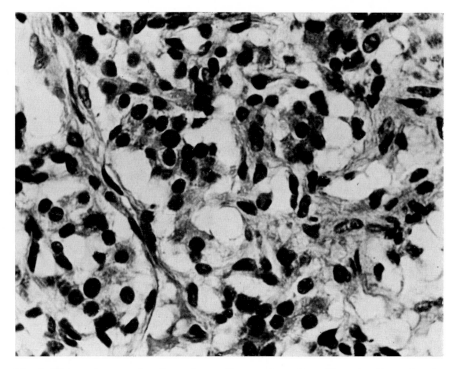

Fig. 3. Glomus tumour of ordinary type with vascular pattern. Haematoxylin-erythrosin-saffron. × 160.

Spontaneous regression of a carotid body tumour has not been reported, and radiological treatment is of questionable value. Most surgeons are of the opinion that operative removal of the tumour is the treatment of choice, especially as subadventitial dissection of the tumour has been possible in the majority of cases. A partly conservative attitude has been advocated by some authors, who restrict their radical surgery to definitely malignant cases. The reason for this conservatism is the high morbidity and mortality rate follow-ing sacrifice of the common or internal carotid arteries, about 30% and 12% respectively. Thus, the risk of damage and of death from the surgical intervention might be higher than that from the disease itself. Today, I think that we escape these surgical hazards by improved diagnostic and surgical procedures. The cerebral collateral circulation is evaluated preoperatively, and facilities for reconstructive vascular surgery are available, if required, when the operation is performed.

The adequacy of the cerebral collateral circulation is estimated before operation by carotid angiography, by electroencephalography and by direct measurement of internal carotid artery pressure.

If the carotid on the affected side is digitally occluded, angiography of the other side will reveal whether collateral circulation exists across the circle of

Table 1. *Carotid body tumours, Rikshospitalet, Oslo 1960–1968.*

Case		Sex	Age (yrs) Year of treatment	Symptoms and findings	Duration	Treatment	Comments
1.	S. H.	♂	66 1960	Lump in the neck. Parapharyngeal growth with displacement of tonsil. Noradrenaline production. Angiography: displacement of int. and ext. carotid arteries	1 year	Extirpation.	Intracarotid pressure reading during operation. Postop. vagus paralysis. Died 1961 of pneumonia.
2.	A. M.	♂	42 1962	Lump in the neck.	1 year	X-rays.	Glomus tumour in contralateral middle ear.
3.	E. E.	♂	40 1963	Lump in the neck.	2 years	Extirpation. Lymph node dissection. X-rays.	Malignant tumour with metastases to lymph nodes and skeleton. Death from metastases 1965.
4.	K. H. H.	♂	76 1963	Lump in the neck.	2 months	Extirpation. Lymph node dissection. Postop. X-rays.	Malignant tumour with lymph node metastases. Sudden death 1966. No signs of recurrence.
5.	H. B.	♀	52 1963	Lump in the neck. Angiography: displacement of carotid, vascular network.	6 years	Extirpation.	Hypothermia. Continuous EEG and intracarotid pressure reading during operation.
6.	E. H.	♀	16 1964	Lump in the neck, pulsating. Parapharyngeal growth with displacement of tonsil. Vocal chord paralysis. Angiography: displacement of carotid, vascular network.	10 years	Extirpation. Resection of carotid bifurcation.	Hypothermia. Continuous EEG and intracarotid pressure reading during operation. Internal carotid small.
7.	J. K.	♀	70 1964	Lump in the neck.	4 years	Extirpation.	Recurrence following removal of carotid body tumour 10 years previously.
8.	O. O.	♂	54 1966	Lump in the neck, suspicious of malignancy. Angiography: displacement of carotid.	4 months	Extirpation. Resection of carotid bifurcation.	Continuous EEG and intracarotid pressure reading during operation. Wall of int. carotid ruptured.

Willis. The demonstration of a crossed cerebral circulation is greatly reassuring in the preoperative selection of the patient who might require ligation of the common or internal carotid. On the other hand, the failure to demonstrate collateral circulation is a reason to avoid carotid ligation, and to be prepared to restore arterial continuity by a vascular graft.

Electroencephalography combined with temporary interruption of the carotid blood flow is also a useful method. The results of the EEG are compared with and evaluated against the arteriographic findings.

Probably, the most accurate means of determining the adequacy of the collateral flow is by direct measurements of internal carotid pressure before and during temporary occlusion of the common carotid (e.g. Sweet, Sarnoff and Bakay, 1950, Johnson, 1953, Crawford, De Bakey, Blaisdell, Morris and Fields, 1960). Direct pressure readings that drop less than 50 % of preocclusion values indicate an adequate cerebral flow and a favourable prognosis. If the pressure falls by more than 60 % of the preocclusion value, the carotid bifurcation should not be sacrificed unless carotid continuity is restored by a graft (e.g. Johnson, 1953, Westbury, 1959–60). Direct pressure reading can also be obtained during the operation, after exposure of the tumour and the carotid arteries.

EEG is also performed during operation, after exposure of the common carotid artery and direct manual interruption of the blood flow. Lack of alteration of the EEG tracings indicates an adequate collateral circulation. In the patients where the carotid had to be sarcified, a correlation was found between the EEG tracings and the subsequent clinical course.

Summary

Approximately 700 cases of carotid body tumours have been reported. Illustrated by 8 personal cases, the clinical features and biological properties of these tumours are reviewed. Attention is drawn especially to a possible production of catecholamines. Diagnosis and therapy are discussed. Examination of the collateral cerebral circulation before and during the operation is stressed.

References

Berdal, P., Braaten, M., Cappelen, Chr., Jr., Mylius, E. A. & Walaas, O., *Acta Med. Scand., 172,* 249 (1962).

Berdal, P., Braaten, M., Cappelen, Chr., Jr. & Mylius, E. A., *Acta Otolaryng.* (Stockholm), Suppl. 188, 211 (1964).

Crawford, S. W., De Bakey, F. W., Blaisdell, C. C., Morris, G. C. Jr. & Fields, W. S., *Surgery, 48,* 76 (1960).

Engström, H. & Hamberger, C.-A., *Acta Otolaryng.* (Stockholm), *48,* 390 (1957).
Glenner, G. G., Crout, J. R. & Roberts, W. C., *Arch. Path.* (Chicago), *73,* 230 (1962).
Johnson, H. C., *Surgery, 33,* 537 (1953).
Kipkie, G. F., *Arch. Path.* (Chicago), *44,* 113 (1947).
von Leden, H., *Z. Laryng. Rhinol. Otol., 44,* 260 (1965).
Lubbers, J., *Nederl. T. Geneesk., 81,* 2566 (1937).
Reese, H. E., Lucas, R. N. & Bergman, P. A., *Ann. Surg., 157,* 232 (1963).
Romanski, R., *Amer. J. Path., 30,* 1 (1954).
Sweet, W. H., Sarnoff, S. J. & Bakay, L., *Surg. Gynec. Obstet., 90,* 327 (1950).
Westbury, G., *Brit. J. Surg., 47,* 605 (1959–60).
Zacks, S. L., *Amer. J. Path., 34,* 293 (1958).

The surgical approach to the external part of the base of the skull related to the anterior and medial cranial fossa

By Siegfried Zehm

Department of Otolaryngology, University Hospital, Würzburg, Germany

The surgical approach to the base of the skull related to the anterior and medial cranial fossa is based on skin incisions in the face. The exposure depends on how much of the structures of the face can be dissected or removed, and has limitations to a certain degree of tissue loss and to its moral and functional capacity.

Two main routes are available. 1. Using the middle face, going through the antrum and the ethmoids (Zange) or the maxilla (Moser)—with or without preservation of the orbital content—suitable for exposing the anterior part of the base of the skull, which permits extension into the sphenoid sinus and nasopharynx (Zöllner) as well as into the orbit itself (Mennig).

2. Using the lateral part of the face, going through the mandible and the zygoma, which opens a space directly underneath the base of the skull related to the medial cranial fossa.

Regarding route 1, there are no difficulties in exposing the dura of the anterior cranial fossa by techniques using surgery of the nasal sinuses and the orbit itself. In comparison with this, the part of the skull related to the medial cranial fossa, except the middle part around the nasopharynx, is awkward to approach and difficult to expose. For years it has been considered a relatively inaccessible area. This is due to the fact that this area is situated underneath the skull at the extreme posterior and lateral position of the maxilla, interlaced with abundant and important nerves, blood vessels and muscles.

This area underneath the base of the skull as a whole extends between the maxilla and the prevertebral fascia, the mandibular joint and the nasopharynx. It includes the Eustachian tube, the internal carotid artery, extreme laterally the jugular vein with its associated nerves and, last but not least, the anatomically much smaller pterygoid fossa. With this in view, I regard this area under clinical aspects as the so-called "retromaxillary space" (Fig. 1).

Attempts at the intraoral approach or by the mid-face exposure (Moser) and the aim of preservation of the orbital content, either by sharp dissection or cautery excision, are encumbered by the constriction of limited exposure of this area and the danger of haemorrhage that is difficult to control. Even

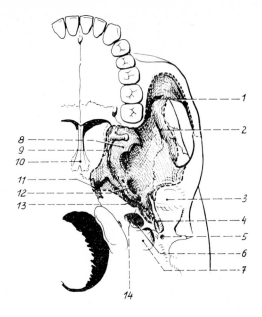

Fig. 1. Retromaxillary Space. 1. infra-orbital sulcus, 2. infraorbital crist, 3. glenoid fossa, 4. styloid process, 5. stylomastoid foramen, 6. carotid canal, 7. jugular fossa, 8. lateral pterygoid plate, 9. medial pterygoid plate, 10. pharyngeal tuber, 11. lacerated foramen, 12. oval foramen, 13. spinae foramen, 14. sphenoid spine.

large composite resections at the maxilla, the orbit and the zygoma (Mündnich, McCarten) are limited by their mid-face approach at the level of the external pterygoid muscle, because of the danger of damaging the internal carotid artery and the mandibular joint. Lacerated joint tissue will develop scar formation, and causes further immobilization of the mandible.

When, in combination with maxillectomy, a partial resection of the mandible proves to be necessary—in a case like this shown as a recurrent adenoma—we advise performing this operation primarily starting on the lateral face. By splitting the lower lip in the midline and lengthening the incision anteriorly to the external ear, a flap can be mobilized to give an adequate exposure to the hyoid and styloid area, the parotid gland, the mandible and even to the maxilla.

This actually is a part of the approach to the retromaxillary space, introduced by Conley in 1956 for the management of primary benign and malignant tumours of this area, and situations associated with the failure of irradiation and the development of recurrent cancer of the tonsil and the associated area. As you may realize, the retromaxillary space can be entered and combined with resections of the maxilla. The internal carotid artery and the jugular vein always stay posteriorly and can be separated, if necessary.

It should be emphasized that the benign tumours of this area are mainly located in the pocket between the internal pterygoid muscle and the mandible and may be removed by splitting the mandible temporally at its angle without running into complications. By preserving the continuity of the mandible, the cavity created can be closed primarily and dressed under continuous suction

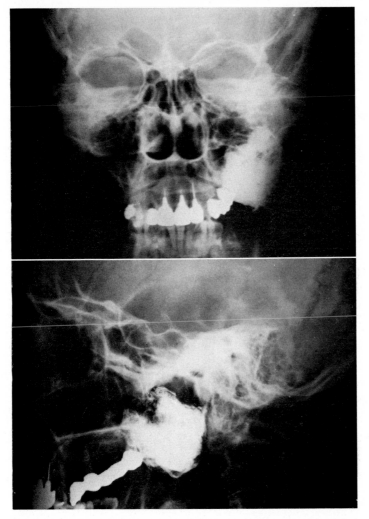

Fig. 2. X-ray contrast of the retromaxillary space — frontal and lateral view.

for a few days. When the ascending ramus of the mandible is resected—in a case of a primary malignant tumour—the cavity is drained into the oral cavity for further control, as it is demonstrated on these X-rays (Fig. 2). It requires hygienic measures until it has healed by second intention.

With the extension of the skin incision right in the temple area of the scalp, the elevated flap gives an adequate exposure to the temporal and infratemporal fossa by cutting the temporalis muscle and the zygomatic bone, displacing them towards the mandible. This incision can also be used single in order to receive information from a biopsy from this particular area.

At the same time, in a composite operation the isolation of the parotid gland should be accomplished with the facial nerve intact. This is carried out

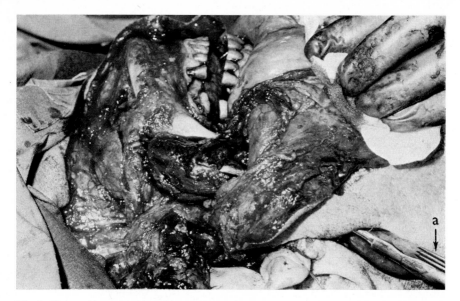

Fig. 3. The working tunnel is achieved, demonstrated by the instrument (a).

by freeing it along its internal aspect, thus creating a bridge of glandular tissue, containing the facial nerve extending from the styloid area anteriorly into the cheek. An adequate working tunnel can be achieved underneath this bridge to perform osteotomy of the ascending ramus of the mandible and free its head from the glenoid fossa (Fig. 3). Dissections follow towards the oval foramen; the mandibular branch of the fifth cranial nerve is excised, the pterygoid muscles are cut at the base of the skull and at the pterygoid plate, which is also removed.

Bleeding is controlled either by ligating the external carotid artery prior to the excisional operation, or ligating the principal branches encountered in the resection. Bleeding from the venous pterygoid plexus is stopped by small transfixions. If the primary lesion is on the lateral wall of the nasopharynx, the Eustachian tube will be resected in its cartilaginous part, and particular care should be taken to preserve its function and to prevent stenosis by inserting a polyethylene tube into its stump temporarily (Fig. 4).

The most extensive exposure of the medial cranial fossa can be obtained when a temporal bone resection is included in the prior excisional operation. As you will see in this 54-year-old man, he underwent an extensive composite operation at the time when he was treated before with appr. 8000 R Co[60] therapy for a malignant adenoma. He was suffering from severe pain, a blockage of his jaw, complete facial paralysis and a swelling of his right lateral face. A neck dissection was done, including an area of heavily irradiated skin in combination with resection of the temporal bone, the zygoma,

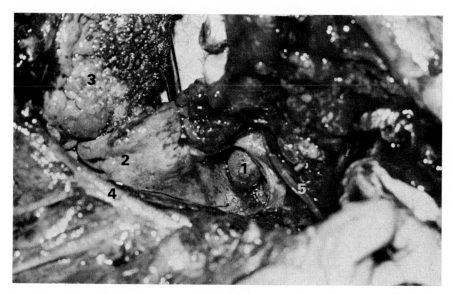

Fig. 4. Nasopharynx open, polyethylene tube running from the nasal cavity in the retained Eustachian tube. 1. posterior end of the right inferior turbinate, 2. retained soft palate on the right side, 3. base of the tongue, 4. hypoglossal nerve, 5. polyethylene tube.

the mandible and the styloid process. The dura of the posterior and medial cranial fossa can be seen free up to the bend of the internal jugular vein and internal carotid artery, where they start running into the cranium. Furthermore, you see the infratemporal fossa, the oval foramen, into the pterygoid fossa and the medial pterygoid plate. In such an extensive exposure, one should keep in mind the importance of rehabilitation of this wound by plastic procedures. Histologically, the tumour was found to be a cylindroma primarily located at the inside of the mandibular joint, extending into the middle-ear cavity.

With this presentation, I was trying to demonstrate the different ways of approach to the base of the skull particularly related to the medial cranial fossa. The named routes have been found desirable and effective in the management of primary benign and malignant tumours. The patients are grateful for the relief of pain, the ability to open the mouth and the resume of normal eating habits.

Summary

The surgical approach to the base of the skull related to the anterior and medial cranial fossa is designed by two main routes going through the face. Exposing the anterior cranial fossa of the base of the skull, techniques are used on the experience of surgery of the nasal sinuses and the orbit itself. In comparison to the exposure of the medial cranial fossa, there are no difficulties as regards limitations in preserving the orbital content, but it can always be extended into the sphenoid sinus and the nasopharynx of the orbit itself.

To expose the medial cranial fossa, an approach on the lateral face is desirable, since this part of the base of the skull is very much related to the area underneath it, which is called the retromaxillary space. This area is awkward to approach and by the constriction of a limited exposure combined with the danger of haemorrhage that is difficult to control. The approach therefore starts by splitting the lower lip in the midline, makes the skin incision in a curve anteriorly to the external ear, and can be extended to the temple area of the scalp. In resecting the ascending ramus of the mandible and the zygoma, the exposure can lead under conditions of a composite resection to the infratemporal area, glenoid cavity, oval foramen, to the pterygoid area directly to the nasopharynx. The internal carotid artery and the jugular vein always stay posteriorly and can be separated, if necessary.

The most extensive exposure can be obtained when, with the prior excisional operation, a temporal bone resection is combined. Then the bone can be freed to the dura of the posterior and medial cranial fossa closely around the knee of the internal carotid artery and the jugular vein. The resulting raw area has to be covered and managed by plastic procedures.

References

Conley, J. J., *Ann. Surg., 144,* 39 (1956).

McCarten, A. B., *Amer. J. Surg., 106,* 696 (1963).

Mennig, H., *Arch. Ohr. Nas. Kehlkopfheilk., 187,* 397 (1966).

Moser, F., *Mschr. Ohrenheilk., 99,* 536 (1965).

Mündnich, K., *Z. Laryng. Rhinol. Otol., 33,* 125 (1954).

Wustrow, F., *Die Tumoren des Gesichtsschädels,* Urban & Schwarzenberg, München–Berlin (1965).

Zange, J., *Operationen im Bereich der Nase und ihrer Nebenhöhlen,* in: Handbuch d. Ophthalm. Op.-Lehre von R. Thiel. Georg Thieme Verlag, Leipzig, 1091 (1950).

Zehm, S., *Die Topographie des retromaxillären Raumes in chirurgischer Sicht,* Habil.-Schrift, Würzburg (1966).

Zöllner, F., *Z. Laryng. Rhinol. Otol., 31,* 1 (1952).

Treatment of advanced cancer of the ethmoid sinuses

By Alfred S. Ketcham, William G. Hammond, Paul Chretien, and John M. Van Buren

Surgery Branch, National Cancer Institute, N.I.H., Bethesda, Maryland, U.S.A.

Although less than 1 % of human neoplastic disease arises in the paranasal sinuses, malignant tumours of this anatomical area remain an enigma to the oncologist. The relative inaccessibility of the sinuses to adequate examination and the ease with which a tumour, arising in a sinus, erodes into adjacent sinuses through the paper-thin bony partitions, may lead to rather extensive local tumour growth without exhibiting any external manifestations of cancer. The frontal lobe of the brain is separated from the ethmoids by only the easily transgressed and traumatized cribriform plate through which pass the olfactory fibers. Tumour rising in or eroding into the ethmoid sinuses therefore has easy access to the anterior cranial fossa. Surgical excision of this superior limit of the ethmoid is fraught with the severe complication of dural perforation resulting in cerebral spinal fluid leakage. Radiotherapy has thus become the popular mode of therapy (Gibb, 1957) for ethmoid tumours, since the complications of osteoradionecrosis of the thin bony partitions of the paranasal sinuses have been more easily handled than has the tumour recurrence which often results from attempted resection of the entire ethmoid sinus by the transfacial approach (MacComb and Martin, 1942).

The cribriform plate can rarely be resected by the usual transfacial approach without creating cerebral complications (Frazell and Lewis, 1963). While 80 % of paranasal tumours arise in the maxillary antrum (Salem *et al.,* 1963, Tabah, 1962) it is our experience that many of these tumours, when finally recognized, have eroded into the ethmoids. It was recognized in 1953, (Smith *et al.,* 1954) that an *en bloc* resection could best be done by elevation of the frontal lobe of the brain and transcranial mobilization of the cribriform plate. By so doing the medial orbital walls (lateral ethmoid partition) can be resected in continuity via the conventional transfacial approach (Ketcham *et al.,*1963, Van Buren *et al.,* 1968).

The refinements in the technique of *en bloc* resection of paranasal sinus cancer by the combined intracranial transfacial approach have been developed in a selected group of 35 patients. This 11-year experience serves as the nucleus of this report.

Material

Every patient admitted with cancer of the paranasal, orbital, and posterior naso-pharyngeal area has been evaluated for possible diseases extension into adjacent anatomical areas. Patients were eliminated for consideration of surgery when distant metastases were demonstrated or when there was evidence of central nervous system involvement. Despite the fact that, radiographically, sinus involvement by tumour can be easily confused with sinusitis or blockage of adjacent areas due to tumour (Salinger, 1961, Martin, 1957, Divine *et al.*, 1957) particular reliance has been placed upon transverse and sagittal tomography. When tomograms (Dodd *et al.*, 1959) stereoscopic Water views, and anterior, posterior, and lateral skull films suggested that there was invasion of the sphenopalatine fossa as evidence by significant erosion of the pterygoid plates, or when the posterior confines of the sphenoid sinuses were eroded, then operative intervention was not chosen as a treatment of choice. Orbital wall erosion has been no deterrent to the combined surgical approach but has indicated the necessity of removing the unilateral orbital contents, *en bloc* with the involved paranasal sinuses. Forty-one patients have undergone the cranial portion of this procedure, 6 of whom exhibited either massive intracranial involvement of the brain or complete but previously unrecognized erosion of the entire posterior extension of the planum sphenoidale. The remaining 35 patients have undergone the entire combined procedure in a definitive attempt at *en bloc* cancer resection.

Twenty-three of the 35 patients had some form of carcinoma, and ten patients had different types of sarcoma. There were also 2 patients with esthesioneuroblastoma (Table 1).

Table 1. *Incidence of type of cancers in 35 patients all of which involved the ethmoid sinuses.*

Carcinoma	
(23 of 35)	
Epidermoid	10
Adenocarcinoma	4
Undifferentiated	3
Transitional cell	3
Adenoid-cystic	2
Basal cell	1
Sarcoma	
(10 of 35)	
Fibrosarcoma	2
Rhabdomyosarcoma	3
Chondrosarcoma	2
Leiomyosarcoma	1
Undifferentiated	2
Esthesioneuroblastoma	2

Ten of the 23 carcinoma patients and 5 of 10 sarcoma patients had received definite treatment, either radiation and/or surgery, previous to admission.

Combined operative procedure

Therapeutic blood concentrations of antibiotics are obtained by 12 hours of preoperative intravenous antibiotics. Antibiotic administration is continued intravenously throughout the operative procedure and for 7 to 10 days postoperatively. Operative skin preparation and draping techniques leave the entire head and neck area exposed, as well as the anterior thigh on the same side of the patient on which the facial exposure is to be made. This allows ready access to the donor site for the split-thickness skin graft which will be taken to cover the intraoral nasal operative defect. Airway intubation through a preliminary tracheostomy is directed to the contralateral side of the patient so that the anesthesiologist is completely free of the operative field. This conveniently allows 3 surgeons to work about the head and neck area.

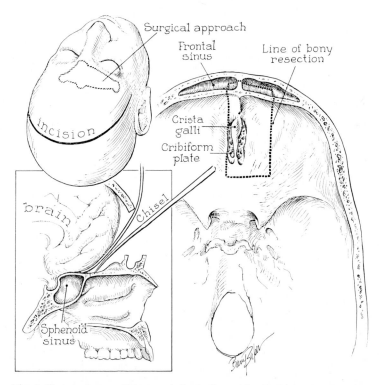

Fig. 1. The craniotomy defect made in the frontal bone will usually be much smaller than depicted. The bony dissection about the cribiform plate may be somewhat more symmetrical on either side of the cribiform area, so as to include both medial orbital walls. Very often the posterior line of dissection will enter into the sphenoid sinus.

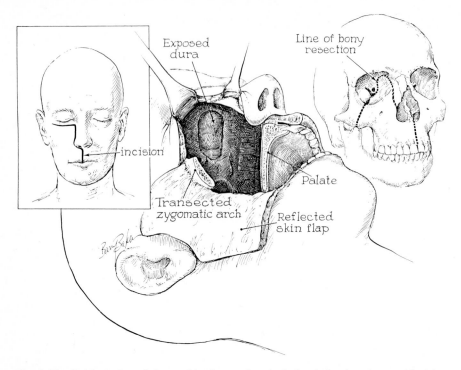

Fig. 2. The facial portion of the combined procedure is depicted showing the usual incision in skin and bone. Exposed dura is intensified high in the facial defect and will be covered with split skin graft. If the orbital contents are to be left intact, the skin incision need not extend horizontally across the lower eyelid.

A coronal scalp incision within the hairline allows the frontal skin flap to be elevated and turned down over the face (Fig. 1). A large burr hole is made in the frontal bone, and often this burr hole will enter the superior portion of the frontal sinus. Experience has demonstrated the infrequent necessity to make a series of burr holes, as depicted in Fig. 1, and actually elevate an entire frontal bone flap. Spinal fluid is then withdrawn by the anesthesiologists from a preoperatively placed lumbar spinal catheter. This facilitates frontal lobe retraction with a half inch ribbon brain retraction. By both blunt and sharp dissection, the dura is progressively separated from the skull base to include elevation from the crista galli and cribriform plate back to exposure of the planum sphenoidale (Ray and McLean, 1943). By osteotome dissection, the cribriform plate in its entirety, is mobilized with this bone transection being carried up onto the medial portion of the orbital roof. If orbital exenteration is to be carried out, this bony dissection is carried further over the orbit than when simple medial orbital wall removal is anticipated. Posterior osteotome dissection is directed across the planum sphenoidale into the posterior ethmoid cells, or more often, into the anterior portion

Table 2. *A review of complications resulting from the combined cranial facial exenteration in 35 patients having cancer involving the ethmoid sinus.*

Infection	Patients
Meningitis	4
Skull flaps (3 removed)	9
Graft slough, complete	2
Cellulitis, periorbital	10

Neurological	Patients
Transient confusion	9
Diabetes insipidus	2
CNS leak (16 healed)	18
Hematoma	1

Miscellaneous	Patients
Oedema (transient)	21
Diplopia (disabling 0)	7
Bleeding	3

of the sphenoid sinus. With this bone mobilization completed, the scalp skin flap is returned to its normal site and the transfacial approach carried out.

A modified Weber-Ferguson incision allows the cheek flap to be retracted laterally (Fig. 2). Osteotome incisions are made through the medial line of the maxillae and palate, across the zygomatic arch to communicate with the inferior orbital fissure, and upward along the lateral nasal bone to communicate with the anterior cranial fossae defect. If the orbital structures are to be sacrificed it may be helpful to do so through the intracranial approach. Transoral curved osteotome dissection across the pterygoid plates frees the specimen posteriorly and allows mobilization of the entire specimen. With some pressure being applied through the intracranial defect upon the bone of the cribriform area, the specimen is delivered down through the facial defect. The nasal septum is retained, if tumour so allows, although the vomer and its superior attachement are removed with the specimen. After careful inspection of the specimen, appropriate marginal biopsies of the operative defect, rather than the specimen itself, are taken for evaluation of tumour infiltration at the wound margins by frozen section. Through the transfacial approach, any small rents in the dura are meticulously closed. The spinal fluid which had been removed through a preoperatively placed spinal catheter is then reinjected and any further dural leaks are closed. A large split-thickness graft is taken from the thigh and carefully placed into this large operative defect thus lining the exposed dura, the sphenopalatine area, bone, and under-surface of the cheek flap. The graft is stabilized by a minimal number of sutures and held in place by cornish wool packing. A plastic button is placed over the enlarged frontal burr hole and the scalp and facial incisions closed.

In those instances where tumour has been found to erode through the cribriform plate, as in 7 of the 35 patients, a segment of dura was excised and left attached to the tumour-infiltrated cribriform area. On 5 occasions it was necessary to close this dural defect with an isolated temporal fascial graft. Four of these patients developed meningitis postoperatively, 2 of whom died and 2 of whom were successfully controlled without residual neurologic deficit.

All patients are immediately fitted with an intraoral maxillary prosthesis as soon as the split-thickness skin graft has sufficient stabilization. This is usually on the 5th or 7th postoperative day when the packing is removed. There are often areas of exposed bone and tissues from incomplete skin graft take but in no instances have these areas failed to re-epithelialize with time.

The large intraoral defect is kept cleansed by the patient, with spray irrigations, although meticulous cleansing is usually no longer necessary after 3 months postoperatively.

Complication and results

The complications (Ketcham et al., 1966) of this aggressive procedure are listed on Table 2. Since decreasing the size of the craniotomy to that of an enlarged burr hole, no patient has developed infection of the craniotomy site. It has been found necessary, in avoiding cellulitis and infection in both the immediate and the later follow-up period, to completely exenterate the frontal sinuses and establish dependent drainage. While it is not uncommon for the patient to leak spinal fluid for a few days, this has stopped spontaneously in all patients by the 17th day, except in the postoperative death at 59 days.

Of the 35 patients, there were 2 postoperative deaths in meningitis.

There are 30 patients in whom longer follow-up for eradication of cancer is possible. The 5-year survival rate in the 30 patients discharged with hope for cure is 23%, or 7 of 30.

Discussions

The advantages of the combined cranio-facial procedure, over the usual transfacial approach, can fully be appreciated by those surgeons who have experienced the usual unsatisfactory attempt to remove tumour within the ethmoid sinuses. This procedure allows: (a) evaluation of intracranial disease, (b) protection of the brain, (c) avoidance of cerebral spinal fluid fistula, (d) improvement of hemostasis, (e) facilitation of en bloc resection of tumour.

It must be emphasized that this procedure is carried out in selected patients after a meticulous roentgenographic survey of the bony anatomy of the skull.

Transverse and sagittal tomography has become an integral part of this evaluation. Admittedly, the 45% overall survival of 16 patients who were alive 2–11 years postoperatively, may not be as significant as the 23% 5-year survival in 7 patients. However, a more optimistic view is developed when one considers that 17 patients were living and free of disease 2 years after their operation, the time when those who eventually died had evidence of lethal disease, and 13 of those 17 are presently living without evidence of disease, a minimum of 3 years following surgery.

The usual site of disseminated disease has been pulmonary metastases, but the most common reasons for failure must be attributed to our inability to determine the extent of tumour invasion in the sphenopalatine fossa and within the sphenoid sinuses themselves.

The cosmetic results of this operation are extremely gratifying. If the facial flap can be held in its normal contour by prosthesis insertion before fibrosis develops, the only significant cosmetic alteration is loss of the orbital contents in those patients who required orbital exenteration (21 of the 35 patients). The fitting of an intraoral operative hard palate prosthesis has been facilitated by always attempting to leave the soft palate intact. In the edentulous patient, snug palate prosthesis fitting is sometimes difficult. If one or more teeth can be left on the opposite maxilla, little difficulty is then encountered and these patients can return to normal speech and eating habits.

At the completion of the operative procedure, it is relatively routine to insert, through the low neck, a cervical esophagostomy (Ketcham *et al.,* 1962). Through a No. 18 French plastic or rubber tube, placed just lateral to the midline of the neck, adequate nutrition can be maintained from the first day postoperatively. This feeding technique averts food accumulating in the operative defect, thereby predisposing to odor and infection.

Summary

A combined intracranial transfacial operative approach to the paranasal sinuses allows *en bloc* tumour resection of the ethmoid sinuses. This procedure has the advantage of allowing evaluation of intracranial extension of disease, protection of the brain, avoidance of spinal fluid fistula, adequate hemostasis, facilitation of resection, and true *en bloc* tumour resection, all resulting in improved long-term survival from ethmoid sinus cancer.

References

Devine, K. D., Scanlon, P. W. & Figi, F. A., *JAMA, 163,* 617 (1957).
Dodd, G. D., Collins, L. G., Egan, R. L. & Herrera, J. R., *Radiology, 72,* 379 (1959).

Frazell, E. L. & Lewis, J. S., *Cancer, 16,* 1293 (1963).

Gibb, R., *Proc. Roy. Soc. Med., 50,* 534 (1957).

Ketcham, A. S. & Smith, R. R., *Amer. J. Surg., 104,* 682 (1962).

Ketcham, A. S., Wilkins, R. H., Van Buren, J. M. & Smith, R. R., *Amer. J. Surg., 106,* 698 (1963).

Ketcham, A. S., Hoye, R. C., Van Buren, J. M. & Johnson, R. H., *Amer. J. Surg., 112,* 591 (1966).

MacComb, W. S. & Martin, H. E., *Amer. J. Roentgen., 47,* 11 (1942).

Martin, H., *Surgery of Head and Neck Tumors,* Paul B. Hoeber, Ind., New York, 311 (1957).

Ray, B. S. & McLean, J. M., *Arch. Ophtha!.* (Chicago), *30,* 437 (1943).

Salem, L. E., Saharia, M. & Travezan, R., *Amer. J. Surg., 106,* 826 (1963).

Salinger, S., *Arch. Otolaryng.* (Chicago), *73,* 196 (1961).

Smith, R. R., Klopp, C. T. & Williams, J. M., *Cancer, 7,* 991 (1954).

Tabah, E. J., *Amer. J. Surg., 104,* 741 (1962).

Van Buren, J. M., Ommaya, A. K. & Ketcham, A. S., *J. Neurosurg., 28,* 341 (1968).

General discussion

Denecke to Fluur and Eneroth

Nach der Tumor- und Nervenresektion an der Schädelbasis treten Beschwerden beim Schlucken auf. Aspiration ist die Folge. Nach unseren Erfahrungen reicht die Operation nach Kaplan zu deren Korrektur nicht aus. Ich korrigiere den Schluckakt deshalb durch eine plastische Operation an Pharynx, Ösophagus, Velum palatinum und Larynx (Arch. Ohr. Nas. Kehlkopfheilk., *178,* 538 (1961) und HNO 9, 351 (1961)). Durch den Eingriff am Larynx wird gleichzeitig die heisere Stimme beseitigt.

Björk to Fluur

Seven years ago, Hamberger, assisted by Diamant, arranged at Karolinska Sjukhuset a course on diseases of the salivary glands. In his introduction, Hamberger told us about a method for management of parotid mixed tumours once used by the skilled surgeon Hybinette and the famous radiologist Berven. Hybinette opened the tumour, leaving the capsule unremoved, and Berven afterwards gave X-ray treatment to the patients. The results had been strikingly good. Soon after this course, I happened to see two cases of large parapharyngeal mixed tumours. In the first case, extracapsular enucleation could be performed. In the second case, such a procedure seemed to be very hazardous, since the tumour extended from the level of the cricoid up to the base of the skull. I remembered what Hamberger had told us in Stockholm. After tonsillectomy, the tumour capsule was opened and enormous masses of typical mixed tumour were evacuated as carefully as possible; the capsule was left in place and X-ray treatment was given afterwards. The observation time is short indeed, but today the status almost resembles that seen after an ordinary unilateral tonsillectomy, showing no signs of recurrence.

Fluur

I would like to add the following to what I have said previously. If you are taking a biopsy specimen through the mouth, you will get scar tissue, which makes extirpation of the tumour much more difficult. Therefore, I advise you to make a puncture biopsy only through the mouth or from the outside.

Zehm to Eneroth

We are surveying 10 benign tumours of this particular area, and I would like to add to your outline another kind of tumour histologically called haemangiopericytoma, which we have found once and removed.

Ogura to Eneroth

How were the 5 carotid body tumours presenting as parapharyngeal tumours recognized before surgery?

Eneroth to Zehm

In the present material, there was no case of a haemangiopericytoma involving the parapharyngeal space. In the literature, about 300 cases of haemangiopericytoma are described—most of them localized to the trunk and extremities. In an analysis of operated head and neck tumours at the Department of Otolaryngology, Karolinska Sjukhuset, during the last 10-year period, 8 tumours proved to fulfil the histological criteria of haemangiopericytoma. Four of these tumours were localized to the nose. Differential diagnosis between haemangiopericytoma and other vascular tumours, such as haemangioendothelioma, paraganglioma, vascular fibrosarcoma etc., can be difficult. For this reason, it is not improbable that a parapharyngeal tumour denoted as a heamangiopericytoma can be a paranglioma (e.g. glomus tumour)—a tumour much more common in this region.

Eneroth to Ogura

As concerns the parapharyngeally growing carotid body tumours—5 of the 12 cases in the material—all were correctly diagnosed preoperatively, i.e., owing to carotid angiography being performed in these cases. The present material, however, contains totally 12 carotid body tumours. A correct cytological diagnosis was made in 6 of the 10 cases in which aspiration biopsy was performed. Phlebography of the internal jugular vein—a method denoted as retrograde jugularography—was performed in 6 of the 12 cases, and in 5 cases a displacement with or without compression of the internal jugular vein was seen. Carotid angiography was performed in 9 of the 12 cases, and with a correct diagnosis in every case. These 9 patients were thus operated on under the preoperative diagnosis of carotid body tumour. In the remaining 3 patients, the carotid body tumour was diagnosed first at operation. Carotid angiography and retrograde jugularography were not performed in these 3 patients, and the tumours were cytologically denoted as neurofibroma, neurofibrosarcoma and thyroid carcinoma, respectively. As no failure in the preoperative diagnosis of carotid body tumours was made with carotid angiography—9 of 12 cases—this method is consequently the best for diagnosing this type of tumour.

Krajina to Berdal

In the last 8 years at the Ear, Nose and Throat Clinic in Zagreb, we had 6 cases of carotid body tumours. In 3 cases we could not separate the tumour from the arterial wall. Histologically, the tumour was closely related to the arterial wall. Regarding irradiation, we used it in 2 cases, where the surgical procedure was stopped. In these cases, the tumour diminished 2 or 3 months later and subjective disturbances were less. The total dose was about 2000 rads, which is sufficient for producing fibrosis in the tumour.

Moberg to Berdal

A comment regarding the information that 20 % of the carotid body tumours are malignant. (1) The histological appearance—even in proven malignant cases—does not show the general morphologic features of malignancy, e.g. pleomorphism of mitotic activity. (2) This tumour grows in an expanding manner, sometimes without a capsule. It is then possible that the tumour may expand to a lymph node and overgrow it, but this is not a metastasis in the ordinary sense. (3) A comparison between the number of proven malignant carotid body tumours with the number of benign tumours is usually made in surgical series. The figure for the benign tumours will then be too small, since—very likely—small tumours are not diagnosed or operated on. (4) The number of proved malignant carotid body tumours is today some 30 cases. If 20 % of all carotid body tumours were to be malignant, it would mean that only some 150 carotid body tumours had been diagnosed throughout the world.

If these considerations are taken into account, the figure of 20 % appears much too high.

Berdal to Moberg

About 20 % malignant cases is an estimated incidence. Perhaps this figure is too high. However, in our series of 8 patients, there were 2 cases of malignancy. Some weeks ago I discussed this question with Professor Dargent (Lyon). In his experience, the incidence of malignant carotid body tumours is even higher than 20 %.

House to Zehm

Preliminary report on temporal bone resection. The entire middle ear has been removed *en bloc* in a patient 3 months ago by removing the temporomandibular joint, locating the carotid artery in the middle fossa, and then drilling off the anterior aspect of the carotid canal. The carotid artery is then slipped out of the canal, and the temporal bone dissected free from the middle and posterior fossa dura.

Zehm to House

This is an important point that Dr. House just mentioned, and for which I want to thank him. The patient demonstrated underwent this extensive bone removal at the base of the skull, including the foramen of the internal carotid artery and the internal jugular vein. Both were freed up to the dura of the middle cranial fossa. In view of the shortness of the time, I cannot go into further details as I should like to do. Therefore, I want to thank again for this comment.

Siirala to Ketcham

How did you get the frontal lobe to collapse to be able to create the beautiful approach to the anterior fossa? What did you do to avoid postoperative oedema of the brain?

Grahne to Ketcham

You mentioned that 20% of your patients were still alive after 5 years. I wonder if there were cases of cylindroma among them. If there were, you may perhaps expect recurrences even after 5 years. We know that we cannot definitely cure cases of cylindroma, despite the fact that they often are alive 5 years or more after the operation.

Ogura to Ketcham

Would you comment on 2 questions: (1) What did you mean by 70% failure in the 35 cases you operated upon? Were these irradiated or operative failures? (2) Do you believe that preoperative irradiation has any place before surgery?

Ketcham

Frontal lobe retraction is easily accomplished if spinal fluid is removed through a preoperatively placed lumbar spinal catheter. As the frontal lobe is dissected from its bony confines, and assisted by a ribbon retractor, it falls posteriorly to allow cribriform plate exposure.

Brain oedema has been directly related to the length of the neurosurgical procedure and, in turn, to the trauma to the frontal lobe caused by the elevation and retraction. In this series of patients, it has not been a significant complication.

Our patients are most often failures to irradiation or surgery before being referred to us for treatment. It is these unfortunate treatment-failure patients who are prone to postoperative complications.

We are not using preoperative radiation unless it be in locally far advanced cases, in whom we doubt our ability to successfully resect locally—then such patients are placed in a controlled blind-study protocol. I am not aware that there is yet available valid information which indicates the true role of preoperative radiation in the treatment of head and neck cancer. Of prime importance, to those who are using preoperative radiation or chemotherapy, is the realization that the subsequent surgery must be as encompassing and essentially identical in its scope as to what it would have been without preoperative treatment.

Chairman's summary of session VI

A. Miehlke

My talk will be a short one, because you certainly will understand that the moderator's task of summarizing the different types of tumours of the base of the skull which we have just heard about is quite a difficult one, for the simple fact that it is not easy to find common points of view. There are, however, two exceptions to this simple statement.

1. Dr. Eneroth managed to specify 5 out of 32 of his cases of parapharyngeal tumours as carotid body tumours—that is, tumours which Professor Berdal has been talking about, and which demand our greatest attention.

2. The treatment of these tumours—like tumours of the pterygoid area or the parapharyngeal space in general—means a highly difficult, if not to say dangerous surgery.

Therefore, let me make a few comments on aspects of the surgical technique. I think that you agree with me, Dr. Berdal and Dr. Krajina, that the approach between the adventitia and media of the carotid artery from the posterior aspect of the carotid bulb is the key-point in the surgical treatment of carotid body tumours. This corresponds to the experience I have made.

With regard to the surgery of tumours in the pterygoid or parapharyngeal area, I would like to state the following. As Dr. Zehm just pointed out, it was Dr. John Conley who, in 1956, inaugurated the lateral approach to the intratemporal and pterygoid area, in other words, to the retromaxillary region, as Dr. Zehm calls it. It is the great advantage of this approach that it allows grasping and embracing the tumour in a wide manoeuvre from the side, while the parotid gland and the facial nerve can be saved. And so I think that we have to be very grateful to Dr. Fluur for giving us such a useful review of this area's so complicated anatomy.

This external surgical approach has been found desirable and effective in the management of primary benign and malignant tumours of this region. The special approach may be part of a large composite resection of the lateral neck, pharynx, mandible and part of the tongue, as Dr. Zehm demonstrated, and as Dr. Conley described in his first paper, or it may be limited to a typical single surgical step, aimed at the direct resection of tumours in this particular area.

Furthermore, I would like to add to Dr. Ketcham's paper on extensive surgery in the ethmoid carcinomas that this procedure reminds me, in principle, of Unterberger's approach in the extradural management of extensive fractures of the base of the skull in its frontal area, and that we have needed this route for a long time. It is, indeed, a very helpful technique. May be, we will hear something more about it in the following session.

I would not like to finish my short comment without expressing the moderator's gratitude to Professor Hamberger for this magnificent symposium, and for your warm hospitality extended to all of us.

SESSION VII

TRAUMA OF THE SKULL BASE

Clinic, classification and treatment of frontobasal fractures

By Franz Escher

Department of Otolaryngology, University Hospital, Berne, Switzerland

Although the subject of frontobasal injuries has been treated in the extensive report in the French ORL Society by Aubry, Calvet, Piquet and Terracol in 1963, and in the outstanding survey of W. Kley in the German Society in 1968, it seems important to analyze these problems in this symposium again. We rhinologists have a missionary obligation to spread our knowledge and our activity in this field, and to prove that our co-operation with the neurosurgeons, the ophthalmologists and the maxillary surgeons is of great value, a fact which is not yet accepted everywhere. You will see that I am in perfect agreement with all active rhinologists, especially with the opinion of my friend W. Kley.

My report is based on personal experience of over 20 years, and concerns the two periods 1947–1959 (first report 1960) and 1960–1968 (June). It deals with altogether 82 open frontobasal fractures, of which 77 necessitated a surgical intervention.

In Table 1, you can see a clear augmentation of admissions in the second period, 52 cases in 8 1/2 years against 30 in the first 12-years period. This is due to two facts. The number of these injuries increases, and a greater number of these patients are directed to our clinic. The percentage of late admissions is the same in both; this will be treated later.

Overlooking the whole problem, three fundamental aspects emerge, i.e.,

1. the social problem
2. the problem of general medicine
3. special medical and surgical problems (assessment of a case, choice of treatment, surgical technique).

1. The social problem

More than 2/3 of the injuries are caused by traffic accidents (Table 2), more than 4/5 being young people in full activity (Table 3). If you consider how often these patients are physically and mentally damaged for their whole life, you will support all intentions of preventive medicine against the battlefield on the roads.

Table 1. *Frontobasal fractures, endocranium open.*

	Frontobasal fractures	Surgical intervention		
		Early op. 1st–30th day	Later op.	Total
1947–1959	30	21	6	27
1960–1968 (June)	52	39	11	50
Total	82	60	17	77

Table 2. *Cause of 51 open frontobasal fractures (1960–1968).*

Traffic	35
Direct trauma, blow projectile	8
Fall	8

Table 3. *Age of 52 cases (1960–1968) with open frontobasal fractures.*

–15 years	10
15–30	22
30–50	12
over 50	8

2. The problem of general medicine

Four fundamental principles can be mentioned for the practitioner:

a) The intact integument does not mean that no injury is behind it.

b) The extent of the injury is always greater than one might judge from the X-ray picture.

c) The presence or absence of concussion of the brain is of no importance when judging the gravity of the injury (Table 4). More than 50 % of the cases show no signs of concussion, or only a short concussion without amnesia.

Observed examples: A football player continues the match after a collision, with a massive rhinorrhoea. Another patient walks by himself to the out-patient department having a brain prolapse into the frontal sinus.

d) The therapy of an open frontobasal fracture must be an active one. Thirteen out of 17 late interventions had to be performed for late meningitis in patients who had no surgical treatment before.

Table 4. *Concussion of the brain. 68 cases open frontobasal fractures to evaluate.*

No signs of concussion	18
Short concussion without amnesia	20
Remarkable concussion with amnesia	11
Deep coma, shock contusion	19

3. Special medical and surgical problems

The *cardinal symptoms* are the following:

a^1 rhinorrhoea
a^2 pneumocranium
a^3 brain substance visible
a^4 late meningitis (Table 5)

a^1 *Rhinorrhoea.* As Table 5 shows, rhinorrhoea is the most frequent symptom. It may be isolated or associated with other symptoms (Table 6). If it is abundant, the situation is clear, but it is not seldom that only a systematic and meticulous research can display it, and fix the area of escape.

Beside the well known use of

the overhanging position
the Queckenstedt test
the pressure test
chemical analysis of the cerebrospinal fluid

the scintigram and the fluorescein coloration of the cerebrospinal fluid may help. It is recommended to tamponade both nose lumina with cotton, and to control it after removing for determination of the side of the escape.

It is to be noted that the transitory rhinorrhoea is as frequent as the persistent one. Sometimes rhinorrhoea appears after meningitis. On the other hand, it also may stop after it. The fact that a certain number of cases of rhinorrhoea are detected only during the operation is very important.

a^2 *Pneumocranium.* This symptom appears in different forms:
External pneumocephalus, which may be combined with skin emphysema.
The rare extradural pneumatocele.

Table 5. *Cardinal symptoms in 52 cases of open frontobasal fractures (1960–1968).*

Rhinorrhoea		
Rhinorrhoea only	17	
comb. other symptoms	11	
only during op.	6	total 34
Pneumocranium		
Pneumocr. only	4	
comb. other symptoms	3	total 7
Brain substance visible		
before operation	8	
only during operation	8	total 16
Late meningitis		total 8

Table 6. *Rhinorrhoea 1960–1968, 34 cases of 52.*

Immediate	
transitory	7
persistent	7
After interval	3
Combined with	
pneumocranium	1
prolapse of brain	5
meningitis	3
After meningitis	2
During operation only	6
Total	34
Stopped after meningitis	1

The intradural forms

— subdural: the air moves with the position of the head,

— subarachnoidal: the air diffuses in the sulcus and the cisterns,

— intraventricular: corresponding to a ventriculogram,

— intracerebral: the air enters a traumatic brain cavity.

Intradural pneumatocele is a sure sign of the opened endocranium. In the pure form without other symptoms, the fissure of the dura producing the valve effect must be very small. In four of these cases, we did not find the split in the dura during revision, in spite of a focus of bone chips around the exposed dura.

a^3 *Brain substance visible.* This symptom need not be discussed if it is clear. But one may be anxious; it may be hidden and can be proved only during operation (in 8 of 16 cases in our series). This applies especially to the fronto-orbital type, with a prolapse into the orbit.

a^4 *Meningitis,* late form, early form (Table 7)
Late meningitis is often the only and most dangerous sign of an earlier frontobasal fracture. This trauma may be forgotten; the longest interval between

Table 7. *Meningitis 1947–1968, 30 cases of 82 fractures.*

Early meningitis 1st–30th day			Late meningitis after months/years			
Before operation	After operation		Without op. before	Operated before		
	N	R		N	R	N + R
9	4	1	13 (9 of these 13 cases, 2–5 attacks)	1	1	1

N = neurosurg., R = rhinolog.

the injury and the meningitis amounts in our observation to 18 years. Repeated meningitis is extremely typical of the traumatic origin. Nine of 13 cases had 2 to 5 attacks. Thirteen of a total of 16 cases had no previous surgical treatment, which proves the importance of primary active therapy. It is to be noted that 2 of these traumatic cases of meningitis were caused by meningococci; one of the patients had in one attack pneumococci in the cerebrospinal fluid, in the other meningococci. Even in a meningococcal meningitis, therefore, we have to envisage a traumatic genesis.

Early meningitis may spread in the first 24 hours after the injury, before an intervention is undertaken. If meningitis occurs after the operation, we have to admit that the endocranium was already infected. It must be pointed out that we observed 4 cases of early postoperative meningitis after neurosurgical intervention and plasty of the dura. In all these cases, an infected zone with bone chips in the ethmoid was discovered at the rhinological exploration. In similar cases, therefore, rhinological exposure of the upper paranasal cavities should follow the neurosurgical procedure. An area that is not drained and not cleaned in the neighbourhood of a duraplasty always presents a potential focus of endocranial infection.

b) *Classification*

Considering the variability of the injuries, it may seem illogical to make any classification. But for the surgical procedure, it is a help to make some groups, it is also a valuable help in systematic teaching. We therefore divide the lesions into 4 types, namely:

b^1 the extensive type
b^2 the localized type
b^3 middle face rupture from the base
b^4 fronto-orbital type

b^1 *Extensive type* (Fig. 1). These extensive injuries—des grands blessés in French literature—cover nearly half of all the cases. They are mostly caused by great force, especially in traffic accidents. These cases need the full attention of all interested groups of surgeons, as the assessment of the brain lesion is their first task. All the following types (b^2–b^4) may be included or associated. No precise general directives for therapy exist. An individual plan for the intervention has to be established for each case in collaboration with neurosurgeons, ophthalmologists and maxillary surgeons.

b^2 *Localized type* (Fig. 2). This type is often caused by direct trauma: blow, projectile and fall. This injury is mostly suitable for rhinological intervention; the dura rupture lies mainly on the crista galli and the cribriform plate, some-

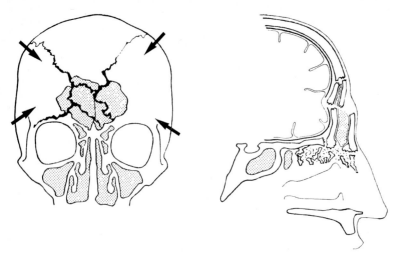

Fig. 1. Frontobasal fracture, extensive type.

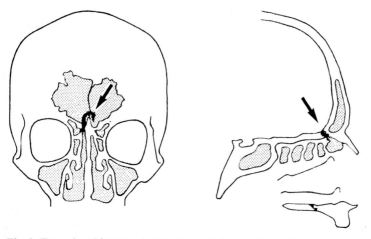

Fig. 2. Frontobasal fracture, localized type (crista galli; cribriform plate).

times in the sphenoid. It must be mentioned that this type can be produced by contre-coup through a fall on the occiput.

b³ *Middle face rupture from the base* (Fig. 3). The full force bounds against the middle face below the front, the profile of the face is pushed back. Consequently, there arises a wide zone of bone splinters on the skull base, beside the maxillary fracture. Rhinorrhoea may occur only at the moment of drawing back the maxillary for reposition and fixation.

In these cases, a meticulous inspection of the base, a duraplasty and removal of all splinters, combined with sufficient drainage, is indicated.

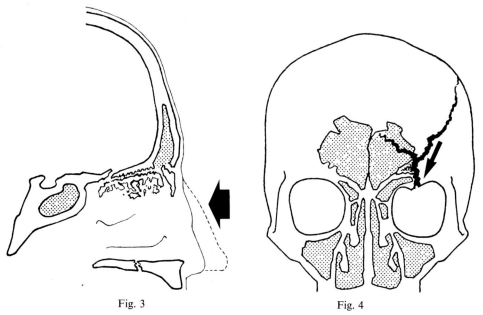

Fig. 3   Fig. 4

Fig. 3. Frontobasal fracture, middle face rupture from the basis. Push back. "Dish face".
Fig. 4. Frontobasal fracture. Latero-orbital type.

b⁴ *Fronto-orbital type* (Fig. 4). Although the pure form of this type is not frequent, it is worth being separated from the others. In these cases we notice the poorest symptomatology. Rhinorrhoea does not exist, the dura rupture is behind the contents of the orbit, the natural tamponade prevents an infection for a long time. When it arises, it generally starts from an orbital ethmoid cell, producing a late complication. In connection with this, I want to emphasize the striking frequency of non-pneumatized frontal bones. In 8 of all 52 frontobasal fractures, i.e., in about 15 %, we find this phenomenon, the normal average being 4–5 %. It seems that a non-pneumatized frontal bone has a minor resistance. It splits like porcelain. This is of special importance for the fronto-orbital type.

c) *Surgical procedure*

c¹ *Time of the intervention* (Table 8). As a general rule, we admit that the operation should be done as early as possible, as soon as the general state permits it. This is the best protection against endocranial infection. No alteration of the tissue with formation of scars and granulations is present. The cosmetic restoration should be as definite as possible, on condition that the safety is guaranteed. A compromise is sometimes necessary, especially if the anterior wall of the frontal sinus must be removed. This is illustrated by Table 8. An example of a primary restoration in a completely destroyed orbit

Table 8. *Operative procedure in 77 cases, 1947–1968 (June).*

Early operation	R	N	N+R simult.	N+R alternat.	Total	
1st–10th day	28	4	13	5	50	
11th–30th day	9	–	1	–	10	60
Later operation after months and years	14	–	2	1		17
Total	51	4	16	6		77

and frontal bone, rupture of the dura and brain prolapse which took 9 hours' operation, is demonstrated.

c^2 *Competence for the surgical procedure.* I would like to emphasize the excellent collaboration with the team of our neurosurgeon, Professor Markwalder. Whenever the frontal region is damaged, with suspicion of an opened air cell system, we discuss the procedure together. Of course, the neurosurgeons treat rhinorrhoea in their own way, too, or in cases of decompression for haematoma and concussion of the brain, the frontal sinus region or the base may be reached. These cases do not figure in our statistics.

If a combined neurosurgical and rhinological intervention is necessary, we prefer to do it simultaneously; an alternating two-stage operation being indicated, the rhinological generally following the neurosurgical intervention.

The scheme for the incisions published by W. Kley corresponds to our view. The neurosurgical incision can also be used for the extradural procedure of Unterberger.

The next figure shows the procedure according to the fracture type. The neurosurgical or the combined neurosurgical-rhinological route is in most cases reserved for the extensive type, but even in this group a certain number of cases are managed by rhinological intervention alone (Table 9).

Table 9. *Classification and surgical procedure in 50 open frontobasal fractures (1960–1968).*

	Extensive type	Localized type	Middle face rupture from the base	Fronto-orbital type
Number of cases	24	16	6	4
N	3	—	–	–
N+R	8	1	–	–
R+O	2	—	–	–
N+R+O	1	—	–	–
R	10	15	6	4

N = neurosrg., O = ophthalmol., R = rhinolog.

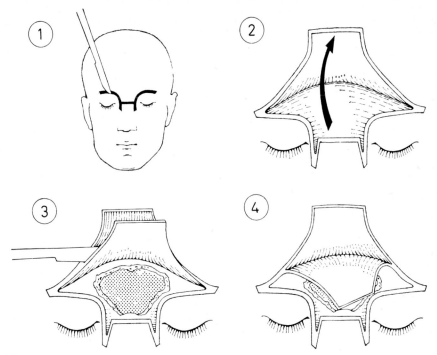

Fig. 5. Incision and use of a turned galea-periosteum flap.

In all the other types we used, with one exception, the rhinological procedure.

c[3] *Technical principles of the rhinological procedure.* At this moment I cannot enter into details.

Two fundamental goals have to be attained:

1. definite closure of the dura
2. removal of all remains of bone splinters and chips, of destroyed mucosa, combined with perfect drainage in the nose cavities, as protection against endocranial infection.

This may be achieved by

— free transplantation of galea-periosteum or fascia lata between the dura and the borderline of the bone,

— closure of the bone hole by a free piece of bone,

— overlapping of the area with a free or fixed and turned galea flap (Fig. 5),

— use of the periorbita according to Peiper,

— use of an anesthesia tube with a cuff for inflating and pressing the transplant against the wall (Fig. 6),

— use of mucosa of the middle turbinate or the septum for epithelization (Fig. 7).

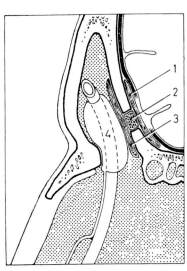

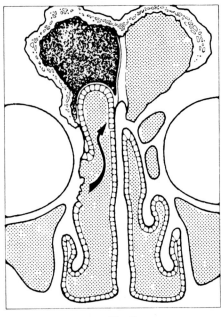

Fig. 6   Fig. 7

Fig. 6. Closure of a hole in the posterior frontal wall. 1. Free fascia graft between dura and hole. 2. Piece of bone in the hole. 3. Free fascia on the outside. 4. Compression with an anaesthesia tube.

Fig. 7. Epithelization of the bottom of a filled frontal sinus with the mucosa of the middle turbinate.

With accumulated experience, the possibility of modifying details of the technique is increasing. In each individual case, one must decide whether a removed bone can be implanted again, or whether or not an anterior frontal wall has to be removed. One thing is obvious: the rhinological route provides a perfect view of the base of the skull, from the frontal sinuses to the sella turcica, as it is well known from transsphenoidal hypophysectomy. If one first takes the route of security and after that the cosmetic view, the rhinological surgery in frontobasal fractures must be and is successful.

References

Aubry, M., Calvet, J., Piquet, J. & Terracol, J., *Les traumatismes des cavités annexes des fosses nasales et leurs séquelles,* Librairie Arnette, Paris (1963).
Kley, W., *Arch. Ohr. Nas. Kehlkopfheilk., 191,* 1 (1968).

Neurosurgical aspects of liquorrhoea

By Lennart Herlin

Department of Neurotraumatology, Karolinska Sjukhuset, Stockholm, Sweden

Until the last 10 years, a selected material with traumatic brain injuries was admitted to the Neurotraumatological Clinic, Karolinska Sjukhuset, namely cases which were referred to the clinic after treatment for some time at other hospitals, where cerebrospinal fluid (CSF) rhinorrhoea had initially been diagnosed. Almost all of these cases were in good condition, with only slight brain injuries, but with obvious CSF leakage either through a fractured frontal sinus or through the ethmoid sinus. A problem from that time was that a fracture through a thin cribriform plate was not always easy to see at radiography, sometimes not even after tomography.

Fractures through the frontal sinus could be studied at radiography, and a density of the ethmoid cells most often revealed the CSF leakage when it passed through a fractured cribriform plate. We experienced no practical difficulties in detecting the lesions on surgical treatment. At this time we had little experience of CSF leakage through the sphenoid sinus.

We did not believe in spontaneous healing of CSF leakage through the nose. However, this was due to the fact that the cases were selected, as I mentioned above.

Although surgical closure of fistulas with CSF rhinorrhoea is usually advisable to prevent infection, dural repair is essentially a prophylactic operation. Experience has shown that the optimal time for repair in the majority of the cases is not in the acute phase after injury, but when both the local and general condition of the patient is satisfactory. The initial operation for compound fractures involving risk of CSF rhinorrhoea is therefore often best limited to a minimum, with removal of any loose bone and careful scalp suture. In a series published by Lewin (1966), only 6 of 108 cases were operated on in the first 10 days after the injury. However, it is impossible to formulate rigid rules as to when surgery should be performed in the individual case. During the past 2 years, full surgical treatment of severely damaged patients was made acutely in several cases.

Initially, like the majority of other authors, we considered it advisable to give preventive antibiotic treatment.

The principle for surgical closure of a CSF fistula through the frontal or the ethmoid sinus is to take up a bone flap and open the dura. The frontal lobe is elevated by brain spatulas, so that the dural split can be completely explored from the inside.

Infectious fibrous tissue may proliferate, together with the sinus mucosa adhering to the arachnoid and to damaged brain tissue. This abnormal tissue often forms a loose string adherent to the bony defect, and permeable to the CSF. It must be completely resected during surgery, before the dural tear is covered from the inside by a fascia lata graft or by pieces of pounded muscle. Extradural covering of the dural tear is not effective. In the cases with leakage through the cribriform plate (usually on one side only), the covering of the dural tear from the inside is sufficient to stop the leakage.

In the cases with CSF rhinorrhoea through the frontal sinus, one often finds a comparatively large volume of brain laceration near the frontal pole. The dura may lack area, thus making a tight suture impossible. Its covering with beaten muscle may be insufficient. To secure a permanent stop of CSF leakage, loose pieces of the walls of the frontal sinus are removed, and the mucosal sac is extirpated. Thereafter, the frontonasal duct is plugged with muscle pieces. Usually, the frontal sinus is separated into a left-sided and a right-sided sinus by a medial bony wall, but there may be a defect in this wall. Therefore, it is advisable to plug the ducts on both sides. In cases where the frontal sinus is fractured only by a fissure and not open for exposure, it is opened by chisels through its posterior wall.

CSF leakage through the middle fossa

Traumatological cases with CSF leakage through the middle ear and the external acoustic meatus often constitute severe cases of brain concussion.

However, the CSF leakage almost always ceases spontaneously after a short time. Surgical treatment in order to close a CSF fistula in this group of patients has become necessary only when a small area of circumscript bone has been fractured and driven deeply into the middle fossa like a nail.

Typical cases with severe injuries from the past 2 years

I. *Male, 40 years old*. Motor car collision accident with crush injury of the facial skeleton, including the upper and lower jaw and teeth. The frontal sinus on both sides was crushed, and wide open to the nasal cavity. The cribriform plate was fractured and loosely displaced in elevation, together with the fractured ethmoid sinus on both sides. There was a laceration of the right frontal lobe. The right eye was broadly ruptured. There was a large dural defect.

The maxillar, zygomatic and nasal bones were first fairly well repositioned, using cerclage and Kirchner's steel rods. Thereafter, a frontal bone flap was turned open on the right side and a frontal lobe resection was performed. The open defects between the brain and nasal cavity were covered with large muscle pieces. The dura was covered from the inside by a large piece of muscle, and then sutured as tightly as possible. It was then covered with muscle also from the outside.

In the period following the brain operation, there was CSF leakage which gradually decreased and ceased after about a month. The patient has recovered very well.

Recently, we have had 4 other very severe traumatic brain lesions with a broad connexion through fractured frontal and ethmoid sinuses from the brain to the nasal cavity. In all of them, CSF leakage stopped some time after the surgery.

II. *Woman, 20 years old*. Car collision accident. The patient struck her head on the front window-frame. There were thin fractures in all three regions of the frontal, the ethmoid and the sphenoid sinus without obvious displacement. The sense of smell was lost. There was CSF leakage bilaterally through the nose. In the early skull X-rays, small air bubbles were seen intracranially near the posterior extent of the sphenoid sinus, in which a fluid level was present. The leakage stopped spontaneously after about a week. No rhinorrhoea has recurred in the almost 2 years that have passed.

During the same period we have had one other similar case in which CSF leakage through the sphenoid sinus stopped spontaneously.

III. *Male, 53 years old*. Accident of unknown nature. X-rays showed a fracture through the clivus and the sella turcica, with displacement of the walls of the sphenoid sinus. There was profuse CSF leakage. A semiconscious condition was considered due to a kind of brain stem lesion.

This patient was operated on at the Clinic of Otorhinology. The sphenoid sinus was reached from an incision between the upper lip and the gum. After evacuation of its mucous sac, the sphenoid sinus was packed with a large piece of muscle wrapped in fascia lata.

The postoperative course was uneventful and the patient recovered.

In cases of CSF leakage through the sella region and sphenoid sinus, dural exploration from the inside is risky, since brain damage may arise due to compression of the frontal lobe, stretching of the hypothalamic region and lesion of the optic chiasm.

Regarding the technical localizing of the fistula responsible for the CSF leakage, I refer to the recent work of Ommaya *et al.* (1968).

It has happened more than once during the past 2 years that an initial traumatic CSF leakage stopped spontaneously. It is not clear how to evaluate beforehand whether or not traumatic CSF leakage will show tendency to stop permanently by itself.

It seems to be preferable to stop CSF fistulas via the sphenoid sinus through a transsphenoid approach.

References

Gurdjian, E. S. & Webster, J. E., *Cerebrospinal fluid rhinorrhea and otorrhea. Pneumocephalus. Compound depressed fracture of the frontal sinus neighbourhood. In Operative Surgery,* Williams & Wilkins, Baltimore, 180 (1952).

Lewin, W., *Clin. Neurosurg., 12,* 237 (1966).

Ommaya, A. K., Di Chiro, G., Baldwin, M. & Pennybaker, J. B., *J. Neurol. Neurosurg. Psychiat., 31,* 214 (1968).

Transmaxillary approach to the skull base in treatment of liquorrhea

By Jan Wersäll

Department of Otolaryngology, Karolinska Sjukhuset, Stockholm, Sweden

A patient with a permanent or intermittent fistula between the subdural space and the nose or paranasal sinuses is threatened by severe illness and death, due to meningitis and meningoencephalitis.

Defects in the posterior wall of the frontal sinus are, as a rule, easily repaired after exploration of the frontal sinus and suture, or covering of the dural defect with muscle fascia transplants. Dural lesions in the bottom of the anterior middle cranial fossa reaching the ethmoidal sinus, the sphendoid sinus or the nasal cavity may be considerably more difficult to cure. Many of these lesions can be reached through the transfrontal approach. When the lesion is located close to the sphenoidal sinus or in the sinus, the possibilities of reaching the lesion through this approach are, however, small. In recent years, lesions of this type have been treated in our clinic through a transmaxilloethmoidal approach with good results.

Indications

Transmaxillary operation in liquorrhea is indicated in all cases with dural lesions reaching the ethmoid sinuses, the nasal cavity or the sphenoid sinus.

Preoperative examination of the patient

X-ray tomography in three planes will usually reveal the localization of a fracture or a defect in the bone. Intralumbal injection of 1 ml of 5 % sodium-fluorescein will give an intense fluorescence of CSF for about four days after the injection, and will enable identification of CSF and often localization of the side and sometimes origin of the flow (Kirchner and Proud, 1960). This method is to be preferred to injection of dyes, which might cause arachnoiditis.

In some cases, air may be seen on the X-ray picture replacing the CSF close to the fistula (Kirchner and Proud, 1960).

Operative technique

The extension of exploration of the skull base is varied, depending on the location of the dural lesion. A wide opening of the frontal wall of the maxillary sinus and complete resection of its medial bone wall are essential for a satisfactory view of the operating field. Although partial exenteration of the posterior ethmoid cells may be sufficient to reach the frontal wall of the sphenoid sinus, the vomer often has to be fractured and pushed over to the other side in order to get sufficient space. When the fracture is located in the posterior ethmoid or sphenoid sinus, the frontal wall of the sphenoid sinus should be opened, and the whole sinus explored on both sides after extraction of the mucosa and of the middle wall of the sinus. Even in cases where the defect is located in the middle ethmoidal region, or in the middle or posterior part of the cribriform lamina, opening of the anterior wall of the sphenoid sinus, will give a better support for the graft (Fig. A, B). The mucosa over a wide area around the fracture line is removed, to form a raw bleeding surface for the graft. Bone fragments should be removed only when they are clearly displaced. A large muscle graft is taken from the lateral part of the quadriceps muscle. The graft is packed into the sphenoid sinus and over

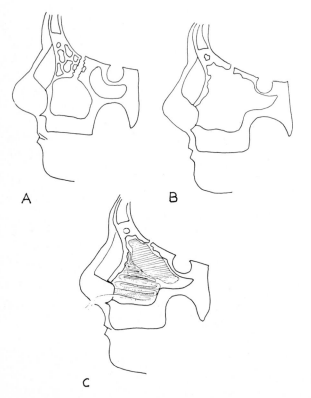

A

B

C

Fig. A–C

the bone fissure or defect in such a way that a large area around the defect is covered by graft. A packing of 3-cm linen ribbon is pressed against the graft, and the whole ethmoidal and maxillary sinus on that side is packed. The packing is pulled through the nose via an incision in the mucosa of the lateral nasal wall (Fig. C).

Postoperative treatment

In view of the risk of postoperative meningitis, the patient should be treated with large doses of a broad-spectrum antibiotic and several million units of penicillin for a week after the operation. The packing is withdrawn successively during the 5th to 8th day.

A certain crust formation after the operation may appear during the first postoperative weeks, and may require daily irrigation of the nose with sterile saline for the first weeks after removal of the packing.

Case reports

A 39-year-old woman with permanent liquorrhea since 1959 possibly related to a slight skull trauma in 1956. X-ray tomography revealed a slightly displaced fracture through the base of the skull, anterior to the sphenoid. When she was referred to our clinic, the patient had been operated on three times via the transfrontal approach with fascia transplantation over the defect without result. In February 1963, the patient was operated on by transmaxilloethmoidal exploration of the base of the skull. A thin fracture line appeared across the ethmoid, anterior to the sphenoid. A muscle graft was applied over the fracture, after removal of the mucosa over a wide area around the fracture. Three weeks after operation, a few drops of fluid appeared in the nose, but the patient has subsequently had no liquorrhea or other symptoms of a dura defect.

A 21-year-old man with a fracture through the pyramid and the sphenoid sinus after a skull trauma in February 1964. Intermittent liquorrhea till September 1964, when the sphenoid sinus was explored through the transmaxilloethmoidal route. A fracture was found to pass through the sphenoid bone from one side of the sphenoid sinus. The sphenoid sinus and the posterior ethmoidal region were packed with a muscle fascia graft, and the patient has had no liquorrhea since the operation.

A 53-year-old man fell from his bed in January 1968. He suffered a fracture through the clivus into the sphenoid sinus, which was diagnosed with X-ray tomography. Constant liquorrhea and repeated attacks of meningitis after the trauma. He was operated on in February 1968 by transmaxilloethmoidal exploration of the sphenoid sinus. Bone fragments which were pressed into the fracture line of the posterior wall of the sphenoid sinus, were removed, as well as all the mucosa of the sphenoid sinus. The defect was packed with a large muscle fascia graft. No liquorrhea or meningitis occurred after the operation.

A 66-year-old woman with a large defect in the ethmoid and frontal bone after repeated operations for a frontal bone meningioma since 1962. There was a large communication to the nasal cavity, and profound liquorrhea. Exploration of the defect was performed via the transmaxillary route, and the defect was packed with a large fascia muscle graft. No recurrence of liquorrhea occurred after operation.

A 46-year-old man with an operated and irradiated plasmacytoma of the sphenoid bone. Liquorrhea occurred before treatment in 1963, and disappeared after transmaxilloethmoidal operation in 1963. Recurrence of the liquorrhea took place in 1967, when a small fistula was found on the posterior wall of the sphenoid sinus at new exploration. New packing with muscle and fascia stopped the leakage.

Discussion

Several reports of closure of dural lacerations causing cerebrospinal rhinorrhea with the transfrontal intracranial route have been published since the first successful operation by Dandy (1926). The early literature was reviewed by Hirsch (1952). The first extracranial operation was reported by Dohlman (1948), who used a flap taken from the middle turbinate for closure of a fistula in the ethmoid region, approached via the anterior transethmoidal route.

Hirsch (1952) used a septal mucosa flap to cover a CSF fistula in two cases, after hypophysectomy via the septal route. Aboulker (1966) reported 15 cases of treatment of dura lesions via the transethmoidal route.

Our own experience from several hundred cases of hypophysectomy have shown that a muscle flap from the quadriceps muscle gives adequate cover of the sella region after hypophysectomy. The transmaxillary approach to the base of the skull gives a wider exposure, under a more appropriate angle of exploration, than any other approach for treatment of any process in this region. It leaves no defect in the bones of the brain capsule, and little postoperative trouble for the patient. Even the fistulas in the posterior ethmoidal region and in the sphenoid sinus can be sufficiently exposed, and the method gives excellent postoperative results.

References

Aboulker, P., Le Beau, J., Sterkers, J. M. & Elbaz, P., *Ann. Otol., 83,* 27 (1966).
Dohlman, G., *Acta Otolaryng.* (Stockholm), *67,* 20 (1948).
Briant, T. D. R. & Snell, D., *Laryngoscope, 77,* 1390 (1967).
Hirsch, O., *Arch. Otolaryng.* (Chicago), *56,* 1 (1952).
Kirchner, F. R. & Proud, G. O., *Laryngoscope,* 70, 921 (1960).

General discussion

Mennig to Wersäll

In my experience, I believe too that the rhinosurgical approach to the base of the skull is not only useful for the interventions on the pituitary gland, both for tumour removal and hypophysectomy, but also for the treatment of liquorrhoea. In the case I will present here, the neurosurgical means had not succeeded in stopping cerebrospinal fluid after a Thorkildsen operation, though the neurosurgeon had operated twice. First we tried to localize the fistula by the technique of Kirchner and Proud with fluorescein; it appeared to be in the sphenoid region. On exploring the sella turcica by the transethmoidal-transsphenoidal approach, we found a defect of bone in the anterior wall of the sella turcica and there a fistula in the dura; in this way we obtained complete healing.

Wersäll to Mennig

This is well in agreement with out own findings.

Chairman's summary of session VII

H. Diamant

The three papers now read have concerned a very important topic in modern society, namely, some of the results of the modern hectic traffic. It is quite clear that most of the fractures of the base of the skull are caused by motor accidents. I think that one of the reasons why we, as oto-rhinologists, must show interest in these lesions is the fact that we often meet them in hospitals where there are no neuro-traumatologists. Furthermore, many of the fractures are in the field of rhinology, and easily accessible, as you have already heard from Dr. Wersäll. Active treatment seems to be absolutely necessary in cases with recurrent or so-called late meningitis. The same applies to cases where, in clinical experience, meningitis seems imminent.

As Dr. Herlin pointed out, many more cases are coming under our hands, because of good transport and acute handling. This means that a certain reluctance is necessary. It is very often rather difficult to estimate the right time for intervention. Many cases have to be thoroughly discussed between rhinologists and neurosurgeons before any active action is taken.

Of course, those cases where brain tissue is visible have to be treated promptly. The sight of brain tissue in itself is very disturbing to most doctors, and the patients cannot be left alone. These difficult cases may also come to others than neurosurgeons, and as an otologist you have at least to be familiar with them.

Treatment of liquorrhoea can, as you have heard, be performed from above and from below, and I am sure that the results are nearly as good. How good they are can only be estimated by a prospected continuous study. And for such we have to wait.

This short survey of mine is to be regarded as an introductory comment on further discussions on the topic of fractures of the base of the skull. Such a discussion has then to be taken up in the next symposium, perhaps called "traumatic lesions of the neck and head", arranged by Professor Hamberger in the same excellent way as this one.

Closing address

By Bengt Gustafsson

Department of Medical Symbiosis Research, Karolinska Institutet, Stockholm, Sweden

The main intention of the Nobel donation has been to promote better international understanding and good will. It is therefore well in accordance with Nobel's wide interests in international activities that the Nobel Foundation has started the series of Nobel symposia. It is evident from the early documents concerning the Nobel Prize and letters from Alfred Nobel that he was very interested in practical medicine. One of his first donations went to a new children's hospital.

He also discussed blood transfusion methods using tubes "made of a molten mass of borax and sodium fluoride, or of borax and sodium silicate. Tubes of such material ought to be able to prevent coagulation without modifying any more corpuscles than those coming in direct contact with them. It is nevertheless probable that the time element is an important consideration and that perhaps blood changes ten times more during the second second than during the first."

The fact that one of the Nobel symposia covers a subject like the disorders of the skull base region is a tribute to the memory of a man of such understanding of the difficulties and importance deriving from the invention of new medical methods for the promotion of clinical medicine. I congratulate you on a very successful meeting, and I wish you further luck with your important work, which is of such direct benefit to mankind.